D0855505

Endocrine Pathophysiology:

A Patient-Oriented Approach

616.407
En25d2

Endocrine Pathophysiology:

A Patient-Oriented Approach

JEROME M. HERSHMAN, M.D.

Professor of Medicine,
UCLA School of Medicine,
Chief, Endocrinology Section,
Medical Service,
Veterans Administration Wadsworth Medical Center
Los Angeles, California

Second Edition

Lea & Febiger *Philadelphia*

Lea & Febiger
600 Washington Square
Philadelphia, PA 19106
U.S.A.

/ Library
/ I.U.P.

616.407 En25d 2

C.1

First Edition, 1977
  Reprinted, 1978
Second Edition, 1982

Translations:
  First Edition—
    Spanish Edition by Nueva Editorial Interamericana, S.A. de C.V.,
    Mexico, D.F., Mexico—1981

Library of Congress Cataloging in Publication Data
Main entry under title:

Endocrine pathophysiology.

  Bibliography: p.
  Includes index.
  1. Clinical endocrinology.   2. Physiology,
Pathological. I. Hershman, Jerome M. [DNLM:
1. Endocrine diseases—Physiopathology.   WK100
H572e]
RC649.E52   1982   616.4'07   82-7183
ISBN 0-8121-0840-X   AACR2

Copyright © 1982 by Lea & Febiger. Copyright under the International Copyright Unio
rights reserved. This book is protected by copyright. *No part of it may be reproduced i*
manner or by any means without written permission from the publisher.

PRINTED IN THE UNITED STATES OF AMERICA

Print Number: 3   2

Preface

The purpose of this volume is to give medical students an understanding of the pathophysiology of endocrine diseases. The authors assume that the student has taken an introductory course in endocrine physiology and biochemistry, so the review of basic endocrinology in each chapter covers only those topics most relevant to clinical medicine.

Endocrine disorders mainly involve either excessive or decreased secretion of specific hormones. The text presents methods of testing specific glandular function with static measurements of hormone levels and effects, with dynamic stimulation tests for evaluation of hypofunction of the endocrine gland, and with dynamic suppression tests for diagnosis of hyperfunctional states.

Systematic discussions of endocrine pathophysiology elucidate the symptoms and signs of endocrine diseases. The chapters also present the principles of therapy for each disorder and relevant clinical pharmacology. Descriptions of endocrine pathology have been kept to a minimum.

Case studies of patients with endocrine disorders illustrate the clinical findings and diagnostic methods. Questions pertaining to these patients test the reader's understanding of the material and emphasize clinical concepts. The answers to the questions appear in a separate section at the end of the text. Students at the UCLA School of Medicine have found that this patient-oriented approach more actively involves them and aids comprehension.

In the five years since the first edition appeared, there have been significant advances in understanding endocrine disease. These advances have been incorporated into each chapter, and obsolete material has been deleted. The new chapter on calcium and phosphate and metabolic bone disease emphasizes the recent, exciting developments on the role of vitamin D in bone physiology and disease.

Although this volume is aimed primarily at medical students, residents in medicine, internists, and family physicians may find it useful as a succinct review of current concepts in clinical endocrinology.

JEROME M. HERSHMAN

Contributors

GLENN D. BRAUNSTEIN, M.D.
Professor of Medicine,
UCLA School of Medicine,
Director, Division of Endocrinology,
Cedars-Sinai Medical Center,
Los Angeles, California

HAROLD E. CARLSON, M.D.
Associate Professor of Medicine,
UCLA School of Medicine,
Assistant Chief, Endocrinology,
Wadsworth VA Medical Center,
Los Angeles, California

INDER J. CHOPRA, M.D.
Professor of Medicine,
UCLA School of Medicine,
Los Angeles, California

JACK W. COBURN, M.D.
Professor of Medicine,
UCLA School of Medicine,
Director, Nephrology Training Program,
Wadsworth VA Medical Center,
Los Angeles, California

MAYER B. DAVIDSON, M.D.
Professor of Medicine,
UCLA School of Medicine,
Director, Diabetes Program,
Cedars-Sinai Medical Center,
Los Angeles, California

DELBERT A. FISHER, M.D.
Professor of Pediatrics and Medicine,
Harbor-UCLA Medical Center,
Torrance, California

ALAN M. FOGELMAN, M.D.
Professor and Chief, Division of Cardiology,
UCLA School of Medicine,
Los Angeles, California

ALLAN R. GLASS, M.D.
Assistant Professor of Medicine,
Uniformed Services University of Health Sciences,
Bethesda, Maryland,
Staff Endocrinologist,
Walter Reed Army Medical Center,
Washington, D.C.

DAN A. HENRY, M.D.
Assistant Professor of Medicine,
UCLA School of Medicine,
Los Angeles, California,
Co-director, Hemodialysis Unit,
Oliveview Medical Center,
Van Nuys, California,
Attending Nephrologist,
VA Medical Center,
Sepulveda, California

JEROME M. HERSHMAN, M.D.
Professor of Medicine,
UCLA School of Medicine,
Chief, Endocrinology Section,
Wadsworth VA Medical Center,
Los Angeles, California

SOLOMON A. KAPLAN, M.D.
Professor of Pediatrics,
UCLA School of Medicine,
Los Angeles, California

Contributors

CHARLES R. KLEEMAN, M.D.
Factor Family Foundation,
Professor of Nephrology and Medicine,
Director, Center for Health Enhancement,
UCLA School of Medicine,
Los Angeles, California

BARBARA LIPPE, M.D.
Professor of Pediatrics,
UCLA School of Medicine,
Los Angeles, California

DAVID H. SOLOMON, M.D.
Professor of Medicine,
UCLA School of Medicine,
Los Angeles, California

RONALD S. SWERDLOFF, M.D.
Professor of Medicine,
UCLA School of Medicine,
Chief, Division of Endocrinology,
Harbor-UCLA Medical Center,
Torrance, California

MICHAEL TUCK, M.D.
Associate Professor of Medicine,
UCLA School of Medicine,
Los Angeles, California,
Chief, Endocrinology Section,
VA Medical Center,
Sepulveda, California

ANDRE J. VAN HERLE, M.D.
Professor of Medicine,
UCLA School of Medicine,
Los Angeles, California

RICHARD WEITZMAN, M.D.†
Assistant Professor of Medicine,
Harbor-UCLA Medical Center,
Torrance, California

ADA R. WOLFSEN, M.D.
Associate Professor of Medicine,
Associate Chief of Endocrinology,
Harbor-UCLA Medical Center,
Torrance, California

†Deceased

Contents

Contents

CHAPTER 1

Principles of Clinical Endocrinology

Jerome M. Hershman

Clinical disorders of endocrine glands are mainly of two types: hyperfunction and hypofunction. Hyperfunction denotes excessive secretion of the hormone. The clinical findings, i.e., the signs and symptoms, of the disorder reflect how oversecretion affects target tissues. Hypofunction denotes deficient secretion of the hormone; the resulting signs and symptoms occur because the amount of this hormone is insufficient to achieve its normal effect on target tissues.

The concept of hyperfunction and hypofunction of endocrine glands implies that these states differ from normal hormone secretion. Unfortunately, the range of normalcy of many hormone measurements overlaps both deficiency and excess of hormonal production and hormonal blood levels. Single baseline values rarely can be used to establish a definitive diagnosis. The physiologic concept of feedback control also serves as a basis for diagnosing hyperfunction and hypofunction of endocrine glands and allows each hormone system to be considered dynamically.

NEGATIVE FEEDBACK

Pituitary tropic hormones, e.g., thyroid-stimulating hormone (TSH) or adrenocorticotropic hormone (ACTH), stimulate the target organs (thyroid or adrenal in this case) to release the target gland hormones (thyroxine (T_4) and triiodothyronine (T_3) or cortisol). In turn, elevated levels of the target gland hormone feed back on the pituitary to inhibit secretion of the tropic hormone. The corollary is that the pituitary detects low levels of the target gland hormone and thus increases its tropic hormone secretion, which causes increased secretion of the target gland hormone. Consider the examples of TSH-T_4 and T_3 or ACTH-cortisol in terms of a need to increase the output of the target gland hormone. Application of this concept to all hormones aids understanding of clinical diagnostic tests.

An x-y plot of tropic versus target gland hormone levels in the blood (Fig. 1–1) illustrates useful dynamic concepts and aids understanding of clinical jargon. Consider the possible levels of ACTH-cortisol or TSH-T_4 and T_3 based on Figure 1–1.

Hypothalamic hormones, secreted into a portal venous system that reaches the pituitary directly, regulate secretion of the pituitary hormones. For each pituitary hormone, a hypothalamic releasing hormone (or factor) exists, and for some pituitary hormones, hypothalamic factors inhibit release of the pituitary hormone. The hypothalamic hormones are useful diagnostic tools for testing the response of the pituitary gland and the target glands. Various chapters detail the clinical application of the hypothalamic hormones and the stimuli that alter their secretion.

CATEGORIES OF ENDOCRINE FUNCTION TESTS

Measurement of the basal level of hormone in blood or urine may be satisfactory for making a diagnosis of hyperfunction or hypofunction when the disorder is severe, especially when the tests illustrate normal feedback relationships; e.g., low T_4 in serum and high TSH in serum indicate primary hypothyroidism.

Stimulation Test. Evaluation of secretory reserve by a *stimulation* test is useful for diagnosing hypofunction and for detecting impaired secretory reserve.

Suppression Test. These tests are useful for diagnosis of hyperfunction because the hyperfunctioning gland by definition is not operating under normal control mechanisms; suppression may be abnormal quantitatively or quali-

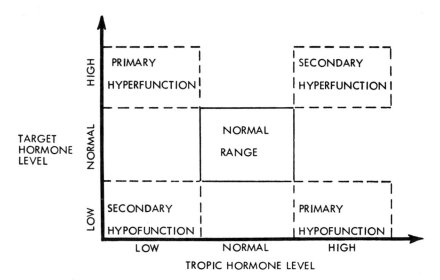

Figure 1–1.   Tropic (pituitary) hormone blood level versus target hormone level to illustrate abnormal functional states.

tatively. By negative feedback control the pituitary gland may be "reset" to respond to high levels of the suppressing hormone, e.g., pituitary ACTH secretion in Cushing's disease, which is discussed later. On the other hand, the gland may be autonomous and secreting without any control, e.g., an adrenal adenoma causing hypercortisolism.

Table 1–1 shows the general scheme of interpretation of suppression and stimulation tests.

TYPES OF HORMONE MEASUREMENTS

These techniques are usually applied to blood serum (or plasma) and urine; rarely are they applied to tissue extracts.

Bioassay. It should be specific; often it is not sensitive for physiologic levels of hormones; moreover it is tedious and expensive.

Chemical Measurement. This procedure measures the hormone, e.g., plasma cortisol by fluorimetry, or it measures a physiologic consequence, e.g., blood glucose as an index of insulin secretion.

Radioimmunoassay. A specific antibody is used to recognize the hormone, but the antibody may also detect a biologically inactive portion of the molecule. Because these assays are so sensitive, they are used extensively to measure blood levels of hormones.

Radioreceptor Assays. These biologically specific tests may be highly sensitive, e.g., using thyroxine-binding globulin as a specific receptor of T_4, or plasma membranes of target organs as receptors for peptide hormones.

Table 1–1. General Scheme for Interpretation of Suppression and Stimulation Tests

Evaluation of hyperfunction		
Baseline hormone level or secretion rate	Suppression test	Interpretation of function
Normal	Normal	Normal
Elevated	Normal	Normal
Elevated	Nonsuppressible	*Hyperfunction
Evaluation of hypofunction		
Baseline hormone level or secretion rate	Stimulation test	Interpretation of function
Normal	Normal	Normal
Low	Normal	Normal
Low	Nonstimulable	Hypofunction
"Low normal"	Nonstimulable	†Impaired reserve function

*Degree of hyperfunction varies from mild to severe.
†Patient may be asymptomatic or have symptoms and signs of hypofunction.

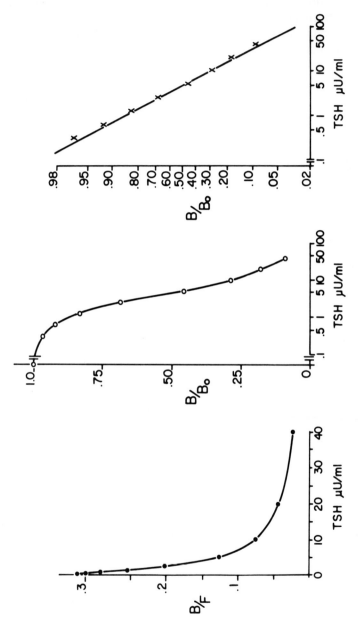

Figure 1–2. Standard curves for the radioimmunoassay of TSH plotted in three different ways: (left) bound/free labeled TSH versus TSH concentration; (middle) bound/bound at 0 dose (B/Bo) versus TSH concentration, log scale; (right) B/Bo on a logit scale (logit $y = \ln\frac{y}{1-y}$) versus TSH concentration, log scale.

Metabolic Effects. This test checks the hormone's effect on a target tissue, e.g., speed of reflex contraction to assess the effect of thyroid hormone.

Clinical Assessment Only. In some cases, there is no readily available bioassay, or the clinical situation may provide all of the bioassay data needed; e.g., normal menstrual cycles indicate integrity of the hypothalamic-pituitary-gonadal axis in women.

The inside cover contains a table of normal hormone concentrations. These values differ slightly among laboratories, depending on the details of methodology. Minor departures from the values in the table are found in some chapters. For the student, pathophysiologic concepts are more important than sharply defined (but often arbitrary) limits of normal.

TERMS

The following terms are used commonly in clinical endocrinology.

Primary Hyperfunction. Hypersection of a hormone usually due to tumor or disease of an endocrine gland itself.

Secondary Hyperfunction. Hypersecretion of a hormone produced by excessive stimulation from its tropic hormone or its physiologic stimulators; no disease of the gland per se.

Primary Hypofunction. Hyposecretion of a hormone due to disease of the gland of secretion.

Secondary Hypofunction. Hyposecretion of a hormone due to lack of a tropic hormone or lack of the physiologic stimulators.

Suppression Test. Administration of the suppressor to test autonomy of hormonal secretion.

Stimulation Test. Administration of the specific stimulator to test hormonal secretory reserve of the gland.

Secretion Rate. Amount of hormone secreted per unit of time.

Production Rate. Amount of hormone produced outside the gland plus that amount secreted by the gland per unit of time.

Half-Life in Blood. Time for blood level of hormone to fall to half of its original value.

Protein-Bound Fraction of Hormone. That percentage of hormone bound to its specific plasma binding protein and therefore considered to be physiologically inactive.

Free or Unbound Fraction. That percentage of the plasma hormone not protein bound—the physiologically active fraction, presumably.

RADIOIMMUNOASSAY

In the radioimmunoassay of hormones, the following reaction occurs:

$$H + Ab \rightleftharpoons H\text{-}Ab$$

$$*H + Ab \rightleftharpoons *H\text{-}Ab$$

where H is the unlabeled hormone (antigen), *H is the radioactive hormone tracer, Ab is the antibody to the hormone, and H-Ab (or *H-Ab) is the hormone-antibody complex. *H and Ab are added to the reaction tube in fixed amounts. H represents the hormone in the standards or unknown serum. The antibody has the same affinity for *H as for H. At equilibrium, the amount of *H bound to Ab (*H-Ab) varies inversely with the amount of hormone (H) added to the tube. With large amounts of H, *H represents a small proportion of total hormone (H + *H), and the antibody binds only a small proportion of the tracer hormone. The *H-Ab complex is separated from the free (unbound) *H and measured in a radioactivity counter.

The data for the standard curve are plotted as shown in Figure 1–2, a radioimmunoassay of TSH. In this assay, varying concentrations of TSH are added to make up the standard curve, and TSH labeled with ^{125}I is the tracer. The TSH bound to the antibody is separated from the free TSH, and the bound labeled TSH (*H-Ab) is counted. The result is often expressed as a ratio of bound counts, B, for a given sample to counts bound at 0 hormone concentration, Bo. Unknowns can be read from each of the standard curves in the different plots. For example, in Figure 1–2, an unknown serum containing a concentration of 5 μU/ml would give a B/F (Bound/Free = *H-Ab/ *H) of 0.126 equivalent to 5 μU/ml (left panel). In the plot of B/Bo versus log TSH (middle panel), the B/Bo of 0.45 also indicates a serum TSH of 5 μU/ml. The straight line representation of the plot of the logit of B/Bo versus log TSH (right panel) has computational advantages because it gives a straight line for the standard curve.

The principal advantage of radioimmunoassay is its great sensitivity, which depends on the high affinity of the antibody for the hormone. These systems can detect hormone concentrations in serum of 10^{-7} M to 10^{-12} M in various assays. Although the assays are generally specific for the given hormone, they may also measure hormone metabolites or precursors devoid of biologic activity. In fact, the recognition sites of the antibody may be directed against a biologically inactive portion of the hormone molecule. This disadvantage may be overcome by replacing the antibody with a naturally occurring biologic receptor for the hormone. Radioreceptor assays presently under development are the next generation of hormone assays.

CHAPTER 2

Pituitary Disease

Harold E. Carlson

EVALUATION OF ANTERIOR PITUITARY FUNCTION

As described in Chapter 1, the function of an endocrine gland is usually assessed by means of specific stimulation and suppression tests, which make use of known normal responses to perturbation in homeostatic regulatory mechanisms. For the pituitary gland, such tests are commonly used to evaluate the secretory status of most of the individual hormones. The following sections briefly cover the structures and functions of the pituitary hormones, along with the factors (both physiologic and pharmacologic) that alter and regulate their secretion. Table 2–1 summarizes clinically useful pituitary stimulation and suppression tests.

Human Adrenocorticotropic Hormone (ACTH)

ACTH is a single-chain polypeptide of 39 amino acids whose principal function is the stimulation of cortisol production by the adrenal cortex. Like most polypeptide hormones, ACTH appears to act by binding to a specific cell membrane receptor and activating adenylate cyclase, which raises intra-

Table 2–1. Clinically Useful Tests of Pituitary Function

Hormone	Stimulation test	Suppression tests
ACTH	Insulin hypoglycemia Metyrapone	Dexamethasone administration
TSH	TRH	T_3 or T_4 administration (not standardized)
LH/FSH	LRH (LH-RH) Clomiphene	Testosterone or estrogen administration (not standardized)
GH	Insulin hypoglycemia Arginine infusion L-dopa	Glucose tolerance
PRL	TRH Chlorpromazine	None

cellular levels of cyclic adenosine monophosphate (cAMP). This action initiates a series of biochemical events culminating in cortisol synthesis and release.

Normally, ACTH secretion (and, hence, cortisol secretion) is episodic, with many secretory pulses occurring throughout the day and night. These pulses appear to be larger and more frequent during the early morning hours resulting, on the average, in a peak of both ACTH and cortisol blood levels at about 6:00 to 8:00 A.M. and a low point in the late afternoon or evening. This 24-hour rhythm is basically determined by the sleep-wake cycle, and adjusts over a period of 2 to 3 weeks to changes in the pattern of sleep and activity.

When pathologic hypersecretion of ACTH is present, blood levels of ACTH and cortisol (if the adrenal glands are intact) are often elevated in the basal state, and the elevation persists in the face of large doses of exogenous glucocorticoid. Such suppression tests, generally using the administration of dexamethasone, are discussed in detail in later sections dealing with the adrenal cortex (Chap. 4). Normal feedback mechanisms lead to secondary hypersecretion of ACTH in patients with primary adrenal failure; in this instance, the elevation of plasma ACTH is readily suppressed by replacement of the missing glucocorticoid.

Several factors stimulate ACTH release:

1. Corticotropin-releasing hormone (CRH), the hypothalamic substance thought to be the final common pathway for most stimuli to ACTH secretion; it has recently been isolated in pure form.
2. Low plasma levels of glucocorticoid.
3. A variety of stresses, e.g., exercise, anxiety, pain, and anesthesia.
4. Hypoglycemia.
5. Bacterial pyrogens.
6. Vasopressin.

Since all probably act by increasing hypothalamic secretion of CRH, they depend on an intact hypothalamus *and* pituitary for a normal response. Vasopressin may act directly on the pituitary corticotrophs, according to some studies.

Procedures commonly used to stimulate ACTH secretion in the clinical evaluation of pituitary function include:

1. Hypoglycemia. Regular insulin, 0.1 or 0.15 U/kg body weight, is injected as an intravenous bolus. The blood sugar drops by at least 50% of its initial level 30 to 45 minutes after injection, provoking ACTH and cortisol secretion, which peaks 60 to 90 minutes after insulin administration. A normal plasma cortisol response consists of a rise of at least 7 μg/100 ml, reaching peak levels of at least 20 μg/100 ml (Fig. 2–1).

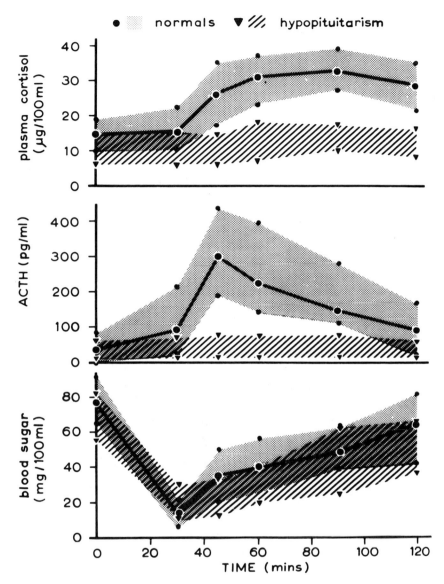

Figure 2–1. Blood sugar, plasma cortisol, and ACTH responses to intravenous insulin in normal subjects and patients with hypopituitarism; the insulin was given at 0 min. The mean responses in normal subjects are shown by the continuous solid lines, while the shaded areas give the range of the observed responses. (From Donald, R.A.: J. Clin. Endocrinol. Metab., 32:225, 1971.)

2. Metyrapone. Oral or intravenous administration of metyrapone, an adrenal inhibitor that blocks the 11-hydroxylase reaction (the final step in cortisol synthesis), lowers plasma cortisol and consequently increases ACTH secretion. This increase in ACTH stimulates the adrenal gland

and results in an accumulation of cortisol precursors behind the 11-hydroxylase block. Normally, the immediate precursor of cortisol, 11-deoxycortisol (also known as compound S) is secreted in increased amounts and can be easily measured in blood or urine. In one commonly used procedure, 3 g metyrapone are given orally at bedtime; serum or plasma compound S and cortisol are measured at 8:00 A.M. the next morning. A fall in serum cortisol to less than 5 μg/100 ml indicates a valid test, and a serum compound S of at least 8 μg/100 ml is a normal response (Fig. 2–2).

With both procedures (hypoglycemia and metyrapone administration), adrenal end products are used as an index of ACTH secretion because the direct measurement of ACTH in plasma is difficult. Therefore, if the responses to either hypoglycemia or metyrapone testing are deficient, it is also necessary to demonstrate that the adrenal glands themselves are capable of responding to ACTH; for this purpose, exogenous ACTH (natural or synthetic) is administered, and plasma or urine steroid responses are measured.

Recent improvements in the methods of ACTH radioimmunoassay have resulted in the availability of reliable plasma ACTH measurements, which have simplified the etiologic diagnosis of adrenal insufficiency: patients with primary adrenal insufficiency have low plasma cortisol levels and elevated plasma ACTH, whereas those with adrenal failure secondary to hypothalamic-pituitary disease have low or low-normal plasma ACTH levels despite low

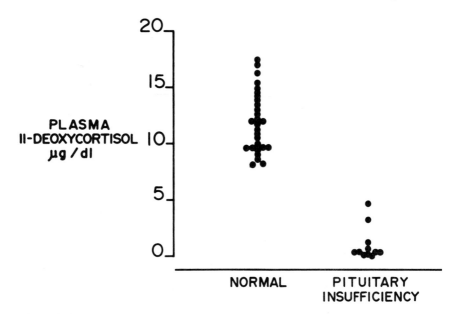

Figure 2–2. Plasma 11-deoxycortisol (compound S) levels following administration of metyrapone to normal subjects and to patients with hypopituitarism. In this test, 2 or 3 g metyrapone were given at bedtime, with measurement of plasma 11-deoxycortisol the next morning.

circulating cortisol concentrations. Provocative tests are still needed to document a more modest loss of ACTH reserve.

Thyrotropin

Thyroid stimulating hormone (TSH) or thyrotropin, with a molecular weight of about 28,000, is one of the three glycoprotein hormones produced by the pituitary; the others are luteinizing hormone (LH) and follicle-stimulating hormone (FSH). In addition to its carbohydrate content, TSH consists of a specific single-chain peptide beta subunit combined with a single-chain peptide alpha subunit; this alpha subunit is virtually identical to the alpha subunit found in the other pituitary glycoprotein hormones, LH and FSH, and also in the placental glycoprotein hormone, human chorionic gonadotropin (HCG). Thyrotropin acts via cyclic AMP to stimulate production of the thyroid hormones, thyroxine (T_4) and triiodothyronine (T_3). Serum levels of TSH, measured by radioimmunoassay, are stable throughout the day and night, with only a modest increase in the late evening hours.

Primary hypersecretion of TSH is rare; most of the cases described appear to result from TSH-secreting pituitary tumors. In normal individuals or in those with TSH hypersecretion secondary to thyroid failure (i.e., primary hypothyroidism), TSH secretion may be suppressed by administering T_3 or T_4, which act directly on the pituitary. Somatostatin, dopamine, and large amounts of glucocorticoid also decrease serum TSH levels. Since low serum levels of T_3 and T_4 normally activate feedback mechanisms to increase TSH secretion, secondary hypersecretion of TSH occurs in primary hypothyroidism. Thus, pituitary or hypothalamic disease should be suspected if the serum TSH is not elevated in the presence of documented hypothyroidism; the absence of palpable thyroid tissue in a hypothyroid patient should also alert the physician to the possibility of TSH hyposecretion because TSH is necessary for the maintenance of thyroid size. In human infants, serum TSH is strikingly elevated within an hour after birth and gradually falls to normal adult levels over the first week of extrauterine life.

Thyrotropin-releasing hormone (TRH) is a hypothalamic tripeptide, pyroglutamyl-histidyl-prolinamide. When TRH is given intravenously to normal individuals, a prompt rise in serum TSH occurs, usually peaking about 30 minutes after TRH administration (Fig. 2-3). An exaggerated response to TRH occurs in patients with primary hypothyroidism, while blunted or absent responses may be seen in hyperthyroidism and in hypopituitarism. In hypothalamic disease, hypothyroidism may coexist with a low or normal basal level of immunoreactive TSH; this TSH shows reduced bioactivity, however. The TSH response to TRH is usually present in hypothalamic hypothyroidism and may be delayed and prolonged. The TRH test is the best test for evaluating the adequacy of TSH secretion.

Gonadotropins

Both LH and FSH are glycoprotein hormones that appear to be secreted by the same pituitary cell. Each consists of the same nonspecific α subunit

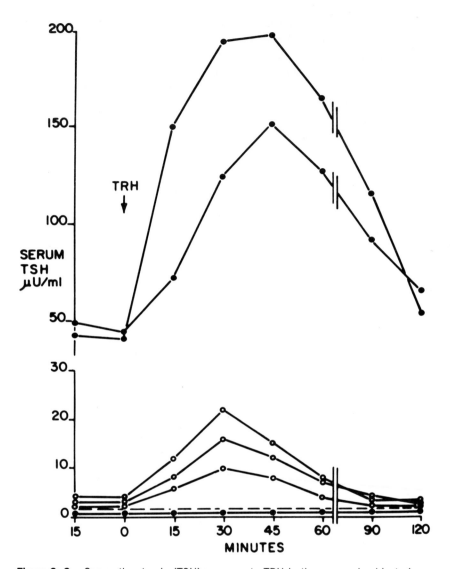

Figure 2–3. Serum thyrotropin (TSH) response to TRH in three normal subjects (open circles), two hypothyroid patients (solid circles), and one hyperthyroid patient with undetectable serum TSH (below dashed line). (From Hershman, J.M.: N. Engl. J.Med., *290*:886, 1974; reprinted, by permission, from The New England Journal of Medicine.)

combined with a unique β subunit that confers hormonal specificity. Each hormone interacts with specific receptors in the gonad, stimulating cyclic AMP production and resulting ultimately in the complex events of gonadal function.

Primary hypersecretion of LH or FSH is rare; when it occurs, it is usually due to secretion of these hormones by a pituitary tumor. Secondary hypersecretion, resulting from gonadal failure, is common and occurs in all normal women after menopause. The secretion of LH and FSH is normally suppressed by elevated serum levels of testosterone or estrogens in both men and women. A poorly characterized product of the testicular germinal epithelium, called inhibin and possibly arising from the Sertoli cells, also appears to suppress FSH secretion and may be important in the normal feedback regulation of this hormone.

Hyposecretion of LH and FSH occurs with many pituitary and hypothalamic diseases. Normally, the secretion of LH and FSH is stimulated by low levels of serum androgens and estrogens, and that of FSH by low serum levels of inhibin in the male. A hypothalamic factor, designated gonadotropin-releasing hormone (GnRH) or LH-releasing hormone (LH-RH, also abbreviated LRH or LRF), is secreted into the hypophyseal portal circulation and causes the release of both LH and FSH from the pituitary (Fig. 2–4). LH-RH, a decapeptide, has been isolated, sequenced, and synthesized. Because this single releasing factor is believed to promote the secretion of both LH and FSH, it is likely that other factors (such as circulating androgens and estrogens) play an important role in modifying the response to LH-RH and thus in modulating the secretion of LH and FSH. Intravenous injection of LH-RH, with subsequent measurement of serum LH and FSH, is the most convenient direct test of pituitary gonadotropin secretion.

Clomiphene, a weak synthetic estrogen, is able to bind to hypothalamic receptors for gonadal steroids and block their normal feedback effect; this lack of feedback results in increased secretion of LH and FSH in normal individuals (Fig. 2–5). A combination of both LH-RH and clomiphene testing may be used, in theory, to differentiate hypothalamic from pituitary causes of hypogonadism; in pituitary disease, responses to both clomiphene and LH-RH are deficient, while normal responses to LH-RH are seen in hypothalamic disease, with absent responses to clomiphene.

Growth Hormone (GH)

GH is a single-chain polypeptide with a molecular weight of about 22,000. Although its principal physiologic effect is stimulation of growth of bone and cartilage (via another peptide, somatomedin), GH also generally stimulates protein anabolism, promotes lipolysis, enhances absorption of dietary calcium, and antagonizes the action of insulin. Somatomedin is thought to be synthesized by the liver and perhaps by other organs; the presence of a normal amount of circulating GH is necessary for normal somatomedin production. Somatomedin promotes growth of cartilage by stimulating the uptake of amino acids and the synthesis of DNA, RNA, and protein in this tissue; GH itself has no stimulating effect on cartilage. GH is secreted in bursts throughout the day, usually following physiologic events such as meals, exercise, or sleep. The secretion of GH by the pituitary is under both stimulatory and inhibitory control by the hypothalamus. GH-releasing factor has recently been

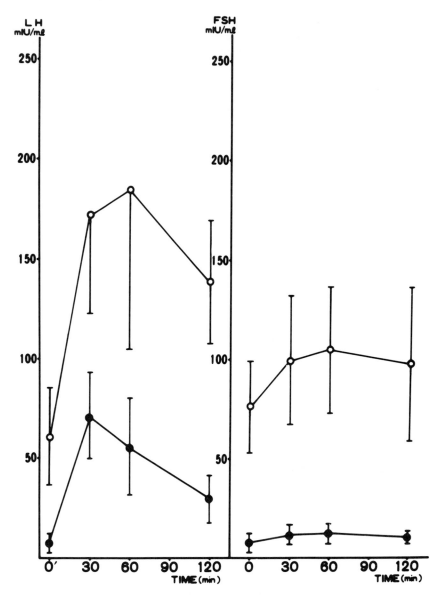

Figure 2—4. Serum LH and FSH responses to LH-RH in 14 normal menstruating women (solid circles) and 7 postmenopausal women (open circles); values shown are mean ± SD. (From Hashimoto, T., et al.: J. Clin. Endocrinol. Metab., 37:910, 1973.)

isolated, and somatostatin, a hypothalamic peptide of 14 amino acids, has been shown to inhibit secretion of GH, as well as secretion of TSH.

Sustained hypersecretion of GH produces overgrowth of bone and some tissue and leads to acromegaly in adults and gigantism in children, in whom the epiphyses of the long bones are still open and capable of further growth

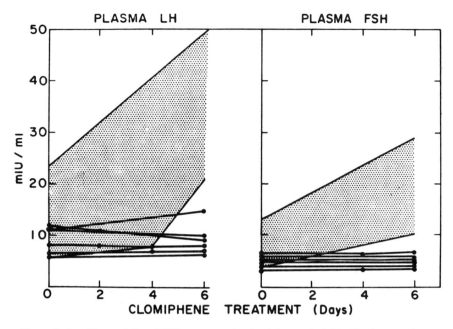

Figure 2–5. Plasma LH and FSH responses to clomiphene administration in normal men (shaded areas) and patients with isolated gonadotropin deficiency (solid lines). (From Bardin, C.W., et al.: J. Clin. Invest., *48*:2046, 1969.)

In normal individuals, GH secretion is suppressed by elevations in blood sugar. Thus, the standard 100-g glucose tolerance test is widely used to evaluate suppressibility of GH; normally, following a glucose load, the serum level of GH falls to less than 5 ng/ml. Other GH suppressants include somatostatin, elevated serum levels of free fatty acids, and glucocorticoid in excess.

GH hyposecretion is often present in hypopituitarism. Many stimuli cause secretion of GH in normal subjects; some of the more common include hypoglycemia, arginine, L-dopa, vasopressin, glucagon, sleep, exercise, and other stress. Most stimuli seem to be potentiated by estrogens; thus adult women usually respond better than men to any test, and the responses of men and children may be improved by giving pharmacologic amounts of estrogen for a few days. The most commonly used tests for evaluating the adequacy of GH secretion are the insulin hypoglycemia test, the arginine infusion test (0.5 g/kg intravenously over 30 minutes), and the L-dopa test (500 mg orally); the simultaneous administration of propranolol enhances GH responses to L-dopa by blocking β-adrenergic pathways that inhibit GH. All 3 tests give approximately equivalent results in young adults of normal weight (Fig. 2–6). Obesity blunts or abolishes the GH responses to all tests. A normal GH response to any test is the achievement, at any time during the test, of a GH

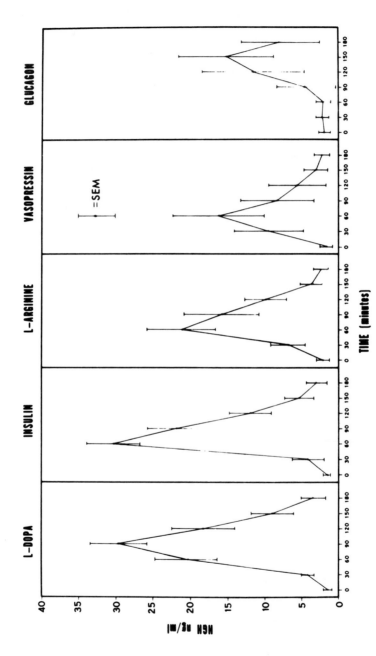

Figure 2–6. Serum growth hormone responses to 5 different stimuli in 20 normal subjects; mean ± SEM is shown. (From Eddy, R.L., et al.: Am. J. Med., 56:179, 1974.)

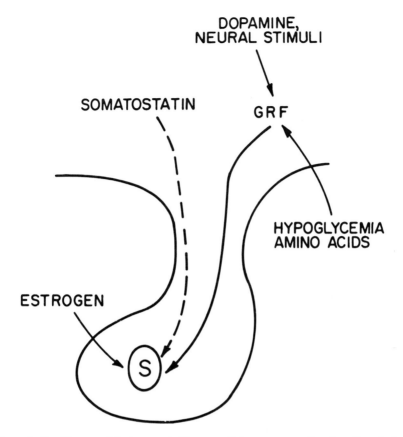

Figure 2–7. Diagram of factors controlling growth hormone secretion from the pituitary somatotroph (S). Solid arrows indicate stimulatory effects while dashed arrows signify inhibition. GRF indicates growth hormone releasing factors.

level in the serum of at least 7 ng/ml. Figure 2–7 illustrates the normal mechanisms controlling GH secretion.

Prolactin (PRL)

A single-chain peptide with a molecular weight of about 22,000, PRL appears to exert its main physiologic action on the breast, where it promotes milk production; the role of PRL in males, in children, and in nonlactating females is currently unclear. In both sexes, a marked elevation of serum PRL normally occurs during sleep, especially in the early morning hours. The primary hypothalamic control of PRL secretion is inhibitory; although the nature of the PRL-inhibiting factor(s) has not yet been determined, its secretion appears to be under dopaminergic control. Dopamine itself probably functions as the major PRL-inhibiting factor.

Hypersecretion of PRL may be due to secretion by pituitary tumors, to blockade of PRL-inhibiting factor action caused by drugs such as phenothiazines, or to hypothalamic destruction; it may also be idiopathic. Hypersecretion of PRL may be asymptomatic or may result in galactorrhea (inappropriate lactation) or hypogonadism. Normally, serum PRL is suppressed by PRL-inhibiting factor, by dopaminergic drugs or their precursors, and by elevated levels of thyroid hormones.

Hyposecretion of PRL may be found with hypopituitarism of varying origins. In normal individuals, PRL secretion is stimulated by phenothiazines and other dopamine antagonists, tactile breast stimulation, stress, low serum levels of thyroid hormones, and TRH; the role of TRH in the physiologic regulation of PRL is unclear. All stimuli to PRL release appear to be potentiated by estrogens. Figure 2–8 illustrates the normal mechanisms controlling PRL secretion, while Figure 2–9 demonstrates PRL responses to TRH in a group of normal subjects. As can be seen, serum PRL peaks 10 to 20 minutes after

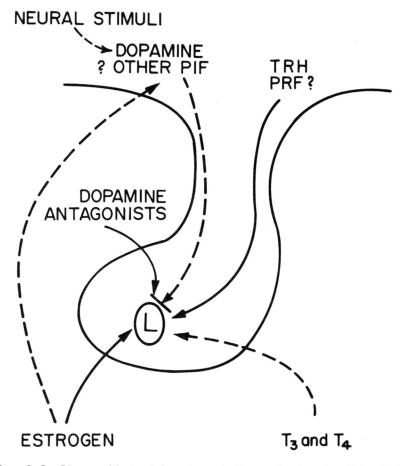

Figure 2–8. Diagram of factors influencing prolactin secretion from the pituitary lactotroph (L). Solid arrows signify stimulatory effects and dashed arrows denote inhibition. PIF and PRF indicate prolactin inhibiting factor and prolactin releasing factor, respectively.

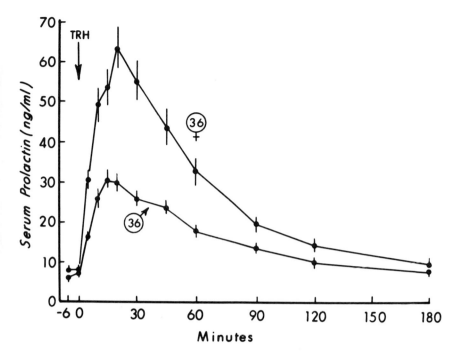

Figure 2–9. Serum prolactin responses (mean ± SEM) to intravenous TRH in normal subjects. Note that the response in women is larger than that in men. (From Jacobs, L.S., et al.: J. Clin. Endocrinol. Metab., 36:1069, 1973.)

giving intravenous TRH; the peak following intramuscular chlorpromazine (not shown) occurs at about 2 hours.

Melanocyte-Stimulating Hormone, and β-lipotropin

Although ACTH has some melanocyte-stimulating activity, the independent existence of a separate melanocyte-stimulating hormone (MSH), distinct from ACTH and other known pituitary peptides in man, is unclear. In general, serum MSH activity appears to parallel that of ACTH.

Recent work has shown that corticotroph (ACTH) cells in the anterior pituitary synthesize a large peptide (MW = 31,000 daltons) that is cleaved into smaller fragments with biologic activity, including ACTH and β-lipotropin. β-lipotropin may in turn serve as a precursor for β-endorphin, a naturally occurring peptide with opiate activity. The remaining fragment of the 31,000-MW precursor contains sequences with MSH activity; the relative importance of these peptides in the control of human skin pigmentation is unknown.

HYPOPITUITARISM

Causes

Hypopituitarism occurs when the secretion of one or more pituitary hormones is deficient. This state may arise from the effects of disease in the hypothalamic centers that control pituitary hormone release or from processes directly affecting the pituitary gland. Hypothalamic lesions, such as tumors (e.g., craniopharyngioma), trauma, histiocytosis X, or sarcoidosis, may decrease secretion of the pituitary hormones that are primarily controlled by releasing factors (i.e., GH, ACTH, TSH, LH, and FSH), while PRL, which is primarily regulated by a hypothalamic inhibitory factor, rises. Some cases of idiopathic or genetic hormonal deficiencies may also be due to deficient or abnormal releasing factors, or to developmental anomalies of midline central nervous system structures.

The pituitary gland itself may commonly be damaged or destroyed by a variety of conditions, including tumors, trauma, infarction (called Sheehan's syndrome when occurring in the postpartum period), surgical procedure, or radiation. Other less common lesions resulting in pituitary destruction include hemochromatosis, granulomas (histiocytosis, sarcoidosis), infections (fungal, tuberculous, luetic, or pyogenic), and aneurysms of the internal carotid artery. The severity of the destructive process causing hypopituitarism varies. Sheehan showed that the classic features of hypopituitarism resulting in death were present when 97% of the pituitary was destroyed. That only 10 to 25% of the pituitary is sufficient for normal hormone secretion implies that the reserve for pituitary hormone secretion in man is substantial.

In addition to destruction of normal pituitary tissue by invasion and compression, pituitary tumors may reduce blood flow from the hypothalamic-hypophyseal portal system and interfere with the delivery of releasing factors from the hypothalamus. Thus, pituitary tumors may cause "hypothalamic hypopituitarism."

Pathophysiology

The pathophysiology and clinical expression of hypopituitarism are variable and depend on which hormones are lost. Clinical features result from loss of gonadotropins, causing hypogonadism; deficient growth hormone, causing dwarfism in children but no clinical syndrome in adults; lack of TSH, causing hypothyroidism; prolactin deficiency, resulting in failure of lactation; and lack of ACTH, causing adrenocortical insufficiency. The frequency of hormone loss is usually in this order (most frequent to least frequent): GH, FSH-LH, TSH, PRL, ACTH; however, any combination of hormone loss may be found, even an isolated deficiency of only one hormone. Demonstration of hormonal deficiencies may help to establish the diagnosis of hypopituitarism, to explain the cause of puzzling symptoms, and to determine the need for replacement therapy.

Deficiency of GH is a common result of pituitary lesions that produce functional impairment. In the adult, GH deficiency has no significant consequences, but in the child it causes dwarfism. In congenital dwarfism due to lack of GH, failure to grow is evident within the first year of life. Even though size at birth is normal, subsequent growth rate is retarded. Infants and young children with GH deficiency may have fasting hypoglycemia. Puberty tends to be delayed even though gonadotropin secretion is intact. Children with GH deficiency are chubby and round-faced and may lack normal muscular development. When the diagnosis is established, therapy with GH injections is successful, provided it is started before epiphyseal closure.

Children with hypogonadism fail to enter normal puberty. Females have little or no breast development and primary amenorrhea. Pubic and axillary hair do not develop fully. Males have an infantile phallus and small testes (less than 12 ml in volume or 3.5 cm in length in the long axis). Body hair is sparse. When hypogonadism occurs as an isolated deficiency, growth may be delayed but is continuous and excessive, owing to failure of epiphyseal fusion. The adolescent with isolated hypogonadotropic hypogonadism is taller than one with multiple trophic hormone deficiencies and, if diagnosed late, may have developed eunuchoid proportions with an upper segment/lower segment ratio of less than one (measured as top of head to pubic symphysis/ pubic symphysis to floor), and an arm span greater than height. Familial hypogonadotropic hypogonadism may be associated with anosmia; some such patients also have midline central nervous system or somatic defects (e.g., cleft palate). In women, acquired pituitary hypogonadism causes secondary amenorrhea, some atrophy of the breasts, and thinning of pubic and axillary hair. In men, acquired hypogonadism causes atrophy of the testes, decrease in beard and body hair, decreased libido, and impotence.

Lack of TSH secretion causes involution of the thyroid and features of hypothyroidism; the detailed clinical picture is described in the next chapter. Hypothyroid patients complain of fatigue, weakness, slowing of mental and physical performance, cold intolerance, impaired memory, hoarseness, constipation, muscle cramps, paresthesias, and dry skin. Usually, these patients gain weight despite reduced appetite. The skin is infiltrated by mucopolysaccharide so that the patient with myxedema has a puffy face and coarsening of the features. Speech is slow, body hair is reduced, and scalp hair is dry and coarse. Anemia is common; metabolic rate is reduced and hypothermia may be present. Patients with myxedema may eventually lapse into coma and die unless treated.

Lack of ACTH reduces cortisol secretion but does not affect aldosterone secretion. Patients are weak and tired; many lose weight because of decreased appetite. They become hypotensive since cortisol is necessary to maintain normal vascular smooth muscle tone. Urinary output is scanty and ability to excrete a water load decreases, resulting in hyponatremia. In contrast with the excessive pigmentation of primary adrenal insufficiency (Addison's disease), patients with secondary (pituitary) adrenal insufficiency have pale skin and fail to tan because of lack of MSH and ACTH. Response to stress is poor; nausea, vomiting, and diarrhea presage cardiovascular collapse from "adrenal crisis," which leads to death unless glucocorticoid therapy is given. The typical picture of Addison's disease is described in Chapter 4; contrast it with deficiency of ACTH causing a lack of cortisol.

Sheehan's syndrome is postpartum hypopituitarism resulting from ischemic necrosis of the pituitary, which is caused by shock from blood loss sustained at the time of delivery. The pituitary in pregnancy is enlarged and more vulnerable to infarction, which Sheehan believed to be caused by arteriolar spasm from the shock. These women fail to lactate and show rapid mammary involution post partum; they also do not resume menstruation. Normal strength and vigor are not regained after the delivery; the pubic hair shaved for the delivery does not regrow. Hypothyroidism and adrenal insufficiency usually become manifest eventually, but all variations of hormonal loss may occur. The skin is waxy, and fine wrinkles appear about the eyes and mouth.

Diabetes insipidus results from destruction of hypothalamic nuclei, which are the source of vasopressin. Extension of pituitary tumor or other pituitary disease to the hypothalamus may cause diabetes insipidus, so that the symptoms of polyuria, polydipsia, and nocturia must be considered together with manifestations of anterior pituitary insufficiency. Diabetes insipidus is considered more extensively in Chapter 10.

Pituitary Tumors

Pituitary tumors may not cause any endocrine deficiency, but instead may produce the signs of a space-occupying intracranial neoplasm. Symptoms vary depending on the size and location (local spread) of the tumor. Headache is a common symptom; it is usually frontal or orbital, but location and severity are variable. It is attributed to pressure on the diaphragma sellae or the surrounding dura mater. Compression of the optic chiasm causes defects in the visual fields, usually bitemporal hemianopsia, often starting in the superior quadrants. Optic atrophy and total blindness may ensue; if so, the optic discs become white. The tumors may extend superiorly into the hypothalamus and cause a disturbance of appetite resulting in obesity, alteration of consciousness, and disturbances in temperature regulation. Obstruction of the third ventricle causes internal hydrocephalus. Lateral extension can compress the third (rarely the fourth or sixth) cranial nerves, causing diplopia or ptosis. Anterior or inferior extension may result in invasion of the sphenoid sinus and cerebrospinal fluid rhinorrhea.

Skull roentgenograms show enlargement of the sella turcica beyond the normal maximum dimension: anteroposterior length of 15 mm and depth of 12 mm on the lateral skull roentgenogram in adults. Erosion of the sella or clinoid processes or a localized bulge in the sellar contour (called a "double floor" when seen on a lateral skull roentgenogram) may also occur (Fig. 2–10), and is often best seen on sellar tomography. Pneumoencephalography is particularly useful in demonstrating suprasellar extension. In this procedure,

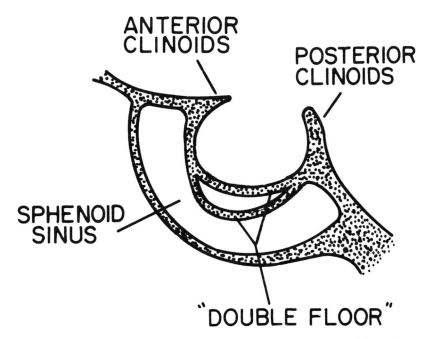

Figure 2–10. Diagram of localized expansion of the sella turcica, which produces a "double floor" when seen in lateral view.

air or oxygen is introduced into the lumbar subarachnoid space; the gas then rises through the cerebrospinal fluid to outline the brain's ventricular system and the subarachnoid cisterns at the base of the brain. Water-soluble radiographic contrast agents may be used in a similar fashion. Arteriography may be needed to delineate lateral extension as well as to rule out aneurysm as a cause of sellar enlargement. Computed axial tomography can usually demonstrate significant suprasellar extension readily; recent technologic improvements have also allowed the visualization of intrasellar lesions in many instances.

It should be emphasized that an enlarged sella turcica does not always mean a pituitary lesion is present. In the *empty sella syndrome,* an incomplete diaphragma sellae allows the arachnoid membrane and cerebrospinal fluid to enter the sella, compressing the normal pituitary gland and, in some cases, enlarging the sella turcica. Pituitary function is usually preserved, and no treatment is required; the condition must be considered in the differential diagnosis of an enlarged sella. Diagnosis of the empty sella syndrome is often made by pneumoencephalography, which shows air in the sella turcica; in many cases, computed axial tomography may suffice to demonstrate cerebrospinal fluid within the sella.

Hemorrhage into a pituitary tumor (pituitary apoplexy) occurs in about 5% of patients. It causes sudden onset of a severe headache and may progress to unconsciousness; blindness may result from compression of the optic chiasm. Paralysis of the oculomotor nerves, often asymmetric, causes deviation of the eyes and pupillary dilatation. Rapid surgical evacuation of the hematoma is usually required for preservation of vision.

Treatment

Hypopituitarism is treated, rather simply, by replacing the missing hormones or the hormones of the affected end organs.

Cortisol

The usual adult replacement is 15 to 30 mg cortisol given orally in divided doses to mimic normal cortisol secretion (e.g., 15 mg at 8:00 A.M. and 10 mg at noon; or 10 mg at 8:00 A.M., 10 mg at noon, and 5 mg at 6:00 P.M.). Patients should be advised to double the dose for minor stressful illnesses, and they must carry identification regarding the need to take cortisol. Large amounts of cortisol (such as 300 mg/day), together with glucose and sodium chloride, are given intravenously for adrenal crisis.

Thyroid

The usual daily maintenance dose in adults is 0.1 to 0.2 mg L-thyroxine given orally as a single dose. It must not be given in hypopituitarism unless cortisol is also given or the adequacy of ACTH secretion assured; otherwise, increased metabolic demands may precipitate an adrenal crisis if the patient cannot respond with increased ACTH and cortisol secretion.

Gonadal Steroids

Men may be treated with a depot testosterone preparation, 200 to 300 mg intramuscularly every 2 to 4 weeks, or methyltestosterone 5 to 20 mg sublingually or 10 to 40 mg orally daily. Methyltestosterone has hepatic toxicity and is not as potent as injected testosterone. Adequate therapy with either preparation restores muscularity, potency, libido, and body hair.

Women may be given a variety of estrogen preparations in a physiologic replacement dosage. In contrast, contraceptive pills are larger than physiologic dosage in order to suppress gonadotropin secretion.

Fertility in men may be achieved by administration of HCG (human chorionic gonadotropin), possibly with addition of a human FSH preparation in proper dosage, but this therapy is difficult. Treatment of women with cyclic administration of human FSH and HCG may result in ovulation so that fertility may be achieved.

Growth Hormone

Children may be treated with human GH by intramuscular injection. Human GH is now readily available commercially.

In some cases (e.g., pituitary tumors), the cause of the hypopituitarism can also be treated; these treatments (usually surgical procedures or radiation) are

Library
I.U.P.
Indiana, Pa.

616.407 En25d2
C.1   25

of major value in relieving and preventing the deleterious local effects of the intracranial mass lesion (e.g., loss of vision or obstruction of the flow of cerebrospinal fluid).

HYPERPITUITARISM

Hyperpituitarism refers to the pathologic overproduction of one or more pituitary hormones *not* secondary to end-organ failure. (This definition thus excludes the TSH overproduction occurring in primary hypothyroidism, for example.) Most cases of hyperpituitarism are due to hormone production by functioning pituitary tumors. Oddly, some pituitary hormones are much more commonly overproduced than others. GH and PRL overproduction are common, ACTH is occasionally overproduced, whereas primary TSH, LH, or FSH overproduction is rare.

Acromegaly and Gigantism

These conditions, resulting from the effects of excess GH, differ only in their age of onset. In the child, when long-bone growth is possible, excess GH greatly increases height, resulting in gigantism; in the adult, following closure of the long-bone epiphyses, bones may grow wider and thicker, and soft tissues may proliferate, leading to characteristic changes in the appearance of the face and extremities. (Acromegaly literally means enlargement of the distal parts of the body.)

The cause of GH overproduction in acromegaly is unclear; in most cases, an autonomously functioning pituitary tumor appears to be the cause, since normal GH secretion may be restored by removal of the tumor. On the other hand, reports of excessive amounts of a GH-releasing substance in acromegalic cerebrospinal fluid have suggested that abnormal hypothalamic regulation of GH secretion may be present and may be responsible for the overproduction of GH (and possibly for the tumor formation) observed. Pathologically, a discrete pituitary adenoma can be demonstrated in most cases. With routine hematoxylin and eosin staining, the cells of the adenoma may be either eosinophilic or chromophobic; however, electron microscopy usually shows specific GH secretory granules in both varieties. Some patients with acromegaly have other endocrine tumors (syndrome of multiple endocrine adenomatosis, type I, with tumors of pituitary, parathyroid and pancreatic islets).

The symptoms of acromegaly derive from the effects of both excess GH and a pituitary tumor; in general, they are more pronounced with longer duration of disease. The nose, jaw, tongue, and soft tissues of the hands and feet are often enlarged (Fig. 2–11). Protrusion of the jaw may result in dental malocclusion; the teeth may also become widely separated. Excessive sweating and oily skin are other common complaints, possibly because of hypertrophy of sweat and sebaceous glands. Bony overgrowth and deformity around joints may result in accelerated osteoarthritis, while soft tissue proliferation in the carpal tunnel of the wrist may compress the median nerve, leading to weakness and paresthesias in the hand. Lactation may be due to the intrinsic lactogenic properties of GH or to the presence of a "mixed" adenoma containing both lactotrophs and somatotrophs. Symptoms of hypogonadism, hypothyroidism, or hypoadrenalism may result from compression or destruction of normal pituitary tissue. Headaches and visual changes occur frequently, owing to the pituitary tumor.

Signs of acromegaly include the changes in appearance just mentioned and visual abnormalities, including extraocular palsies and the classic bitemporal hemianopsia; additionally, hypertension is often seen. Deepening of the voice due to vocal cord thickening is characteristic. Generalized visceromegaly, with enlargement of the heart, liver, and kidneys, is frequent; although the enlarged kidneys may have an increased glomerular filtration rate (creatinine clearance may be 150 to 300 ml/min), the cardiac enlargement may be associated with congestive heart failure. Cardiac and cerebrovascular diseases are responsible for most of the increased mortality in acromegaly. The relative contributions of elevated GH, hypertension, and glucose intolerance to the heart disease remain to be defined.

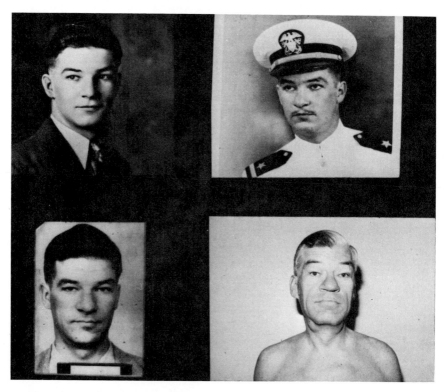

Figure 2–11. Sequential photographs of a patient with acromegaly. Note progressive coarsening of the facial features with time. Patient is seen at 18 years of age in the upper left photo, 22 years in the upper right, 27 years in the lower left, and 53 years in the lower right.

Routine laboratory studies may show glucose intolerance (45% of patients), hyperphosphatemia, and hypercalciuria. Although basal fasting serum GH is usually elevated in acromegaly, stress may produce similar elevations in normal individuals. Since GH secretion is normally suppressed by glucose, the best diagnostic test for acromegaly uses the measurement of GH during a standard oral glucose tolerance test; as previously mentioned, serum GH in normal subjects should be less than 5 ng/ml 1 to 2 hours after glucose, whereas most subjects with acromegaly fail to show this degree of suppression (Fig. 2–12). Many patients with acromegaly also show transient GH stimulation following administration of TRH or LH-RH and suppression after L-dopa; none of these responses are seen in normal subjects. Serum somatomedin levels are usually moderately increased in acromegaly. X-ray studies in acromegaly may show bony enlargement of the jaw, paranasal sinuses, hands, and feet. Soft tissue enlargement may also be seen; the heel pad thickness is measured in this regard and is greater than 20 mm in acromegaly. Skull films often reveal an enlarged sella turcica. Special studies such as pneumoencephalography, computed axial tomography, and carotid angiography are

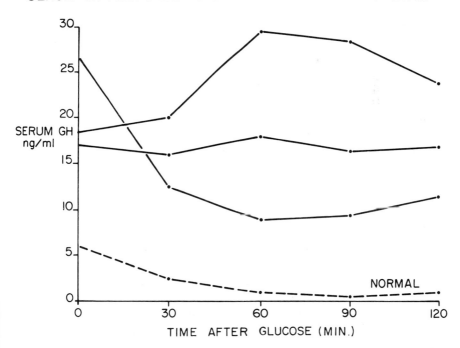

Figure 2–12. Varying patterns of growth hormone responses to an oral glucose load in three patients with acromegaly (solid lines). Although one patient showed partial suppression of serum growth hormone, this did not reach the low levels seen in normal subjects (dashed line).

useful to delineate the size and extent of the tumor and are particularly useful in guiding the neurosurgeon or radiotherapist.

The treatment of acromegaly has been reasonably successful in 60 to 80% of patients through the use of pituitary ablative techniques (surgical procedures or radiation). Although radiation therapy is associated with a slower fall in GH levels (over 1 to 5 years), it is less likely to produce hypopituitarism than is an operation. Promising medical treatments such as somatostatin and bromocriptine administration are being investigated for use when patients are not cured by ablative techniques or when these treatments are unsuitable. Somatostatin must be given intravenously, and its effects on GH secretion last only for the duration of the infusion. Bromocriptine, a drug that has dopamine-like actions and may be given orally, has longer-lasting effects.

Galactorrhea

The inappropriate production of breast milk (i.e., not associated with normal postpartum nursing) is known as galactorrhea; although it may occur in both men and women, it is much more common in women, probably because of their greater breast development. Since lactogenic hormones are necessary for normal milk production, it is not surprising that an excess of one such hormone, PRL, would be associated with galactorrhea; indeed, in many cases of galactorrhea, serum PRL levels are elevated. PRL elevations commonly result from various medications (phenothiazines, reserpine, α-methyldopa), from diseases affecting the hypothalamus or pituitary stalk (since PRL is primarily under hypothalamic inhibitory control), or from overproduction by pituitary tumors.

In cases of pituitary tumors making PRL, the adenoma may be either eosinophilic or chromophobic on routine staining with hematoxylin and eosin, but electron microscopy usually reveals PRL secretory granules. Small pituitary tumors (called microadenomas) producing PRL are usually located in the lateral wings of the pituitary, where lactotrophs are normally concentrated; somatotrophs (and therefore GH secreting adenomas) are found in this same region also.

Apart from the symptoms of a pituitary tumor per se (e.g., headache), excessive PRL secretion may result in galactorrhea, amenorrhea, decreased libido, impotence, and possibly gynecomastia (male breast enlargement); amenorrhea with galactorrhea is probably the most common complaint. Although some of the features of hypogonadism may be due to compression of the normal pituitary by the tumor, in many cases the high levels of PRL may suppress LH and FSH release, probably by suppressing LH-RH secretion. Few signs of excessive PRL production exist; careful breast examination may be necessary to demonstrate minimal galactorrhea. The pituitary tumor may produce visual field defects, extraocular palsies, and signs of hypopituitarism.

Unfortunately, no dynamic testing procedures can reliably differentiate functional (i.e., nontumorous) from tumor-produced hyperprolactinemia. L-dopa administration often suppresses serum PRL in both tumor and nontumor cases. The PRL response to TRH and other secretagogues is often blunted in cases of PRL-secreting tumors, although this reduced response is not universal. Perhaps the most useful procedure is simply multiple measurements of basal serum PRL; persistent elevation of serum PRL to levels above 100 ng/ml (normal male levels are less than 15 ng/ml; normal female less than 20 ng/ml) usually indicates the presence of a PRL-secreting pituitary tumor. Small tumors, of course, may be associated with less severe hyperprolactinemia.

X-ray findings of either generalized or localized sellar enlargement (i.e., a "double floor" on plain films, thinning or bulging of the sellar floor on tomography) provide strong evidence to support the diagnosis of pituitary tumor. As with other pituitary tumors, computed axial tomography, carotid angiography, and pneumoencephalography are useful in demonstrating suprasellar and lateral extension.

Both surgical removal and radiation therapy are effective; recently, a promising medical treatment has emerged in the form of bromocriptine administration; this ergot alkaloid suppresses PRL secretion in normal subjects and in patients with functional or tumorous hyperprolactinemia and shrinks PRL-secreting tumors in many patients.

Other Hormones

Primary overproduction of other pituitary hormones is less common. Inappropriate ACTH overproduction occurs in Cushing's disease, usually due to a small ACTH-secreting pituitary tumor. Following bilateral adrenalectomy (an older treatment for Cushing's disease), ACTH secretion increases greatly; the ACTH-secreting pituitary tumor may then enlarge, leading to signs of an expanding sellar mass as well as intense hyperpigmentation due to the intrinsic melanocyte-stimulating action of ACTH or possibly coexistent overproduction of a human MSH. In this situation, known as Nelson's syndrome, serum ACTH levels are often elevated to several thousand picograms per milliliter (normal serum ACTH levels are about 100 pg/ml). The radiologic findings are similar to those for other pituitary tumors, and either neurosurgical removal or radiation therapy may be effective treatment.

A few cases of TSH-producing pituitary tumors have been reported. These tumors result in hyperthyroidism in the presence of elevated TSH levels. Nontumorous hyperplasia of the thyrotrophs sufficient to enlarge the sella turcica may occur in *hypo*thyroidism and needs to be differentiated from a TSH-secreting tumor; the demonstration of hypothyroidism rather than a hyperthyroid state is usually adequate to make this distinction.

Gonadotropin-secreting tumors are also rare; some may arise as a consequence of primary hypogonadism, while others may be associated with normal or increased gonadal function. Gonadotroph hyperplasia may result from primary hypogonadism and may also produce sellar enlargement.

CLINICAL PROBLEMS*

Patient 1. A 34-year-old woman had suffered a severe postpartum hemorrhage 1 year before examination. She had been in shock at least 4 hours and had required transfusion of 2500 ml of blood. Failure of lactation, permanent amenorrhea, some atrophy of the breasts, and excessive fatigue followed the delivery.

PHYSICAL EXAMINATION. This examination revealed a well-nourished woman; temperature was 36.5°C, pulse was 90/min, blood pressure (BP) 90/70, weight was 120 pounds and height was 63 inches. Visual fields were normal by the confrontation method. Oral mucous membranes were normal. The thyroid gland was not palpable, and the areolar pigment was pale. Chest, cardiac, and abdominal examination was normal. Pelvic examination showed decreased vaginal secretions, small uterus, and nonpalpable adnexa. Axillary and pubic hair were diminished. Skin was pale but not dry. Neurologic examination was normal.

LABORATORY DATA

Complete blood count—normal. Urinalysis—normal.

Chest roentgenogram: small cardiac silhouette.

Skull roentgenogram: relatively small sella turcica with lateral cross-sectional area 50 mm^2 (normal, 65 to 140 mm^2).

Serum T$_4$—7 μg/100 ml (normal, 5 to 12 μg/100 ml). Cortisol—4 μg/dl at 8:00 A.M. (normal, 7 to 18 μg/100 ml).

Serum LH—2 mIU/ml (normal, 4 to 20 mIU/ml). FSH—2 mIU/ml (normal, 4 to 20 mIU/ml).

Serum estradiol—20 pg/ml (normal premenopausal female, greater than 25 pg/ml).

The patient was given 0.1 U/kg regular insulin intravenously at zero time for testing GH and ACTH reserve:

Time (min)	Glucose (mg/100 ml)	GH (ng/ml)	Cortisol (μg/100 ml)
0	80	<1	5
30	30	1	5
60	40	2	6
90	60	1	7
120	70	1	7

The patient was next given 500 μg TRH intravenously at zero time:

Time (min)	TSH (μU/ml)	PRL (ng/ml)
0	2	5
30	10	8
45	11	6
60	6	5
90	4	4

QUESTIONS

1. What is the pathogenesis of this disorder?
2. Which hormones are deficient and which appear intact?
3. What would be the hazards of testing her with metyrapone?
4. Because of hypopituitarism, a pneumoencephalogram was ordered. During the procedure, she became cold, clammy, and hypotensive. What would you do to treat her? Was the pneumoencephalogram indicated?

Patient 2. A 51-year-old man came to the emergency room complaining of 4 days of increasing retro-orbital headache and diplopia. Additional history included: 8 years of decreased libido; 3

*Answers to questions in clinical problems are found in the section following Chapter 11.

years of chronic fatigue, cold intolerance, decreased beard growth, and poor tanning of the skin. On close questioning, he admitted to a progressive increase in shoe and ring size over the past 20 years, along with increasing enlargement of his nose, lips, tongue, and jaw.

PHYSICAL EXAMINATION. BP was 100/60 lying and 80/50 standing. The left pupil was dilated and did not react to light. The left eye was deviated laterally and could not be adducted past the midline. Visual fields by confrontation demonstrated a bitemporal hemianopsia. Pubic and axillary hair was scanty. The testes were 2.5 cm in length and were softer than normal. The skin was dry and pale, and appeared thickened. Deep tendon reflexes showed a prolonged relaxation phase. The nose, jaw, zygomata, and lips were prominent; the tongue was large. Soft tissues of the hands and feet were increased.

LABORATORY DATA. Skull roentgenograms showed an enlarged sella turcica; chest roentgenogram revealed a normal cardiac silhouette. Laboratory studies included an unremarkable urinalysis; hematocrit was 35 (normal, 42 to 52); white blood count was 6600, with 6% eosinophils on the differential (normal, 3% or less); serum sodium was 128 mEq/L (normal, 135 to 145 mEq/L); potassium was 4.7 mEq/L (normal, 3.5 to 5.0 mEq/L); plasma cortisol was 3 μg/100 ml (normal, 7 to 18 μg/100 ml); serum calcium was 11.9 mg/100 ml (normal 9.0 to 10.5 mg/100 ml).

Over the next 8 hours, the patient was given fluids and hydrocortisone intravenously; although his BP increased to 120/80, his headache worsened, and vision in the nasal field of the left eye deteriorated. An emergency surgical procedure was performed.

Other laboratory studies (specimens drawn on admission, but results returned postoperatively) included: serum thyroxine—3.1 μg/100 ml (normal, 5 to 12 μg/100 ml); serum TSH—less than 1 μU/ml (normal, less than 6 μU/ml); serum testosterone—189 ng/100 ml (normal male, 300 to 1100 ng/100 ml); serum LH—1.7 mIU/ml (normal, 1 to 15 mIU/ml); serum PRL—4 ng/ml (normal male, less than 15 ng/ml); serum GH—47 ng/ml (normal basal GH, less than 5 ng/ml).

QUESTIONS

1. What chronic processes affected this man's pituitary gland? How long ago did they begin?
2. What acute process was superimposed on this condition?
3. Interpret the history and laboratory findings in relation to these processes.
4. Other similar cases may have elevated serum PRL levels. How would you explain this finding?
5. What kind of operation do you think was performed? Why was a surgical procedure chosen over radiation? What long-term endocrine treatment would you recommend?
6. What other endocrine disorder may exist in this patient? What further diagnostic studies should be done (when the patient can tolerate them)?
7. If surgical intervention had not been necessary, what might have happened to this patient's elevated serum GH over the next few weeks?

Patient 3. This 10-year-old boy had a 4-year history of slow growth, and a 9-month history of intermittent headaches.

PHYSICAL EXAMINATION. The examination revealed a short (3 SD below the mean), mildly obese (sixteenth percentile) prepubertal male with dry skin. The optic fundi showed pale discs, and visual fields revealed bitemporal hemianopsia. A skull roentgenogram showed erosion of the posterior clinoids of the sella turcica and calcification in the suprasellar region. Surgical exploration revealed a large suprasellar cystic tumor, with involvement of the optic chiasm. The cyst was drained and some tumor removed. Pathologic diagnosis was craniopharyngioma. Postoperatively, the patient developed polyuria.

LABORATORY DATA. The following postoperative laboratory studies were obtained:
Serum thyroxine—2.8 μg/100 ml (normal, 5 to 12 μg/100 ml).
Serum T_3 (by radioimmunoassay)—70 ng/100 ml (normal, 80 to 180 ng/100 ml.)
Serum TSH—<1 μU/ml (normal, less than 6 μU/ml).
A TRH stimulation test was performed using 7 μg/kg TRH intravenously:

Time (min)	TSH (μU/ml)
0	<1
15	8
30	18
45	20
60	26
75	22
90	14

Evaluation of GH and ACTH: The patient was pretreated with diethylstilbestrol, 5 mg twice daily for 3 days; regular insulin 0.1 U/kg was given intravenously at zero time, with the following results:

Time (min.)	Blood sugar (mg/100 ml)	Serum GH (ng/ml)	Plasma cortisol (μg/100 ml)
0	80	<2	8
30	38	3.6	
45	55	2.9	
60	60	<2	12

QUESTIONS

1. Why was the patient pretreated with diethylstilbestrol prior to GH testing? What effect may the diethylstilbestrol have on the plasma cortisol concentrations?
2. Can you be sure the patient is GH deficient? What would you do before retesting GH secretion?
3. Explain the results of the TRH stimulation test based on the location of the tumor.

Patient 4. The patient is a 27-year-old white single woman. At age 13, she experienced the onset of 4- to 5-day menses, which recurred regularly for about 6 months; then she began to skip periods, and a year later had ceased having menstrual periods. At about age 13, she began to have breast enlargement and pubic hair growth, and her development of secondary sexual characteristics progressed normally. At 18 years of age, birth control pills were given with resulting withdrawal bleeding, but no spontaneous menstrual periods occurred.

Since age 16, she has frequently experienced milky discharge from both breasts, usually after removing a tight brassiere; she denied any history of breast trauma or excessive manipulation. She has not taken any medication other than birth control pills at any time.

For the past 3 years, she has had frequent occipitofrontal headaches, unrelated to time of day, meals, or other factors. She has occasionally noted spots before her eyes, but denies other visual disturbance except for a transient (5-minute) loss of vision in her right temporal field while driving 5 months ago.

PHYSICAL EXAMINATION. Vital signs were entirely normal. There was no abnormal pigmentation of the skin, plethora, or acne. The eyes showed full extraocular movements, and visual fields were intact to confrontation. No masses were noted in the breasts, but a slight milky discharge could be expressed from each nipple following vigorous palpation.

LABORATORY DATA. CBC, urinalysis, and serum electrolytes were normal. A skull roentgenogram showed that the sella turcica was not enlarged, but a "double floor" existed. Bilateral carotid arteriograms were normal. Pneumoencephalogram was unremarkable except for slight upward bulging of the diaphragma sellae.

Serum FSH—8 mIU/ml (normal, 4 to 20 mIU/ml).
Serum LH—3 mIU/ml (normal, 4 to 20 mIU/ml).
Serum estradiol—20 pg/ml (normal premenopausal female, greater than 25 pg/ml).
Serum thyroxine—6.9 μg/100 ml (normal, 5 to 12 μg/100 ml).
Serum T_3—181 ng/100 ml (normal, 80 to 180 ng/100 ml).
Serum TSH—1.9 μU/ml (normal, less than 6 μU/ml).
Urinary specific gravity after overnight water deprivation was 1.025.
An insulin hypoglycemia test was performed:

Time (min)	Blood sugar (mg/100 ml)	Serum GH (ng/ml)	Serum cortisol (μg/100 ml)	Serum PRL (ng/ml)
0	95	2	17	495
30	44	7	24	565
60	62	22	39	605
90	91	15	30	515

Metyrapone test for ACTH reserve (3 g given orally at bedtime):
At 8:00 the next morning, plasma cortisol—5.2 μg/100 ml, plasma 11-deoxycortisol—28.9 μg/100 ml.

HOSPITAL COURSE. On August 16, 1974, she underwent transsphenoidal resection of a pituitary tumor; postoperatively, diabetes insipidus developed, diminishing spontaneously by the time of discharge on August 24, 1974. Radiotherapy (4500 rads) was given to the sellar region between October 28, 1974, and November 29, 1974. Replacement therapy was given with hydrocortisone (25 mg/day), L-thyroxine (0.2 mg/day), and an oral estrogen preparation, given cyclically. By late November, 1974, galactorrhea had moderately diminished.

The following hormonal measurements were obtained postoperatively:

Date	Serum T_4 (μg/100 ml)	Serum PRL (ng/ml)	Urine osmolality (mOsm/kg)
8/20/74	9.4	170	
9/26/74	3.7	164	433
11/14/74	12.3	100	384

QUESTIONS

1. What is the preoperative status of the pituitary hormones (except PRL)?
2. What is the cause of the amenorrhea and low gonadotropins?
3. When did the disease process begin?
4. Why did diabetes insipidus appear and is it still present?

SUGGESTED READING

General

Linfoot, J.A. (ed.): Recent Advances in the Diagnosis and Treatment of Pituitary Tumors. New York, Raven Press, 1979.

Martin, J.B., Reichlin, S., and Brown, G.M.: Clinical Neuroendocrinology. Philadelphia, F.A. Davis, 1977.

Post, K.D., Jackson, I.M.D., and Reichlin, S.: The Pituitary Adenoma. New York, Plenum Medical Book Co., 1980.

Hypopituitarism

Daughaday, W.H., Herington, A.C., and Phillips, L.S.: The regulation of growth by endocrines. Annu. Rev. Physiol, *37*:211, 1975.

Snyder, P.J., et al.: Diagnostic value of thyrotropin-releasing hormone in pituitary and hypothalamic diseases. Ann. Intern. Med., *81*:751, 1974.

Acromegaly

Levin, S.R.: Manifestations and treatment of acromegaly. Calif. Med., *116*:57, 1972.

Wright, A.D., et al.: Mortality in acromegaly. Q. J. Med., *39*:1, 1970.

Prolactin Overproduction

Frantz, A.G.: Prolactin. N. Engl. J. Med., *298*:201, 1978.

Kirby, R.W., Kotchen, T.A., and Rees, E.D.: Hyperprolactinemia—a review of recent clinical advances. Arch. Intern. Med., *139*:1415, 1979.

Malarkey, W.B.: Prolactin and the diagnosis of pituitary tumors. Annu. Rev. Med., *30*:249, 1979.

Schlechte, J., et al.: Prolactin-secreting pituitary tumors in amenorrheic women: a comprehensive study. Endocr. Rev., *1*:294, 1980.

CHAPTER 3

Thyroid Disease

Jerome M. Hershman, Inder J. Chopra,
Andre J. Van Herle, David H. Solomon,
and Delbert A. Fisher

PHYSIOLOGY AND BIOCHEMISTRY

Biosynthesis of Thyroid Hormones

Biosynthesis of thyroid hormones in the thyroid gland involves three stages occurring in a stepwise manner:

1. The thyroid gland employs an energy-requiring process to trap (concentrate) iodide from the circulation against a gradient.
2. Iodide is oxidized and incorporated into tyrosyl residues in the thyroglobulin molecule to form monoiodotyrosine (MIT) and diiodotyrosine (DIT), which are biologically inactive and serve mainly as precursors of thyroid hormones.
3. Iodotyrosines are coupled within the matrix of thyroglobulin to form thyroid hormones; coupling of two molecules of DIT leads to the formation of thyroxine (T_4); coupling of a molecule of DIT with a molecule of MIT results in the formation of $3,5,3'$-T_3 (T_3) or $3,3',5'$-T_3 (reverse T_3, rT_3). Figure 3–1 shows the structures of the iodothyronines.

Oxidation of thyroid iodide is mediated by a peroxidase. The peroxidase is also involved in coupling of iodotyrosines to form iodothyronines. Peroxidase activity is present mainly in the apical portion of the thyroid epithelial cell. This location of the peroxidase restricts the iodination to the cell-colloid interface and provides the thyroid with a mechanism for minimizing accidental iodination of nonthyroglobulin intracellular protein. Once iodinated, thyroglobulin containing newly formed iodothyronines is stored in the follicular lumen. T_4 is the most abundant iodothyronine in the thyroid. Its concentration in the human thyroid is about 10 to 15 times greater than that of T_3 and about 80 to 100 times greater than that of rT_3. The molar amounts of MIT and DIT in the thyroglobulin are nearly twice that of T_4.

34

3, 5, 3', 5'-THYROXINE
(T₄)

3, 5, 3'-TRIIODOTHYRONINE
(T₃)

3, 3', 5'-TRIIODOTHYRONINE
(reverse T₃, rT₃, T₃')

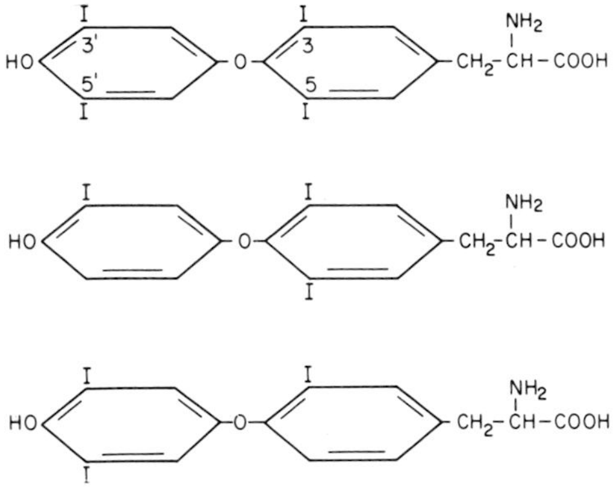

Figure 3–1. Structural formulas of T_4, T_3, and reverse T_3.

The iodothyronines (T_4, T_3, and rT_3) are formed and held in peptide linkage in the matrix of thyroglobulin. Release of iodothyronines involves endocytosis of thyroglobulin from the follicular lumen, and hydrolysis of thyroglobulin by a protease and a peptidase in the epithelial cell to liberate free iodoaminoacids (T_4, T_3, rT_3, DIT, and MIT). Most of the iodothyronines are secreted into the circulation, whereas most of the iodotyrosines are deiodinated intrathyroidally, and the iodide so produced is reused in further synthesis of iodoaminoacids. Thyroid secretory products also include a small quantity of intact thyroglobulin.

Thyroid-stimulating hormone (TSH) stimulates each step in thyroid hormone synthesis, and several agents can inhibit various steps. Certain monovalent ions, perchlorate and thiocyanate, are competitive inhibitors of transport (trapping) of iodide; thionamide drugs, propylthiouracil (PTU) and methimazole, can inhibit the peroxidase enzyme system and block iodination of tyrosine and coupling of iodotyrosines; excessive doses of iodide and lithium carbonate can inhibit release of thyroid hormones. Figure 3–2 summarizes these steps in biosynthesis.

Transport and Peripheral Metabolism of Thyroid Hormones

Iodothyronines (T_4, T_3, rT_3) circulate in human serum bound to three serum proteins, which (in order of decreasing affinity for iodothyronines) are: thyroxine-binding globulin (TBG), thyroxine-binding prealbumin (TBPA), and albumin. The binding of iodothyronines is so strong that normally only a small fraction of circulating iodothyronines is unbound (approximately 0.03% of T_4, 0.3% of T_3, and 0.3% of rT_3) and free to diffuse into the tissues. This small fraction is referred to as the "free" fraction in contrast with total (protein-bound plus free) iodothyronine concentration in serum. The small free fraction is the biologically active fraction of the circulating iodothyronines; the protein-bound iodothyronine serves mainly as a reservoir for making the "free" fraction of iodothyronines available to the tissues. Recent studies

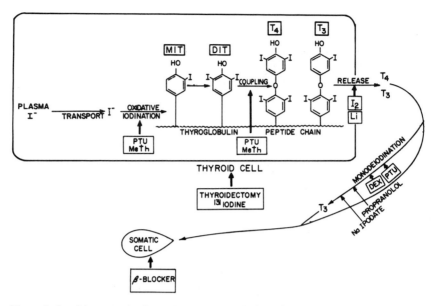

Figure 3–2. Biosynthesis of thyroid hormone and sites of action of agents used in treatment of hyperthyroidism (PTU: propylthiouracil; Meth: methimazole; I_2: stable iodine; β-blocker: propranolol, for example; Li: lithium; Dex: dexamethasone)

Table 3–1.   Mean Euthyroid Values of Serum Concentration, Metabolic Clearance Rate, and Production Rate of Iodothyronines

Iodothyronines	Serum concentration (μg/100 ml)	Metabolic clearance rate (L/day)	Production rate (μg/day)
T_4	8.5	1.0	85
T_3	0.12	27	30
rT_3	0.03	80	32

show that albumin-bound T_4 and T_3 dissociate readily in hepatic and brain capillary beds and may contribute T_4 and T_3 delivered to these tissues.

T_3 is biologically the most active iodothyronine; its calorigenic activity is about 3 times greater than that of T_4. Reverse T_3 (rT_3) has little or no calorigenic activity. Table 3–1 lists the mean values for serum concentrations, metabolic clearance rates, and daily production rates of iodothyronines. T_4 is most plentiful in serum (about 8.5 μg/100 ml), it disappears from the circulation slowly (half-life of approximately 6 days), and its production rate approximates 85 μg/day. T_3 concentration in serum is only about one-seventieth that of T_4, it disappears much more rapidly (half-life of approximately 1 day) than T_4, and its production rate is about 32 μg/day. The serum concentration of rT_3 is small (about 30 ng/100 ml) because it is cleared rapidly from serum; its production rate (about 32 μg/day) is similar to that of T_3.

Normally only about 25% of the daily production rate of T_3 and about 3% of that of rT_3 derive from thyroidal secretion; 75% of the daily production rate of T_3 and nearly 97% of the daily production rate of rT_3 arise from peripheral metabolism of T_4. Both forms of T_3 (T_3 and rT_3) are metabolized further by deiodination to diiodothyronines (T_2s), monoiodothyronines (T_1s), and ultimately to thyronine (T_0). Little information is available on the biologic function of rT_3, T_2s, T_1s, or T_0.

Thyroid hormones (T_4 and T_3) act on many tissues to increase metabolic activity and protein synthesis. Thyroid hormone is essential for normal growth and development. Recent studies show binding of T_3 and T_4 to nuclear receptors. The subsequent biochemical steps by which T_3 and T_4 exert their effects are unclear. There may also be sites of action unrelated to nuclear binding of the hormones. Thyroid hormones have direct effects on energy metabolism in mitochondria and on membrane transport in lymphoid cells. Through their effects on nuclear receptors, thyroid hormones control the synthesis of Na/K-dependent adenosine triphosphatase (ATPase), growth hormone, β-adrenergic receptors, and hepatic α-glycerophosphate dehydrogenase and malic enzyme. The clinical entities of hypothyroidism and hyperthyroidism are dramatic examples of the effects of the thyroid hormones on the intact organism.

THYROID FUNCTION TESTS

Thyroid function tests seek to define: (1) the level of thyroid function (hyperthyroid, euthyroid, or hypothyroid), (2) the cause of any departure from euthyroidism, and (3) the nature of abnormalities of thyroid structure.

The total T_4 or T_3 in serum is measured by radioimmunoassay (RIA). The free fraction of the hormones is measured by equilibrium dialysis of serum that has been labeled with radioactive T_3 or T_4. The dialyzable fraction multiplied by the total T_3 or T_4 yields an estimate of the concentration of free T_3 or free T_4. This method is difficult to perform, so that a simpler test called the T_3 uptake is generally used to estimate the degree to which serum T_3 or T_4 is unbound (free). It is an estimate of the saturation of the binding sites on TBG and the other serum proteins.

T_4 Binding Equations

1. *Dissociation equation*

$$TBG \cdot T_4 \rightleftharpoons TBG + T_4$$

2. *Equilibrium expression*

$$\frac{(TBG)\ (T_4)}{(TBG \cdot T_4)} = K$$

where (TBG) = concentration of unsaturated TBG binding sites
(T_4) = concentration of free T_4
$(TBG \cdot T_4)$ = concentration of TBG-bound T_4

3. *Solve for free T_4*

$$(T_4) = \frac{K(TBG \cdot T_4)}{(TBG)}$$

The equation means that the concentration of free T_4 is proportionate to the bound T_4 (essentially identical to the total T_4) and inversely proportionate to the concentration of unsaturated TBG binding sites (estimated by the T_3 uptake test).

A few essential points should be made about each of the frequently used thyroid function tests.

Serum Thyroxine (T_4)

The test measures the total amount of thyroxine in serum by radioimmunoassay. The normal range is about 5 to 12 $\mu g/100$ ml serum.

Serum T_4 is elevated in hyperthyroidism and is low in hypothyroidism. Because the binding equilibrium of equation 1 is always shifted far to the left, elevation of TBG increases the serum thyroxine. This increase happens during pregnancy or with the administration of estrogen because estrogen increases hepatic production of TBG. Serum thyroxine is low in euthyroid persons who have a low TBG. This reduction occurs in cirrhosis owing to a low synthesis of TBG and in the nephrotic syndrome because of a loss of TBG in the urine. Only rarely is a low TBG congenital.

Free Thyroxine Concentration (FT_4)

The *percentage* of free T_4 (%FT_4) is measured by determining what proportion of a tracer amount of radioactive T_4 added to the patient's serum is dialyzable. Normally, dialyzable T_4 is only 0.03% of the total serum thyroxine (range, 0.025 to 0.035%). The test is more relative than absolute because of considerable variation in the technique between laboratories. Then the free thyroxine may be calculated by:

$$FT_4 = Total\ T_4 \times \%FT_4$$

Normally, its approximate range is 1.0 to 2.5 ng/100 ml. Free T_4 is high in hyperthyroid and low in hypothyroid patients.

Triiodothyronine Uptake (T_3 Uptake) (T_3U)

The results depend on competition for radioactive T_3 between an anion-exchange resin (or other nonspecific binder) and the unsaturated binding sites on TBG in the patient's serum. TBG binds both T_3 and T_4. As the test is usually performed, the patient's serum is incubated with resin and labeled T_3; then radioactivity on the resin is counted. In normal serum, from 25 to 35% of the labeled T_3 attaches to the resin. The resin-uptake of radioactive T_3 is high in hyperthyroidism because the binding sites on TBG are relatively saturated, so more of the exogenous tracer T_3 is available to bind to the resin; it is low in hypothyroidism because the binding sites are relatively unsaturated, so less of the tracer T_3 is taken up by the resin. Figure 3–3 explains the test.

This test is not useful taken alone. Its only value is to allow the serum T_4 to be interpreted in the light of an estimate of unsaturated TBG binding sites, as discussed in the introduction. It should *never* be called a "T_3" or a "T_3 Test" because it in no way measures serum T_3. In fact, since T_3 binds to TBG with one-tenth of the avidity of T_4, changes in serum T_3 have little effect on the T_3 uptake; the test result is essentially determined by serum concentrations of TBG and T_4.

Free Thyroxine Index (FT₄I)

In practice, it is convenient to express the T_3U as a ratio, comparing the patient's T_3U with the T_3U in a normal serum pool run simultaneously. Then, the FT_4I is calculated as follows:

$$FT_4I = T_4 \times T_3U \text{ ratio}$$

As an example, one might look at typical results in a euthyroid woman taking birth control pills.

Results: $T_4 = 15 \ \mu g/100 \ ml$
$T_3U = 20\% \ (normal = 30\%)$
$T_3U \ ratio = \dfrac{20}{30} = 0.67$

Calculation: $FT_4I = 15 \times 0.67 = 10$ (normal = 5 to 12, same as for T_4).

Remember that the FT_4I has essentially the same significance as FT_4; only the numbers and units are different. To show that FT_4I is only an index rather than an accurate measurement of the free hormone, it does not have units.

Serum Triiodothyronine (T₃)

This test measures the total amount of triiodothyronine in serum by radioimmunoassay. (The normal range is about 80 to 180 ng/100 ml.) It is a useful test for mild hyperthyroidism since T_3 rises earlier and more markedly than does T_4 in all common forms of hyperthyroidism. "T_3 thyrotoxicosis" is the name given to hyperthyroidism associated with supranormal serum T_3 and normal serum T_4 concentrations.

Measurement of T_3 concentration is less useful in the diagnosis of many forms of hypothyroidism because an insufficient thyroid remnant, driven by TSH, secretes a hormone mixture high in T_3 relative to T_4. Thus, while T_4 may be distinctly subnormal, T_3 may be within the normal range, and the patient may indeed be hypothyroid.

Serum Free Triiodothyronine Concentration (FT₃)

FT_3 is measured and calculated in the same way as FT_4 and has the same significance. The normal range for the percentage of free T_3 is 0.23 to 0.47%, and the normal range for FT_3 is 240 to 620 pg/100 ml.

A serum free triiodothyronine index (FT_3I) can be calculated by the same manipulation of data for T_3 as was done for T_4. The serum T_3 concentration is multiplied by the T_3 uptake expressed as a ratio of normal (see previous example).

Serum Thyrotropin (TSH)

Serum TSH, which is measured by radioimmunoassay, is particularly useful in the diagnosis of hypothyroidism and for separation of thyroidal from pituitary hypothyroidism. In thyroidal hypothyroidism, levels of TSH are supranormal. In some patients who are euthyroid as a result of compensatory thyroid hypertrophy (e.g., endemic goiter and chronic thyroiditis), serum TSH may be above normal. In pituitary hypothyroidism, serum TSH is usually undetectable.

The method for radioimmunoassay is undergoing improvement. Until now, the normal range has been thought to be up to 10 μU/ml, with a quarter of normal sera having undetectable amounts. With more sensitive methods, all normal persons may have detectable levels and the normal range is 0.5 to 5.0 μU/ml. The level in hyperthyroidism is low.

Thyrotropin-Releasing Hormone (TRH) Test

TRH, a potent tripeptide hormone produced in the hypothalamus, stimulates the thyrotroph cell of the pituitary gland to increase its release of TSH. For testing purposes, the synthetic hormone (usually in a dose of 500 μg) is injected intravenously. The prompt rise in serum TSH reaches a peak in 30 minutes and returns to normal in 90 to 120 miutes. The peak value exceeds 5 μU/ml and is usually less than 35 μU/ml in normal persons. The rise is exaggerated in primary hypothyroidism, but the test is unnecessary since baseline TSH is already elevated. The TRH test may be useful to distinguish pituitary from hypothalamic hypothyroidism (see Chap. 2).

In hyperthyroidism and in persons receiving full or excessive replacement doses of thyroid hormone, no rise in serum TSH occurs after injection of TRH. In patients who have Graves' ophthalmopathy (exophthalmos) but are euthyroid, responses to TRH are either abnormally small or abnormally large, only rarely normal.

Thyroid Uptake of Radioiodine (RAIU)

A tracer dose of radioactive iodide, 123-iodine (^{123}I) or 131-iodine (^{131}I), is given to the patient by mouth. The radioactivity over the thyroid gland is counted at various intervals of time, usually 4 or 6 and 24 hr. The normal 24-hr uptake is about 10 to 35% of the tracer dose.

The thyroid uptake is increased in hyperthyroidism and reduced in hypothyroidism. It is also reduced (1) in euthyroid patients who take drugs or chemicals containing iodine since the pool of iodide in the body is expanded and the tracer is diluted in a larger pool; (2) in patients taking thyroid hormone, which suppresses TSH; and (3) in patients taking antithyroid drugs, which interfere with trapping of iodide (thiocyanate or perchlorate) or organic binding (propylthiouracil or methimazole). Since the average American diet is high in iodine, normal thyroid uptake overlaps that in hypothyroidism. The thyroid uptake of radioiodine is increased in euthyroid patients on a low iodine diet.

Thyroid Suppression Tests

Normal thyroid function is suppressible by giving exogenous thyroid hormone. When 75 μg T_3 is administered daily for 7 days, the patient's 24-hr thyroid uptake of radioiodine falls below 10% of the dose or below half the baseline thyroid uptake (i.e., the uptake before giving the exogenous thyroid hormone). Examples of normal thyroid suppressibility are patients 1 and 2 in Table 3–2. Hyperthyroid patients do not have normal suppressibility. Examples of hyperthyroid responses are shown by patients 3 and 4 in Table 3–2. Note patient 2 whose euthyroidism was associated with a high uptake, suggesting an unusually low iodine content in the diet. Note also patient 3 for the opposite result: a hyperthyroid patient had a normal uptake, presumably due to excessive dietary iodine.

This test carries some risk for older patients or those with cardiac disease because the T_3 administered may cause tachycardia. It is chiefly indicated when all other tests and clinical observations have left the diagnosis in doubt.

Antithyroid Antibodies

One of the hallmarks of autoimmune thyroid disease is the presence in serum of antibodies directed toward thyroglobulin or a thyroid microsomal antigen. The manifestations of autoimmune thyroid disease vary all the way from no clinical manifestations to Hashimoto's thyroiditis to Graves' disease.

Antithyroglobulin antibodies are usually measured by hemagglutination of thyroglobulin-coated tanned red cells. Titers greater than1:16 are considered to be significant.

Antimicrosomal antibodies are also assayed by hemagglutination. Titers greater than 1:100 are significant. About 10% of persons with no evident disease, mainly women, have significant titers.

Thyroid Scan

A scan is not indicated to determine the *level* of thyroid function. Its main purpose is to determine the cause of hyperthyroidism. A well-done scan distinguishes among Graves' disease, hyperfunctioning adenoma, and hyperthyroidism with multinodular goiter. The thyroid scan also shows whether a thyroid nodule concentrates radioiodine to the same extent as the other

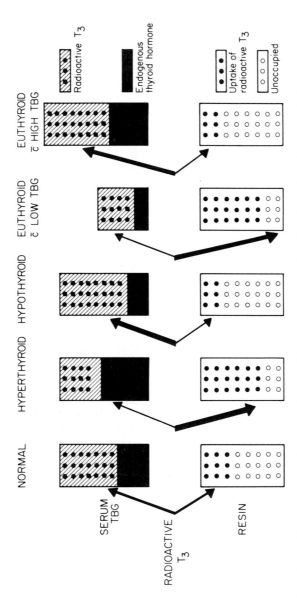

Figure 3–3. T₃ uptake test: diagram of the principle and changes in thyroid and nonthyroid disease. Radioactive T₃ added to patient's serum binds to the binding sites on TBG that are unoccupied by endogenous thyroid hormone, predominantly T₄. The radioactive T₃ not bound to TBG is taken up by the resin. Results of T₃ uptake are expressed as a percentage of the total radioactivity that has been taken up by the resin. Solid dots represent radioactive T₃. (From Chopra, I.J., and Solomon, D.H.: Thyroid function tests and their alterations by drugs. Pharmacol. Ther., C. *1*:367, 1976.)

Table 3–2. 24-Hour Thyroid Uptake

Patient	Before T_3 (%)	After T_3 (%)
1	30	6
2	50	16
3	30	28
4	60	52

thyroid tissue (isofunctional nodule) or whether it is cold (hypofunctional). Figure 3–4 shows typical abnormal thyroid scans.

HYPOTHYROIDISM

Hypothyroidism is the syndrome resulting from a deficiency of thyroid hormones, which causes many metabolic processes to slow down. Symptoms include fatigue, slowing of mental and physical performance, cold intolerance, impaired memory, change in personality (grouchiness or apathy), exertional dyspnea, hoarseness, constipation, muscle cramps, paresthesias, and dry skin. In newborns, hypothyroidism imparts a characteristic picture called cretinism (Fig. 3–5). Cretins show retarded development of the brain, which may be irreversible, and retardation of growth leading to dwarfism. In children, growth retardation, delayed dentition, and delayed bone maturation are characteristic manifestations of thyroid hormone deficiency. Precocious puberty occurs in some children.

Pathophysiology

The skin is infiltrated by mucopolysaccharide so that the face is puffy, especially around the eyes. The features become coarse and the eyebrows thinned. The tongue may enlarge and the vocal cords become thick leading to hoarseness. Retarded cerebration slows speech. Muscle contraction and relaxation (tendon reflexes) are slowed. There is mild weight gain. Myocardial contractility is reduced and the pulse tends to be slow. Heart sounds are distant. Effusions may occur in serous cavities including the pericardium. Atherosclerosis is accelerated because of high serum levels of triglyccride and cholesterol. The rate of degradation of lipids is even slower than the rate of synthesis. The skin tends to be dry and has a yellow tint, possibly due to carotene accumulation caused by a reduced rate of conversion of carotene to vitamin A. Body hair may be lost and not replaced, and scalp hair often becomes dry and coarse. Anemia is common, usually owing to a reduced rate of red cell production. The anemia usually is normochromic and normocytic, but may be macrocytic or microcytic. Menorrhagia secondary to anovulatory cycles may also contribute to the anemia. In some women with primary hypothyroidism, amenorrhea develops and suggests the incorrect diagnosis of hypopituitarism.

The spectrum of severity ranges from severe hypothyroidism with its classic features (called myxedema) to a mild, nearly asymptomatic subclinical dis-

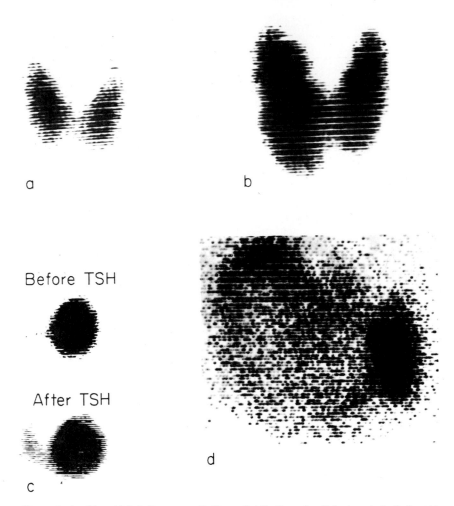

a   b

Before TSH

After TSH

c   d

Figure 3–4. Thyroid Scintiscans. *a*, Uniform distribution of radioisotope in both thyroid lobes of a normal subject. *b*, Distribution of radioactivity in patient with active Graves' disease. Note that the gland is larger and the distribution of radioactivity is uniform. *c*, Autonomous toxic nodule. All the isotope is concentrated in a left-sided thyroid nodule (top). Following injection of 10 IU TSH, the previously suppressed extranodular thyroid tissue becomes visible (bottom). *d*, Large hypofunctional nodule in the right lobe of the thyroid, with normal uptake of isotope in the left lobe. Patient had a biopsy-proved papillary-follicular carcinoma of the thyroid.

order. In the latter instance, sensitive thyroid function tests are necessary to establish the diagnosis. Severe hypothyroidism may progress to myxedema coma, which is usually precipitated by another stressful illness. Such patients are hypothermic because of a marked reduction in metabolic rate, and they have typical features of myxedema. Hypoventilation leads to respiratory acidosis and carbon dioxide narcosis. Some patients experience emotional instability, delusions, hallucinations, and overt psychosis (myxedema madness).

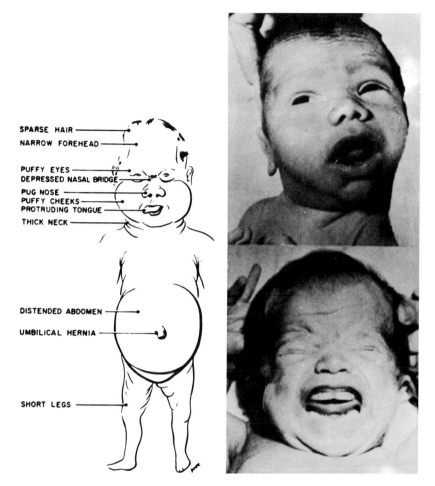

SPARSE HAIR
NARROW FOREHEAD
PUFFY EYES
DEPRESSED NASAL BRIDGE
PUG NOSE
PUFFY CHEEKS
PROTRUDING TONGUE
THICK NECK
DISTENDED ABDOMEN
UMBILICAL HERNIA
SHORT LEGS

Figure 3–5. The photographs on the right show the characteristic cretinoid facies in two untreated hypothyroid infants seven and eight weeks of age. The drawing on the left summarizes the principal physical features of such infants. (From Fisher, D.A: Mod. Treatment, *1*:133, 1964.)

Causes

Hypothyroidism may be either congenital or acquired. The etiologic classification is as follows.

Congenital
1. Thyroid dysgenesis
   a. Thyroid aplasia
   b. Thyroid hypoplasia
   c. Ectopic thyroid (usually hypoplastic)
2. Inborn defects in thyroid hormone synthesis or metabolism
   a. TSH nonresponsiveness
   b. Inability to trap iodide
   c. Inability to organify iodide

(1) without deafness
(2) with deafness
d. Inability to couple iodotyrosines
e. Iodotyrosine deiodinase defect
f. Iodoprotein secretion defect(s)
g. Deficient or abnormal thyroglobulin synthesis
h. Peripheral unresponsiveness to thyroid hormones
Acquired
1. Chronic lymphocytic (Hashimoto's) thyroiditis
2. Idiopathic atrophy
3. Iatrogenic
4. Endemic hypothyroidism
5. Hypopituitarism and/or hypothalamic disease

Congenital Hypothyroidism

Thyroid Dysgenesis. These infants have a deficiency in the volume of thyroid tissue. Most (80%) have a small amount of glandular tissue, often located ectopically, such as at the base of the tongue (lingual thyroid). Screening of newborns by measuring serum T_4 and TSH shows that this congenital disorder occurs in 1 per 4000 births.

Inborn Defects in Thyroid Hormone Synthesis. The patients usually have goiter and may be cretinous, hypothyroid, or euthyroid depending on the severity of the defect. These defects are rare.

TSH NONRESPONSIVENESS. The patients have a small gland with a low radioiodine uptake, hypothyroid function tests, and lack of response to exogenous TSH.

IODIDE TRANSPORT DEFECT. Features include low thyroid uptake of radioiodine, low thyroid concentration of iodine, and salivary I^-/ plasma I^- less than 10. Administration of iodine raises plasma iodide, which, by diffusion, increases intrathyroid iodide and thus permits synthesis of normal amounts of hormone.

ORGANIFICATION DEFECT. Failure of oxidative iodination results in rapid and high uptake of radioiodine, but the radioiodine is not oxidized and organically bound; thus it can be displaced from the gland by thiocyanate or perchlorate. The specific oxidative enzyme system (peroxidase) for organification of iodine is deficient. Some patients with a milder form of this syndrome have nerve deafness. The combination of nerve deafness and familiar goiter is called Pendred's syndrome.

DEFECTIVE COUPLING OF IODOTYROSINES. Radioiodine tracer is taken up rapidly and retained (organified), but the patient's system cannot couple iodotyrosines to form iodothyronines. Thyroidal iodine is primarily in the form of MIT and DIT with only trace amounts of T_4 and T_3. This defect is probably not attributable to a single specific deficiency because the coupling reaction is complex and poorly understood.

DEFICIENT IODOTYROSINE DEIODINASE. Normally MIT and DIT, released by proteolysis of thyroglobulin, are rapidly deiodinated in the thyroid. Little MIT or DIT is secreted. Iodotyrosine deiodinase is present in many organs. Patients with this defect have high MIT and DIT concentrations in the blood.

When they are given labeled MIT or DIT, they excrete the intact molecule in the urine. Synthesis of T_4 and T_3 can occur, but leakage of MIT and DIT depletes iodine stores. This defect is inherited as an autosomal recessive.

IODOPROTEIN SECRETION DEFECT(S). This disorder may be due to defective thyroglobulin biosynthesis or defective thyroglobulin breakdown, or it may be associated with another biosynthetic defect (iodotyrosine deiodinase deficiency) and high TSH activity. An iodinated protein, which resembles serum albumin, can be identified in the thyroid and in the blood of these patients. The iodinated protein is measured as PBI, but unlike T_4 and T_3, it is not extractable with butanol. This protein contains MIT and DIT in peptide linkage. The iodinated albumin is also detectable in small amounts in the serum of patients with other thyroid diseases and in some normal individuals.

DIMINISHED OR ABNORMAL THYROGLOBULIN SYNTHESIS. Patients have goiter, high uptakes of radioiodine, and absence of thyroglobulin in the thyroid.

PERIPHERAL UNRESPONSIVENESS TO THYROID HORMONE. A few families have been reported with deaf-mutism, goiter, stippled epiphyses, and elevated serum T_4. The findings suggest peripheral resistance to the effects of thyroid hormone.

Acquired Hypothyroidism

Hashimoto's Lymphocytic Thyroiditis. This condition is the commonest cause of hypothyroidism. The patient usually has a euthyroid goiter and is asymptomatic. However, in 15 to 20% of cases the patient is hypothyroid and in 5 to 10% hyperthyroid. Acquired idiopathic hypothyroidism after 8 years of age is attributable to Hashimoto's thyroiditis until proved otherwise (see later section).

Idiopathic Atrophy. This disorder is the second most common cause of adult hypothyroidism. It is usually due to lymphocytic thyroiditis. There are small remnants of thyroid tissue with occasional follicles, fibrous tissue, and lymphocytic infiltration. A high proportion of patients have antibodies to thyroid tissue.

Iatrogenic Hypothyroidism. This common disorder occurs after surgical thyroidectomy, after ^{131}I treatment of hyperthyroidism or thyroid cancer, with overdosage of antithyroid drugs (a reversible condition), and with high doses of iodine in susceptible individuals.

Endemic Hypothyroidism Including Cretinism. Patients with this condition and their parents usually have goiter. This syndrome occurs in regions of severe iodine deficiency. Endemic cretins may be hypothyroid or euthyroid in later life, but they retain short stature and the characteristic appearance of cretinism. Mental retardation, deafness, and other neurologic abnormalities may predominate, leading to the term "neurologic cretin."

Hypopituitarism. Lack of TSH may be associated with deficiencies of other pituitary hormones, but unitropic loss of TSH occurs. Most pituitary lesions cause a loss of growth hormone (GH) and gonadotropin before loss of TSH and ACTH. This condition is called secondary or pituitary hypothyroidism. A low serum TSH differentiates it from primary hypothyroidism in which serum TSH is elevated.

Hypothalamic Disease. Organic suprasellar lesions or other processes without a defined organic lesion may cause a deficiency of TRH, alone or in combination with loss of other hypothalamic hormones. The diagnosis is established in hypothyroid patients by finding a low serum TSH that increases after administration of TRH.

Therapy

The treatment of hypothyroidism involves administration of exogenous thyroid hormone. The following are among the preparations available.

	Average daily adult replacement dose
1. Sodium l-thyroxine (synthetic T_4)	100–200 μg
2. Sodium l-triiodothyronine (synthetic T_3)	50–75 μg
3. Preparations of mixed synthetic	50–100 μg T_4
T_4 and T_3 in a ratio of 4:1	+ 12.5–25 μg T_3
4. Thyroid USP (desiccated thyroid, dried thyroid, or thyroid extract)	
A cleaned, dried, and powdered preparation of animal (usually porcine or bovine) thyroid gland previously deprived of connective tissue and fat.	90–180 mg
5. Thyroglobulin	
The final purified product of porcine thyroid gland with a molecular weight of 660,000.	90–180 mg

L-thyroxine is the preferred preparation for replacement therapy because it is more uniform than biologic preparations, its absorption is more reliable, it is easily measured in serum, and most of the circulating T_3 comes from conversion of T_4 to T_3 in tissue. Thus, normal ranges for T_4 and T_3 can be applied to monitor therapy.

The history and physical examination are useful guides to the adequacy of therapy and should be the first approach, but mild hypothyroidism or mild hyperthyroidism cannot be excluded in this way. Measurement of circulating levels of T_4, T_3, and TSH are helpful. With the use of synthetic l-thyroxine or thyroid USP, the serum T_4 should be regulated to the midnormal range. When this regulation occurs, the serum T_3 and TSH levels are generally normal also.

HYPERTHYROIDISM

Hyperthyroidism is a clinical syndrome that occurs when excessive amounts of thyroid hormones in the circulation affect peripheral tissues. The most common cause of hyperthyroidism is Graves' disease, a multisystem disorder characterized by one or more of three pathognomonic clinical entities: (1) hyperthyroidism associated with a diffusely enlarged thyroid gland, (2) infiltrative ophthalmopathy, and (3) infiltrative dermopathy (pretibial myxedema). Hyperthyroidism is the most frequent clinical entity in patients with Graves' disease. When infiltrative ophthalmopathy (or dermopathy) occurs in the absence of hyperthyroidism, the condition is referred to as "euthyroid Graves' disease."

The causes of hyperthyroidism other than Graves' disease include:

1. Hyperfunctioning solitary thyroid adenoma ("hot" nodule).
2. "Toxic" multinodular goiter.
3. Lymphocytic thyroiditis with low thyroid radioiodine uptake.
4. Subacute (granulomatous) thyroiditis (early phase).
5. Ingestion of excessive amount of thyroid hormones (thyrotoxicosis factitia).
6. TSH-producing pituitary adenoma (rare).
7. Trophoblastic tumors (hydatidiform mole, choriocarcinoma) that secrete excessive amounts of chorionic gonadotropin, a weak thyroid stimulator.
8. Thyroid carcinoma (follicular type), usually metastatic.
9. Struma ovarii (ovarian teratoma with thyroid elements).

Etiology of Graves' Disease

The cause of Graves' disease is unknown. The serum IgG of patients with Graves' hyperthyroidism contains a thyroid stimulator that has been detected in a variety of systems. Bioassay of the serum in mice and guinea pigs showed that this stimulator had a longer action than pituitary TSH; this action gave rise to the name, long-acting thyroid stimulator. That the IgG of Graves' patients displaces TSH from its receptor on the thyroid plasma membrane is evidence that it binds to this receptor. This IgG increases adenyl cyclase in thyroid tissue, increases cyclic adenosine monophosphate (AMP), and increases the release of thyroid hormones. Each assay has given rise to a different name for this stimulator; the generic term, thyroid-stimulating immunoglobulin, seems most appropriate. With a sensitive method, such as measurement of the increase of cyclic AMP in thyroid slices, the stimulator can be detected in the IgG of over 90% of patients with active Graves' hyperthyroidism. The lower frequency of detection in other systems is probably attributable to insensitivity of the assays.

Because the thyroid-stimulating immunoglobulins cause the hyperthyroidism, Graves' disease is an autoimmune disorder. The trigger for the excessive production of these antibodies by B-lymphocytes is unknown. There is some evidence that T-lymphocytes (helper cells) stimulate these B-cells, but whether the disorder is primarily due to B-cells or T-cells is unclear.

The cause of the ophthalmopathy in Graves' disease is less clear than that of the hyperthyroidism. Recent work suggests that the following are factors.

1. Exophthalmos-producing IgG's are present in the serum of Graves' disease patients; these immunoglobulins cause exophthalmos in a fish bioassay and stimulate the incorporation of radioactive sulfate into mucopolysaccharide in the harderian (retro-orbital) gland of mice.

2. Deposition in retro-orbital tissues of thyroglobulin-antithyroglobulin complexes. Recent studies suggest that antithyroglobulin antibodies can be detected in nearly all patients with Graves' disease. Scintiscan techniques have also demonstrated the existence of lymphatic channels draining lymph containing thyroglobulin from the thyroid to the retro-orbital areas. Thyroglobulin-antithyroglobulin complexes in the thyroid could be transported to the retro-orbital areas and thus involved in the ophthalmopathy of Graves' disease.

The cause of the dermopathy of Graves' disease is unknown.

Constitutional, Emotional, and Hereditary Factors in Pathogenesis of Graves' Disease

Graves' disease occurs about 6 times more frequently in women than in men. It frequently occurs at puberty, during pregnancy, and at menopause. A history of severe stress (emotional, financial, or physical) precedes the onset of hyperthyroidism in many patients with Graves' disease. The frequency of the disease is about 0.4% in the general population. It may be familial since it is about 20 times more common in sisters of the patients than in the general population. The frequency of histocompatibility antigens HLA-DR3 and HLA-B8 in patients with Graves' disease is much greater than in the general population.

Pathologic Features of the Thyroid in Graves' Disease

The thyroid gland is diffusely enlarged and soft-to-normal in most cases. Microscopically, the follicles are small and lined with hyperplastic columnar epithelium. Colloid is scanty, and marginal scalloping and vacuolization are evident. The nuclei are vesicular and mitoses are frequently seen. Hyperplastic epithelium demonstrates frequent papillary projections into the lumen of the follicles. Vascularity of the gland is increased, and it is generally infiltrated with lymphocytes and plasma cells that are frequently aggregated in the form of lymphoid follicles.

Symptoms and Signs

The clinical features of hyperthyroidism mainly reflect two effects of excessive circulating thyroid hormone levels: (1) increased metabolic activity in various tissues and (2) increased sensitivity of tissues to catecholamines.

Patients complain of nervousness, weight loss despite good appetite, heat intolerance, and increased perspiration. The skin is warm and moist; vitiligo (patchy depigmentation) may occur as an associated, possibly autoimmune disorder. The free margin of the nail is lifted up from its base (onycholysis); instead of the normal convex junction of the free end of the nail with the nail bed, the junction becomes straight or concave.

Cardiovascular manifestations, directly reflecting the effect of thyroid hormone on the heart, are prominent with tachycardia; tachyarrhythmias, e.g., atrial fibrillation and paroxysmal atrial tachycardia; systolic hypertension; and widened pulse pressure.Congestive heart failure is usually related to the tachycardia, increased cardiac work, and sometimes underlying heart disease.

The dyspnea that occurs is related to intercostal muscle weakness and/or increased oxygen utilization. Patients often have increased appetite and mild hyperdefecation, but diarrhea is unusual. Nervousness, emotional lability, and hyperkinesia are common since thyroid hormone affects the nervous system.

Muscle weakness is more marked proximally because of catabolism of muscle protein; muscle wasting may also be striking. Myasthenia gravis or periodic paralysis may coexist. Mobilization of bone mineral leads to osteoporosis, and hypercalcemia occurs in about 10% of patients.

Hematologic manifestations include neutropenia, lymphocytosis, anemia, and increased red-cell mass due to the excess demand for oxygen. Oligomenorrhea, amenorrhea, and decreased libido occur. Gynecomastia is found in 10 to 20% of men and may be related to a high serum estradiol/testosterone ratio.

Ophthalmopathy

Patients with Graves' disease are characterized classically by bilateral proptosis (exophthalmos) that may be asymmetrical; exophthalmos may even be unilateral (Fig. 3–6). Proptosis is due to infiltration of the retro-orbital space with lymphocytes, mast cells, and mucopolysaccharides and to retro-orbital muscle edema and interstitial myositis. Besides proptosis, ophthalmic symptoms may include increased lacrimation, gritty sensation in the eyes, diplopia, and diminution in vision. Clinical findings may include lid lag, lid retraction (leading to a "stare"), conjunctival congestion, conjunctival edema (chemosis), congestion of the lateral rectus muscle insertion, and limitation of extraocular muscle movement, commonly involving the inferior rectus muscle and leading thereby to a diplopia upon upward and lateral gaze.

Approximately 1% of patients develop severe and progressive (malignant) exophthalmos, which may result in exposure keratitis, diminution in visual acuity due to optic nerve involvement, panophthalmitis, and even dislocation of the globe.

Infiltrative Dermopathy

This condition is present in fewer than 5% of patients. It is frequently associated with ophthalmopathy and usually involves the pretibial region of the legs (see Fig. 3–6). The skin is thickened and shiny, violaceous, and difficult to raise into a fold. Microscopically, the dermis is thickened and infiltrated with mucopolysaccharide and cells of chronic inflammation.

Laboratory Diagnosis

Elevated serum levels of thyroid hormones are the hallmark of the diagnosis. Ordinarily, serum thyroxine, serum triiodothyronine, free T_4, and free T_3 are all elevated.

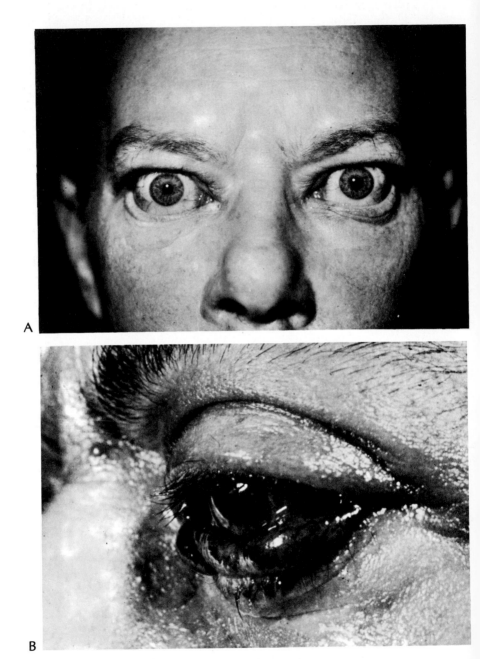

Figure 3—6. *A,* 45-year-old man with Graves' disease showing typical stare and exoph-thalmos. *B,* Severe exophthalmos with periorbital swelling and chemosis in a woman.

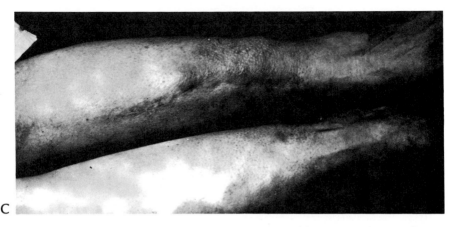

C

Figure 3–6 (Cont'd). *C*, Pretibial dermopathy in a 40-year-old woman who has nodular areas of induration and violaceous thickened skin (right).

Some hyperthyroid patients have an elevated serum T_3 concentration and a normal serum T_4 concentration. This clinical entity, T_3-thyrotoxicosis, may occur in patients who have Graves' disease or "toxic" nodular goiter as the cause for their hyperthyroidism. Thyroid ^{123}I uptake may be normal or high in these patients, but is not suppressible with exogenously administered T_3.

Hyperthyroid patients have increased saturation of thyroid hormone binding proteins in serum as assessed by the T_3 uptake test, which shows an increase in the free T_4 index. Although thyroidal radioiodine uptake increases, it is low in patients who are hyperthyroid owing to ingestion of thyroid hormones (thyrotoxicosis factitia), to subacute thyroiditis, or to lymphocytic thyroiditis. The thyroid scan in Graves' disease shows diffuse uptake of radioiodine. The scan is helpful if a solitary hyperfunctioning thyroid adenoma is being considered as the cause of hyperthyroidism (see Fig. 3–4).

Treatment of Hyperthyroidism

Three definitive modes of treatment are available for hyperthyroidism: drugs, ^{131}I, and surgical thyroidectomy.

Drugs

Thionamide drugs, propylthiouracil and methimazole, inhibit the peroxidase enzyme system of the thyroid gland and reduce synthesis of thyroid hormone. In addition, propylthiouracil (but not methimazole) inhibits monodeiodination of T_4 to T_3 in peripheral tissue. Figure 3–2 illustrates these mechanisms. The usual starting dose of propylthiouracil is 300 to 600 mg/day, given in divided doses every 6 to 8 hours, because the duration of action is short, about 6 to 12 hours. Methimazole is 10 times as potent and has a longer duration of action; the usual starting dose is 30 to 60 mg/day. Improvement of the hyperthyroidism occurs in 2 to 4 weeks allowing reduction of the dose. Side effects are skin rash, arthralgia, abnormal liver function, neutropenia, and, rarely, agranulocytosis. After a course of treatment lasting 12 to 18 months, about half the patients have a lasting remission.

Iodine in a dose of 6 to 2000 mg/day inhibits release of hormone from the gland, probably by interfering with proteolysis of thyroglobulin (see Fig. 3–2), resulting in a rapid fall of serum T_4 and T_3 levels. Iodine may block the peroxidase enzyme system also. Unfortunately, many patients "escape" from these effects in several weeks. Iodine is usually prescribed in large doses (5 to 10 drops of saturated solution of potassium iodide [50 mg/drop] 2 to 4 times daily). Lithium also slows the release of hormone from the gland by interfering with proteolysis of the colloid.

Sympathetic blocking drugs produce significant improvement in many features of hyperthyroidism. The β-receptor blocking drug, propranolol, is the agent of choice because of its rapid onset of action. It reduces tachycardia tremor, nervousness, and perspiration without affecting the secretion of thyroid hormone. It is given in a dose of 10 to 40 mg every 4 to 6 hours.

Radioiodine

[131]I destroys thyroid tissue mainly by the β radiation, which is selectively concentrated in the thyroid follicular cells. The radiation also impairs the ability of residual tissue to replicate and damages the microvasculature. Administration is simple; the patient merely swallows the radioiodine. The usual dose is 2 to 10 mCi. The only significant undesirable complication is permanent hypothyroidism, which appears in 30 to 70% of patients. Although hypothyroidism is recognized more commonly in the first year after treatment, it may not become manifest for many years.

Surgical Procedure

Subtotal thyroidectomy rapidly cures hyperthyroidism. It is carried out when the patient has been made euthyroid with antithyroid drugs to prevent a serious exacerbation of hyperthyroidism ("thyroid storm") in the postoperative period. Stable iodine is given for 10 days preoperatively to control the hyperthyroidism and to reduce the vascularity of the thyroid gland. Unfortunately, a high incidence of serious complications occurs with surgical thyroidectomy: hypothyroidism, hypoparathyroidism from inadvertent removal or damage of the parathyroid glands, and vocal cord paralysis from cutting the recurrent laryngeal nerves. Other complications include hemorrhage necessitating tracheostomy, cosmetic disfigurement, and recurrent hyperthyroidism.

Ophthalmopathy and Dermopathy of Graves' Disease

The ophthalmopathy may be given symptomatic treatment with artificial tears or protective glasses. Glucocorticoids may help in certain cases. Surgical decompression of the orbit may be required in patients with severe ophthalmopathy. For the dermopathy, topical glucocorticoids are frequently helpful.

THYROIDITIS

Thyroiditis probably is the commonest cause of thyroid disease in the United States. The various types are:
1. Acute suppurative thyroiditis
2. Acute (subacute) nonsuppurative thyroiditis
3. Chronic thyroiditis
   a. Chronic lymphocytic (Hashimoto's) thyroiditis
   b. Riedel's thyroiditis
   c. Radiation thyroiditis
   d. Thyroiditis associated with echinococcus disease, sarcoidosis, syphilis, and other disorders

In clinical practice only acute-subacute thyroiditis and Hashimoto's thyroiditis are encountered. Suppurative thyroiditis is a rare disease, and Riedel's thyroiditis is recognized as a fibrous variant of Hashimoto's thyroiditis.

Hashimoto's (Chronic Lymphocytic) Thyroiditis

This disease is the most frequently observed thyroid disorder in the United States. A recent survey in euthyroid, asymptomatic adolescents revealed an incidence of 1.4%. Relative age incidence rates peak at 40 to 50 years, so that the absolute incidence rate may approach 2 to 4% at that time. The disease is characterized by infiltration of the thyroid tissue by lymphocytes and plasma cells so that a moderate-sized, firm, nobby goiter develops. The gland is nontender in most cases, and signs of an infection are absent. The disease usually is detected incidentally by palpation of the goiter, but some patients have thyroid dysfunction.

The origin is not entirely clear, but accumulating evidence suggests that the disease has an immunologic basis. Circulating antibodies against thyroid gland constituents include antithyroglobulin, antimicrosomal, anticytoplasmic, and antinuclear antibodies, which can be detected by agglutination, precipitation, complement fixation, or immunofluorescent techniques. Cell-mediated immunity also is evident. There is a relative increase in "T" cells in circulating blood, and these cells can be shown to be sensitized to thyroid antigens. Lymphocyte-dependent, antibody-mediated cytotoxicity also has been demonstrated.

Certain families tend to develop Hashimoto's thyroiditis. Studies of twins show concordance in identical twins. The tendency of affected families to carry circulating thyroid autoantibodies also is clear, but the precise method of inheritance and the relationship of this characteristic to the thyroiditis are not known. Hashimoto's thyroiditis occurs with increased incidence in patients with chromosomal disorders (Turner's, Down's, and Klinefelter's syndromes). It also occurs in association with other endocrine gland deficiencies of presumed autoimmune origin, including Addison's disease, hypoparathyroidism, diabetes mellitus, and gonadal insufficiency; pernicious anemia and moniliasis may also be found in these patients. These abnormalities occur in various combinations, but only one has been given "syndrome status," i.e., Schmidt's syndrome (Hashimoto's thyroiditis and adrenal insufficiency with or without diabetes mellitus).

Clinically, the patients with Hashimoto's thyroiditis may have euthyroid goiter (70 to 75%), hypothyroidism with or without goiter (20%), or hyperthyroidism. About 30% of patients with Hashimoto's thyroiditis have a nodular goiter.

A number of markers for Hashimoto's thyroiditis aid in diagnosis, especially the presence of circulating antibodies. Antibodies to microsomes are more frequently detectable than antithyroglobulin. The thyroid scan is spotty and uneven because of the lymphoid infiltration of the gland. Iodide organification is abnormal, so that administration of perchlorate discharges a large proportion of the trapped radioiodine (positive perchlorate discharge test). As the disease progresses and thyroid tissue is damaged, the serum TSH increases and eventually the thyroidal response to exogenous TSH is lost.

Hyperthyroidism associated with low thyroid uptake of radioiodine is usually due to lymphocytic thyroiditis. The thyroid is not tender and is only slightly enlarged. Apparently, the inflammatory process causes a "leak" of thyroid hormone into the circulation, but biosynthesis is reduced. The disease is self-limited and usually does not result in permanent hypothyroidism. The pathophysiologic basis for the functional difference between this disorder and Hashimoto's thyroiditis with hypothyroidism is unclear.

No specific treatment exists for Hashimoto's thyroiditis. Some evidence suggests that thyroid hormone suppresses the disease (decreases goiter size and reduces circulating antibody titers), but most observers have not substantiated this hypothesis. Hypothyroidism, once present, is generally permanent and requires treatment with thyroid hormone.

Acute-Subacute Nonsuppurative (Granulomatous) Thyroiditis

This entity usually is referred to as subacute thyroiditis because the course runs from two weeks to several months. It is generally self-limited and of unknown cause, although a viral origin seems most likely. The onset is characterized by fever, malaise, and a firm, tender goiter. Often an upper respiratory infection or a prodrome of malaise, myalgia, and fatigue precedes this condition. The frequent presence of fever and systemic features suggests an infectious process. The disease often occurs in association with viral epidemics, including mumps, influenza, measles, and the common cold; and shows increase in antibodies to a variety of viral antigens including coxsackie, adenovirus, influenza, and mumps.

Antithyroid antibodies occur in 40 to 50% of patients, but the titers are low, peak several weeks after the onset, and disappear after several months. Thus, they probably occur as a result of the disease and are not involved in the pathogenesis. The signs and symptoms can be divided into 3 subgroups: local, systemic and metabolic.

Local Manifestations

These include neck pain, usually in the area of the thyroid and sometimes with radiation to the ears; pain on swallowing; sore throat; and often visible swelling in the area of the thyroid gland. Thyroid tenderness is common.

Systemic Symptoms

Malaise and fatigue are present in 80% of patients. Fever, anorexia, myalgia, occasional chills, and features of an upper respiratory infection also may occur.

Hypermetabolism

This symptom is manifest in about half the patients; they may complain of nervousness, sweating, heat intolerance, tachycardia, insomnia, and increased appetite (sometimes with weight loss). These manifestations presumably relate to the release of thyroid hormones from the severe thyroid cell damage caused by the infectious agent. The serum T_4 and thyroglobulin are increased because of release of T_4 and thyroglobulin. The damaged thyroid cells fail to trap iodine, and the thyroidal radioiodine uptake is reduced early in the disease. The local and systemic symptoms and signs and the elevated T_4 in association with a low thyroid uptake of radioiodine suggest the diagnosis. The hyperthyroidism is self-limited, usually subsiding in two to six weeks. Rarely, there are no local symptoms or thyroid tenderness. Hyperthyroidism with a low uptake of radioiodine raises the suspicion of "silent thyroiditis," which is more often due to lymphocytic thyroiditis.

No specific therapy exists, and antithyroid medication offers little benefit because of the short duration of hyperthyroidism. Symptomatic therapy for the local or systemic discomfort may be helpful. Aspirin or glucocorticoids have been given with apparently good results.

As recovery proceeds, the radioactive iodine uptake increases as the follicular cells resume normal function. The elevated levels of T_4 fall as glandular colloid is depleted and may reach hypothyroid levels if recovery of follicular cell function is delayed. At this point, features of hypothyroidism appear in about one-fourth of the patients, and the diagnosis of Hashimoto's thyroiditis is most strongly considered. Thyroid function eventually returns to normal; however, an enlarged, hard, nontender thyroid gland may persist for weeks or months after the acute phase. In some patients with protracted or recurrent thyroid tenderness, administration of thyroid hormone appears beneficial.

ENDEMIC GOITER

Endemic goiter is defined as enlargement of the thyroid gland to twice the normal size or to 40 g or larger in at least 10% of the population of an area. Endemic goiter still occurs in all continents, even though its incidence in certain areas of the world has decreased because of the prophylactic use of iodine. Sporadic nontoxic goiter is a term used to designate goiter with a lower incidence than that observed in endemic goiter areas. Euthyroid goiters are sometimes covered by the general term, "simple goiter."

Etiology

One of the well-recognized causes is the low daily dietary iodine intake in these regions. The minimal dietary requirement of iodine is around 100 µg/day. Dietary deficiencies of iodine are prevalent in areas where the soil and consequently the water and food supply are poor in iodine. Foods with recognized high iodine content are saltwater fish, shellfish, and chicken. Major areas of natural iodine deficiency include the northwestern and Great Lakes areas of the United States, the mountainous areas of Central and South America, the Alps and the Himalayas, and Central and South Africa. In some of these areas, the incidence of goiter has been greatly reduced by iodine prophylaxis. In certain areas of the world, iodine deficiency is associated with other factors that cause goiter formation. Supporting evidence is that certain fractions of populations subjected to severe iodine deficiency do not develop goiters and that iodine supplementation does not always eradicate the disorder completely.

The pathogenic mechanism for goiter development in iodine-deprived areas is presumed to require increased levels of serum TSH, which causes hyperplasia of thyroid cells in an effort to maintain thyroid hormone homeostasis. The thyroidal hyperstimulation by thyrotropin leads to an increased iodine uptake and enables the gland to accumulate sufficient iodine (despite a low dietary iodine intake) to maintain normal thyroid hormone levels in most individuals. Patients with endemic goiter have a low urinary iodine excretion, an elevated radioiodine uptake, and an elevated serum TSH level. In the compensated state, thyroxine levels are usually low or normal, with a normal or even slightly increased serum T_3 level.

The use of iodized salt in certain areas of the world (e.g., the United States and Switzerland) and the injection of iodized oil in other areas (Republic of Zaire) have reduced both the development of goiter in these areas and the size of existing goiters.

Clinical Features

Clinically the patients are euthyroid in the compensated state. The thyroid can be moderately to grossly enlarged. In childhood the gland is diffusely enlarged; nodule formation develops postpuberally, especially in females. Males are definitely less likely to develop goiter. In the decompensated state, the patients may become hypothyroid. Cretinism is the most severe form of the disorder and is sometimes associated with deaf-mutism.

THYROID NODULES AND THYROID CARCINOMAS

A thyroid nodule is a common deformity of the thyroid gland found during careful physical examination by inspection and palpation. Nodules are not usually associated with alterations in thyroid function in the extranodular tissue. Thyroid nodules may not be detectable clinically when they are less than 1 cm in diameter even though they may be readily found then on pathologic examination of the thyroid gland. For practical reasons, the present discussion deals only with the clinically detectable nodule. Figure 3–7 shows a typical thyroid nodule.

Etiology

Almost all pathologic processes of the thyroid gland can manifest themselves as a nodule. The following pathologic entities frequently cause nodule formation (single or multiple nodules): (1) adenomas (with or without central cystic degeneration), (2) thyroid carcinoma, (3) subacute thyroiditis, (4) chronic lymphocytic thyroiditis, (5) colloid goiter with cyst formation, (6) metastatic cancer to the thyroid, and (7) granulomatous involvement of the thyroid gland.

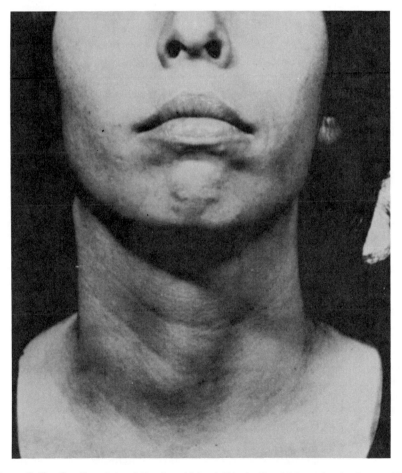

Figure 3–7. Small nodule of the thyroid is visible in the right paratracheal area. The nodule represents a cyst located in the inferior pole of the right thyroid lobe.

Adenomas and Carcinomas

In experimental animals prolonged, increased stimulation of the thyroid gland by TSH, induced by iodine deficiency or antithyroid agents, can be responsible for thyroid hyperplasia and tumor formation of the follicular cells. If x-ray irradiation of the thyroid is performed during dietary iodine deficiency, tumor formation in animals increases. When these tumors are transplanted to histocompatible hosts, the tumors may metastasize and eventually kill their host. In man clinical evidence strongly suggests that the incidence of both benign and malignant tumors increases following exposure to radiation. Patients who were irradiated in the thymic or tonsillar area for thymic or tonsillar enlargement during childhood have a striking increase in the incidence of thyroid tumors (papillary and follicular carcinomas as well as adenomas). Exposure to radiation from fallout of the atomic blomb (β and γ rays) also led to the development of benign and malignant thyroid tumors.

Colloid Goiters

These goiters become nodular in their end stage. The first stage, hyperplasia of the thyroid cells, is followed by colloid accumulation. When the two changes coexist in the gland, the term "colloid goiter" is applied. In the final stage, degenerative changes (infarction, hemorrhage, necrosis) occur and lead to nodularity. These nodules can be distinguished clinically from true adenomas because of the multiplicity of nodules in the colloid goiter.

Metastatic Thyroid Cancer

Secondary metastatic lesions to the thyroid are frequent pathologically but not clinically, presumably owing to the high vascularity of the thyroid gland. One-fourth of patients who die from metastasizing neoplasms have metastases in the thyroid gland. Lymphomas especially of the non-Hodgkin type sometimes involve the thyroid gland.

Granuloma of the Thyroid (Sarcoidosis, Tuberculosis)

These lesions rarely cause thyroid nodularity and should be considered only when a patient with a nodule has a coexisting granulomatous disorder.

Clinical Presentation

Symptoms

Benign or malignant nodules of the thyroid gland are symptomless most of the time and are frequently found on a routine physical examination. If a nodule is large, it can compress the esophagus leading to dysphagia, it can compress the trachea leading to respiratory difficulties, and it can compress the recurrent laryngeal nerve and cause impairment of the voice, such as hoarseness or even vocal cord paralysis. Occasionally, a malignant lesion manifests itself as a painful nodule. As a rule, benign lesions are not painful except in acute or subacute thyroiditis.

Signs

The nodule is usually discovered by inspection and palpation of the thyroid gland (Fig. 3–7). The consistency of nodules varies from soft to firm. The firmness of the lesion has been used as a clue to its possible malignant nature, but unusual hardness is not a reliable sign of malignancy. Of greater importance is the presence of pathologic lymph nodes in the cervical area. This factor may suggest the presence of a thyroid malignant tumor even when no thyroid lesion is palpable.

Pathophysiologic Mechanisms

The exact reason for development of the nodular goiter is still unknown in the majority of cases because the previously discussed mechanisms such as irradiation and iodine deficiency explain only a small percentage of goiters and nodules. The role of subtle changes in the biosynthesis of thyroid hormone has not been fully investigated, mainly because of lack of sensitive and reliable methods for these studies.

Classification of Carcinoma and Adenoma

Differentiated thyroid carcinomas make up approximately 85% of all malignant tumors of the thyroid. Differentiated carcinomas (papillary or follicular carcinomas) are far less malignant than anaplastic carcinomas, which make up 5% of thyroid malignancies. If the papillary or follicular carcinoma is confined to the thyroid gland in a patient less than 40 years old, long-term survival is not reduced. Papillary carcinoma spreads through the lymphatics, and on examination, the lymph nodes are positive for carcinoma. As a rule, follicular carcinomas have a tendency to spread via the hematogenous route and metastasize to lung, liver, bone, and brain.

Medullary carcinoma of the thyroid, also called thyroid carcinoma with amyloid stroma, represents about 5% of all thyroid carcinomas. This tumor is of considerable interest because of its familial incidence in patients with the syndrome of multiple endocrine adenomas (type 2) consisting of medullary thyroid carcinoma, pheochromocytoma, and hyperparathyroidism. Many of the familial patients have mucosal neuromas and a characteristic appearance (long thin face, long extremities, and poor musculature). Sporadic (nonfamilial) cases also occur. The thyroid tumor originates from the parafollicular C-cell and produces calcitonin. High serum concentration of calcitonin serves as a marker for the medullary carcinoma. Stimulation of calcitonin secretion by infusion of calcium to produce hypercalcemia gives an excessive calcitonin response in these patients and aids diagnosis of the tumor in a preclinical phase in afflicted family members. Although the patients have excessive calcitonin secretion, they are not hypocalcemic; their apparent resistance to the metabolic effect of calcitonin may be explained by recent evidence that shows that high concentrations of calcitonin decrease the number of receptors for the hormone.

Separation of Benign from Malignant Lesions

Important factors in the investigation of the patient with a thyroid nodule include a history of irradiation for thymic or tonsillar enlargement in childhood or a family history of thyroid carcinoma (medullary carcinoma). Nodules in men or in young children are more commonly malignant than those in adult women.

The following physical findings suggest malignancy: (1) enlarged lymph nodes in the cervical area, (2) invasion of the surrounding structures by the tumor as manifested by hoarseness and pressure symptoms, and (3) extreme firmness of the lesion.

Thyroid function is usually normal in patients with a malignant tumor of the thyroid. If the patient has hypothyroidism or hyperthyroidism, it is unlikely that the thyroid nodule is malignant, even though a malignant lesion can occur in a gland with active Graves' disease or Hashimoto's thyroiditis.

Roentgenograms of the neck show small dense calcifications (aggregated psammoma bodies) in some malignant tumors of the thyroid. Shell-like calcifications, on the other hand, usually indicate a benign tumor.

Serum calcitonin concentration is increased in patients with medullary carcinoma of the thyroid. Infusion of calcium or pentagastrin leads to a substantial release of calcitonin in these patients and improves the detection of medullary carcinoma in family members.

Thyroglobulin levels in serum are elevated in patients with thyroid carcinoma, but this elevation is not specific for thyroid cancer. Other disorders can cause elevated levels of thyroglobulin, e.g., Graves' disease, toxic adenomas, subacute thyroiditis, and endemic goiters. The test is useful, however, in the diagnosis of recurrent metastatic disease in patients with differentiated carcinomas because a high thyroglobulin level in a patient with previously resected thyroid carcinoma indicates the presence of secreting thyroid tissue (Fig. 3–8).

Aspiration of the nodule with a thin needle yields cellular material that may be diagnostic. The fine-needle aspiration method is often successful for making the diagnosis of colloid goiter, lymphocytic thyroiditis, granulomatous thyroiditis, papillary carcinoma, medullary carcinoma, and anaplastic carcinoma. Unfortunately, the cytologic examination cannot distinguish the common follicular adenoma from a follicular carcinoma. Cystic contents can be aspirated through the needle to "decompress" the cyst.

Scanning of the thyroid gland with radioactive iodine has been widely used in an attempt to distinguish benign from malignant lesions. This approach has failed because at least 80% of the lesions that do not concentrate radioactive iodine are benign.

Thyroid ultrasonography has become an important tool to distinguish the solid from the cystic lesion. Cystic lesions are almost uniformly benign; mixed solid and cystic lesions are sometimes malignant. Most malignant lesions are solid by ultrasonography although not all solid lesions by ultrasonography are

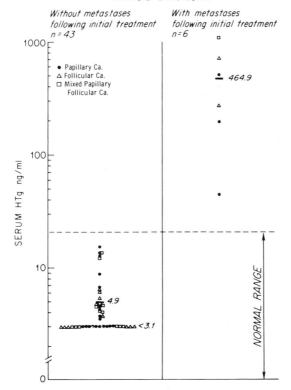

Figure 3—8. Serum thyroglobulin (HTg) levels in patients with differentiated thyroid carcinoma following therapy. The mean serum HTg concentration for patients without evidence of metastases (left panel) and with evidence of metastases (right panel) is indicated by the solid horizontal line. The patients with metastases can be clearly distinguished from the patients without metastases. (From Van Herle, A.J., and Uller, R.P.: J. Clin. Invest., 56:72, 1975.)

malignant. The technique has shown that about 20% of thyroid nodules are cystic. Figure 3–9 shows examples of ultrasonography.

Therapy

Two general forms of therapy have been advocated for the management of thyroid nodules. One approach uses thyroid hormone to suppress TSH secretion in all patients with thyroid nodules because TSH is regarded as a growth factor for the nodule; the second approach advocates surgical removal of all thyroid nodules. In clinical practice, the therapy is individualized; lesions with definite suspicion of malignancy are removed surgically. Nodules that are not likely to be malignant, such as cystic lesions or multinodular goiters, can be treated with doses of thyroid hormone, which suppress TSH secretion, usually 0.15 to 0.25 mg thyroxine daily.

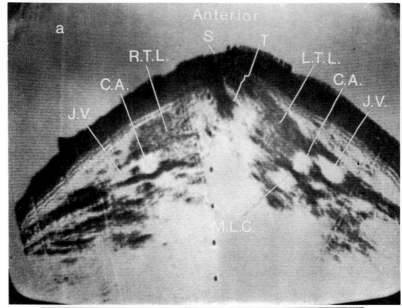

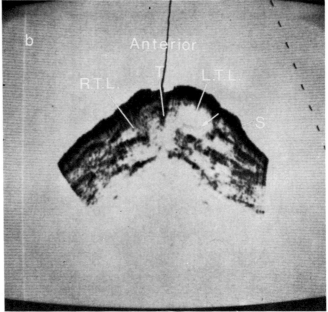

Figure 3–9. *a,* Ultrasonogram of the normal thyroid gland. (S: skin and transducer artifact; T: trachea; L.T.L.: left thyroid lobe and R.T.L.: right thyroid lobe; C.A.: carotid artery; J.V.: jugular vein; M.L.C.: musculus longus colli.) *b,* Ultrasonogram of a thyroid gland containing cyst in the left thyroid lobe. A sediment is clearly visible in the cystic lesion (arrow).

After thyroidectomy for thyroid carcinoma, treatment with radioactive iodine is often given to remove residual malignant or normal tissue, and at subsequent times it is given when functional metastases become evident.

CLINICAL PROBLEMS

Patient 1. A 50-year-old housewife complains of progressive weight gain of 20 pounds in 1 year, fatigue, loss of memory, slow speech and a lower voice, cold intolerance, and ataxia noted during weekend hikes.

PHYSICAL EXAMINATION. On physical examination, her face is puffy, she speaks slowly, her skin is pale, cool, and dry, and it has a yellow tint. Temperature 97°F, pulse 60, regular, BP 120/85. The thyroid gland is not palpable. Tendon reflexes are slowed with a delayed return phase.

LABORATORY DATA. Hemoglobin is 9 g/100 ml, hematocrit (HCT) is 30, white blood count (WBC) is 7000/mm³, red cells are macrocytic, and the differential WBC is normal. Her serum T_4 concentration is 2.3 μg/100 ml, and the serum TSH is 100 μU/ml.

QUESTIONS

1. Which of her clinical features suggest neurologic symptoms from a lack of thyroid hormone?
2. Which laboratory test shows that the patient has primary hypothyroidism rather than hypothyroidism secondary to pituitary disease? Would a skull roentgenogram be indicated?
3. What is the most likely cause of her hypothyroidism, and what test should be ordered to confirm this diagnosis?
4. What is the explanation for her anemia?

Patient 2. A 25-year-old secretary complains of nervousness, weakness, and palpitations with exertion for the past 6 months. Recently, she has perspired excessively in her office and wants to sleep with fewer blankets than her husband. She has maintained a normal weight of 120 pounds but is eating twice as much as she did 1 year ago. She also complains of protrusion of her eyes, excessive lacrimation, and a sandy sensation in her eyes, but no diplopia. Menstrual periods have been regular but there is less bleeding. She has been taking birth control pills for 3 years.

PHYSICAL EXAMINATION. She appears anxious and hyperkinetic. Her pulse is 120/min., BP 130/60. Her skin is warm, moist, and smooth. She has lid lag, normal ocular motility, mild exophthalmos (though measuring only 18 mm bilaterally on the exophthalmometer; normal, less than 20 mm), and slight periorbital swelling. The thyroid is diffusely enlarged to 60 g (3 times normal size), with a prominent isthmus and normal consistency. She has a bounding cardiac apical impulse, a pulmonic flow murmur, and a systolic bruit over the thyroid. She has a fine tremor and rises from a deep knee bend with difficulty. The rest of the examination is unremarkable.

LABORATORY DATA. Serum T_4 is 22 μg/100 ml and serum T_3 is 550 ng/100 ml.

QUESTIONS

1. What is the diagnosis? Are additional diagnostic tests indicated?
2. Calculate her free thyroxine index; her T_3 uptake was 40% (mean normal, 30%).
3. What is the cause of the pulmonic flow murmur? Of the thyroid bruit?
4. What therapy would you prescribe, and what is her prognosis?
5. Is there any contraindication to pregnancy?

Patient 3. A 23-year-old hospital dietician had pharyngitis with a fever of 101°F for 1 week. Two weeks later, she had a recurrence of a mild sore throat, noted swelling of her lower anterior neck, and moderate pain with swallowing.

PHYSICAL EXAMINATION. Her temperature was 100.5°F, pulse 100, BP 120/60. Her pharynx appeared normal. Her thyroid was enlarged to 40 g, the left lobe being slightly larger than the right; the entire gland was tender. There was no cervical lymphadenopathy.

LABORATORY DATA. Thyroid function tests showed serum T_4, 18.1 μg/100 ml; free T_4, index 18; serum T_3, 350 ng/100 ml; thyroid ¹²³I uptake, 2% at 24 hours.

QUESTIONS

1. What are the diagnosis and the cause of the condition?
2. Why is the thyroid uptake of radioiodine so low?
3. What would her serum thyroglobulin be?
4. Is she hyperthyroid?
5. What therapy would you recommend?

Patient 4. A 14-year-old girl is referred for evaluation of a goiter. She is entirely asymptomatic though the family has a history of goiter in the mother, 2 maternal aunts, and her sister.

LABORATORY DATA. Recent thyroid function tests show serum T_4 is 5 μg/100 ml, serum T_3 is 130 ng/100 ml, serum TSH is 14 μU/ml, and thyroid radioiodine uptake is 30% at 6 hours and 18% at 24 hours; scan showed a symmetrically enlarged gland.

PHYSICAL EXAMINATION. Your evaluation reveals no clinical features of hypothyroidism. Her thyroid gland is 40 g, symmetric, and firm; it has "sharp" margins. You order antithyroglobulin antibodies, which return positive at 1:512. Because of her goiter and the thyroid function tests, you prescribe 0.15 mg thyroxine daily. She notes a slight increase in energy and interest in physical activity.

After she finishes the next school year, your reevaluation shows that the thyroid is just palpable. Thyroxine therapy is stopped. Three months later there are no features of hypothyroidism, serum T_4 is 6.5 μg/100 ml, and serum TSH is 3 μU/ml.

QUESTIONS

1. What is the diagnosis for her at age 14?
2. Why is the thyroid uptake higher at 6 hours than at 24 hours?
3. How do you explain the other initial thyroid function tests?
4. What has happened to her 1 year later, and can you give a long-term prognosis?
5. Which endocrine disorders are associated with this one?

Patient 5. A 60-year-old retired coal miner complained of worsening of exertional dyspnea, fatigue, and a lump in the throat. Because of chronic bronchitis, he had been taking 10 drops of saturated solution of potassium iodide 3 times daily (equivalent to 1.5 g iodine per day) as an expectorant for the past year. He also admitted to somnolence, periorbital edema, dry skin, increasing intolerance to cold, and a weight gain of 15 pounds in the past 6 months.

PHYSICAL EXAMINATION. His appearance was myxedematous with dry skin, coarse hair, hoarse voice, and diffuse enlargement of the thyroid to an estimated weight of 50 g; reflexes showed marked slowing of the relaxation phase. The remainder of the physical examination was characterized by stigmata of severe chronic bronchitis.

LABORATORY DATA. Thyroid function tests showed serum T_4 is 1.5 μg/100, FT_4I is 1.2, and TSH is 68 μU/ml. Perchlorate discharge test (2 days after stopping iodide): thyroid uptake 20% at 1 hour, 30% at 3 hours; then 1 g potassium perchlorate was given; uptake fell to 5% after 1 hour. The physician recommended stopping the potassium iodide and prescribed bronchial dilators. Repeat evaluation 3 weeks later showed considerable subjective improvement, increased mental alertness, reduction of thyroid size to between 35 and 40 g, weight loss of 10 pounds, and faster tendon reflexes. At this time, thyroid function studies showed serum T_4 was 4.0, FT_4I was 3.9, serum TSH was 15 μU/ml, 24 hour thyroid uptake was 40%, and perchlorate discharge test was normal. No additional therapy was prescribed, and he continued to improve and became euthyroid during the next 3 months.

QUESTIONS

1. What was the cause of the goiter and myxedema, and what was the pathophysiology?
2. How does one take advantage of this effect of iodine?

Patient 6. A 35-year-old lawyer comes to your office because he discovered a small lump in his neck while shaving 1 week ago. He recently learned that he had received x-ray therapy for recurrent tonsillitis at age 5.

PHYSICAL EXAMINATION. This examination is entirely normal except for a 2-cm firm nodule in the left lower lobe of the thyroid; there is no cervical lymphadenopathy.

LABORATORY DATA. A thyroid scan shows that the nodule is cold; an ultrasonogram confirms that it is solid. Serum T_4 is 9 μg/100 ml, and serum TSH is 3 μU/ml.

1. What are the diagnostic possibilities?
2. Is the history of radiation to the neck important?
3. What additional diagnostic procedures would be helpful?
4. What therapy do you recommend?

SUGGESTED READING

Physiology and Biochemistry

Chopra, I.J., et al.: Pathways of metabolism of thyroid hormones. Recent Prog. Horm. Res., *34*:531, 1978.

DeGroot, L.J., and Niepomniszce, H.: Biosynthesis of thyroid hormone: basic and clinical aspects. Metabolism, *26*:665, 1977.

Greer, M.A., and Solomon, D.H. (eds.): Handbook of Physiology, Section 7: Endocrinology. Vol. III. Thyroid. Baltimore, Williams & Wilkins, 1974.

Lissitzky, S.: Biosynthesis of thyroid hormones. *In* The Thyroid. Physiology and Treatment of Disease. Edited by J.M. Hershman and G.A. Bray. Oxford, Pergamon Press, 1979.

Oppenheimer, J.H.: Thyroid hormone action at the cellular level. Science, *203*:971, 1979.

Robbins, J., et al.: Thyroxine transport properties of plasma, molecular properties and biosynthesis. Recent Prog. Horm. Res., *34*:477, 1978.

Werner, S.C., and Ingbar, S.H.: The Thyroid. 4th Ed. New York, Harper & Row, 1978.

Hypothyroidism

Fisher, D.A., et al.: Screening for congenital hypothyroidism: results of screening one million North American infants. J Pediatr., *94*:700, 1979.

Ibbertson, H.K.: Hypothyroidism. *In* The Thyroid. Physiology and Treatment of Disease. Edited by J.M. Hershman and G.A. Bray. Oxford, Pergamon Press, 1979.

Report of a Committee of the Clinical Society of London to Investigate the Subject of Myxoedema. London, Longmans, Green and Co., 1888.

Stanbury, J.B.: Familial goiter. *In* The Metabolic Basis of Inherited Disease. 4th Ed. Edited by J.B. Stanbury, J.B. Wyngaarden, and D.S. Fredrickson. New York, McGraw-Hill, 1978.

Hyperthyroidism

Brown, J., et al.: Autoimmune thyroid diseases—Graves' and Hashimoto's. Ann. Intern. Med., *88*:379, 1978.

Geffner, D.L., and Hershman, J.M.: Hyperthyroidism. Causes, etiology of Graves' disease, clinical features, general aspects of treatment. *In* The Thyroid. Physiology and Treatment of Disease. Edited by J.M. Hershman and G.A. Bray. Oxford, Pergamon Press, 1979.

Nikolai, T.F., et al.: Lymphocytic thyroiditis with spontaneously resolving hyperthyroidism. Arch. Intern. Med., *140*:478, 1980.

Volpé, R.: Thyrotoxicosis. Clin. Endocrinol. Metab., *7*:1, 1978.

Thyroiditis

Fisher, D.A., et al.: The diagnosis of Hashimoto's thyroiditis. J. Clin. Endocrinol. Metab., *40*:795, 1975.

Glinoer, D., et al.: Sequential study of the impairment of thyroid function in the early stage of subacute thyroiditis. Acta Endocrinol., *77*:26, 1974.

Greenberg, A.H., et al.: Juvenile chronic lymphocytic thyroiditis: clinical, laboratory, and histological correlations. J. Clin. Endocrinol. Metab., *30*:293, 1970.

Volpé, R.: Thyroiditis: current views of pathogenesis. Med. Clin. North Am., *59*:1163, 1975.

Goiter and Carcinoma

Ashcraft, M., and Van Herle, A.J.: Management of thyroid nodules. I. History and physical examination, blood tests, x-ray tests and ultrasonography. Head Neck Surg., *3*:216, 1981.

Ashcraft, M., and Van Herle, A.J.: Management of thyroid nodules. II: Scanning techniques, thyroid suppressive therapy, and fine needle aspiration. Head Neck Surg., *3*:297, 1981.

Astwood, E.B., Cassidy, C.E., and Aurbach, G.D.: Treatment of goiter and thyroid nodules with thyroid. JAMA, *174*:459, 1960.

DeGroot, L.J. (ed.): Radiation-Associated Thyroid Carcinoma. New York, Grune & Stratton, 1977.

Delange, F.M., and Ermans, A.M.: Endemic goiter and cretinism. Naturally occurring goitrogens. *In* The Thyroid. Physiology and Treatment of Disease. Edited by J.M. Hershman and G.A. Bray. Oxford, Pergamon Press, 1979.

Melvin, K.E.W.: Medullary carcinoma of the thyroid. *In* The Thyroid. Physiology and Treatment of Disease. Edited by J.M. Hershman and G.A. Bray. Oxford, Pergamon Press, 1979.

Stanbury, J.B., and Hetzel, B.S.: Endemic Goiter and Cretinism. New York, John Wiley & Sons, 1980.

Thijs, L.G., and Wiener, J.D.: Ultrasonic examination of the thyroid gland. Am. J. Med., *60*:96, 1976.

Van Herle, A.J., and Uller, R.P.: Thyroid cancer. Classification, clinical features, diagnosis and therapy. *In* The Thyroid. Physiology and Treatment of Disease. Edited by J.M. Hershman and G.A. Bray. Oxford, Pergamon Press, 1979.

Walfish, P.G., et al.: Combined ultrasound and needle aspiration cytology in the assessment and management of hypofunctioning thyroid nodules. Ann. Intern. Med., *87*:270, 1977.

CHAPTER 4

Adrenal Disease

Ada R.Wolfsen, Michael Tuck, and
Solomon A. Kaplan

ADRENAL CORTEX

Physiology

Adrenocortical growth and steroid secretion are primarily controlled by the pituitary hormone, adrenocorticotropin (ACTH). Figure 4–1 shows the secretory regulation of the hypothalamic-pituitary-adrenal axis. Corticotropin releasing hormone (CRH) is secreted by the hypothalamus into the hypophyseal-portal system and, upon reaching the pituitary, causes ACTH release; CRH is a 41-amino-acid polypeptide. ACTH is carried by the peripheral circulation to the adrenal where it is bound by specific receptors and causes steroid synthesis and secretion. Hypothalamic secretion of CRH is regulated by neural input from higher brain centers such as the limbic system. This neural input inhibits CRH synthesis and secretion with a 24-hour cycle resulting in a circadian rhythm of ACTH and cortisol secretion. ACTH and cortisol are released in secretory bursts that occur most frequently during the sixth to eighth hours of sleep and cease during the 2 hours prior to sleep.

The circadian rhythm is overcome by stress, e.g., surgical procedure, emotional situations, and hypoglycemia. Hormonal stimuli such as vasopressin, histamine, and angiotensin also release CRH and ACTH. Cortisol from the adrenal inhibits hypothalamic CRH and pituitary ACTH release; this negative feedback can be overcome by stress. ACTH also has a negative feedback effect on CRH release.

ACTH is synthesized as part of a large precursor molecule that is also a precursor for the lipotropins (LPH) and the endorphins. ACTH, β-lipotropin and γ-lipotropin, and β-endorphin are secreted together by the same pituitary cell.

A secretory pulse of ACTH causes the adrenal to release cortisol, adrenal androgens, and aldosterone. ACTH acts by binding to a specific receptor on the surface of the adrenal cell; this binding activates cyclases of the cell,

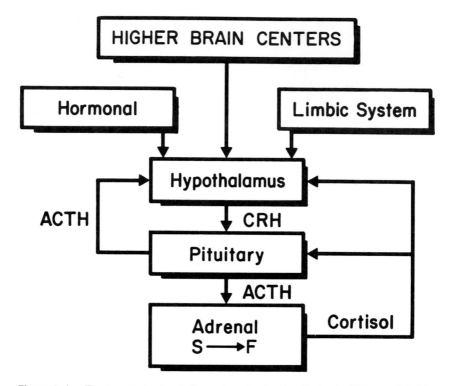

Figure 4–1. The hypothalamic-pituitary-adrenal axis. Hypothalamic CRH, regulated by hormonal input and neural input from higher brain centers, is delivered by the hypophyseal portal system to the pituitary where it causes ACTH release. ACTH acts on the adrenal gland to cause steroid synthesis and secretion. Cortisol and ACTH inhibit CRH release. Cortisol also inhibits ACTH release by the pituitary.

which form cyclic AMP from adenosine triphosphate (ATP) and cyclic guanosine monophosphate (GMP) from guanosine triphosphate (GTP). These cyclic nucleotides stimulate steroidogenesis and adrenocortical growth. In the absence of endogenous ACTH, the adrenal glands atrophy.

Cortisol, once secreted, circulates bound to cortisol-binding globulin (transcortin). Free (unbound) cortisol is available to enter the cell to exert physiologic effects; it is rapidly metabolized by the liver and excreted by the kidney.

All steroids are believed to exert physiologic effects by penetrating the cell to bind to specific cytoplasmic receptors in target tissue. The steroid-receptor complex is transported to the nucleus, binds to a nuclear receptor, and regulates transcription of mRNA from DNA for the synthesis of specific enzymes. Glucocorticoids promote the synthesis of enzymes that regulate the metabolism of carbohydrate, fat, and protein. In muscle and adipose tissue, cortisol is catabolic causing degradation of protein to amino acids and degradation of fat to fatty acids and glycerol. Amino acids and glycerol are used by the liver and kidney as substrates for glucose synthesis. Physiologic concentrations of cortisol are important for permitting normal function of almost all body cells.

Secretion of adrenal androgens is under the control of ACTH and other undefined factors. Adrenal androgens, consisting primarily of dehydroepiandrosterone and dehydroepiandrosterone sulfate, but also androstenedione and testosterone, are metabolized to 17-ketosteroids and measured colorimetrically in the urine.

In contrast to cortisol, of which ACTH is the sole regulatory factor, aldosterone secretion is regulated by three well-defined control mechanisms: the renin-angiotensin system, operating through volume-mediated changes; potassium ion, operating independent of volume; and ACTH. Under most conditions the renin-angiotensin system predominates over the other control factors and operates via changes in extracellular fluid volume (Fig. 4–2). For example, under conditions of volume depletion, renin, a proteolytic enzyme, is released from the juxtaglomerular cells of the renal afferent arterioles. Two intrarenal receptor mechanisms that perceive either changes in volume or sodium ion control renin release. The juxtaglomerular cells respond to increments in renal perfusion pressure; the adjacent macula densa perceives changes in sodium delivery to the distal nephron. Released renin acts enzymatically

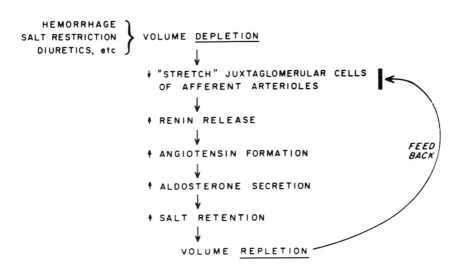

Figure 4–2. Mechanism of aldosterone stimulation by volume depletion. Decreased stretch of the afferent arterioles in volume depletion results in renin release by the juxtaglomerular cells. Renin cleaves its α_2-globulin substrate to form angiotensin I, which is rapidly converted to angiotensin II. Angiotensin II stimulates aldosterone production by the adrenal cortex. Aldosterone acts on the distal tubule to increase sodium retention and restore blood volume, thereby inhibiting further renin release.

on a circulating α_2-globulin substrate to cleave off the decapeptide, angiotensin I. Angiotensin I, which has no known major physiologic function, is rapidly converted (by specific converting enzymes located mainly in the lung) to the octapeptide, angiotensin II. Angiotensin II then stimulates the production of aldosterone in the zona glomerulosa of the adrenal cortex. Angiotensin II is rapidly degraded by several angiotensinases, and a seven-amino-acid heptapeptide metabolite (angiotensin III) is also capable of releasing aldosterone. Released aldosterone acts on the distal tubule to increase sodium retention and restore effective blood volume, thereby shutting off the initial stimulus for renin release.

A second important control factor for regulation of aldosterone is potassium ion. Either infusion or oral ingestion of potassium can increase aldosterone production, and depletion of potassium has the opposite effect. This effect appears to be a direct action of potassium to stimulate aldosterone production in the zona glomerulosa. The exact role of potassium in net aldosterone regulation is uncertain.

Finally, contrasted to its major role in glucocorticoid regulation, ACTH displays only modest effects on aldosterone control. ACTH acutely stimulates aldosterone, but this response is not sustained. In the absence of ACTH, in hypopituitarism or steroid-suppressed subjects, aldosterone response remains relatively intact.

Aldosterone is secreted from the zona glomerulosa cells of the adrenal cortex. With normal sodium and potassium intake, about 50 to 250 μg are secreted daily. Aldosterone is weakly bound to plasma proteins, and is rapidly inactivated by the liver and kidney. As a result, circulating levels of this hormone are low. The acid-labile metabolite of aldosterone in the urine represents approximately 10% of total daily aldosterone production. Plasma levels of aldosterone can be measured by radioimmunoassay. The normal range for plasma aldosterone on a regular sodium intake is 2 to 10 ng/100 ml, and for urinary excretion it is 10 to 15 μg/24 hours. However, these levels are influenced by dietary sodium and potassium, posture, and time of day.

LABORATORY TESTS OF ADRENOCORTICAL FUNCTION (TABLE 4–1)

ACTH. This hormone is secreted in episodic bursts that precede secretory bursts of cortisol. Between 6:00 and 10:00 A.M., plasma ACTH ranges from 20 to 120 pg/ml, and has a half-life ($t^{1}/_{2}$) in plasma of 2 to 5 minutes.

Plasma Aldosterone. On a normal or high-salt diet in the supine position, plasma aldosterone concentrations range from 2 to 10 ng/100 ml. Upright posture and a low-sodium diet (<2 g/day) increase aldosterone through activation of the renin-angiotensin system.

Plasma Cortisol. Its concentration is determined by the adrenal cortisol secretory rate, the concentration of corticosteroid-binding globulin, and the rate of removal of cortisol by the liver. Cortisol is secreted in episodic bursts and has a $t^{1}/_{2}$ in plasma of 60 to 90 minutes. The normal cortisol secretion

Table 4–1. Normal Values

Plasma Concentrations

ACTH (morning)	20–120 pg/ml
Aldosterone (supine)	2–10 ng/100 ml
(upright)	2–5 times supine
(low-sodium diet)	2–5 times increase
Cortisol (morning)	7–18 µg/100 ml
(evening)	2–9 µg/100 ml
Dehydroepiandrosterone sulfate (adult male)	130–550 µg/100 ml
(adult female, reproductive years)	60–340 µg/100 ml

Urinary Excretion Rates

Aldosterone (normal salt)	10–15 µg/24 hr
(low salt)	3–5 times increase
Free cortisol	20–100 µg/24 hr
17-OHCS	3–10 mg/24 hr
17-KGS	<20 mg/24 hr
17-KS (male)	10–22 mg/24 hr
(female)	5–15 mg/24 hr

rate in adults is 7 to 26 mg/day; in children the average secretory rate is 12 mg/m^2/day. Normal plasma cortisol concentrations by radioimmunoassay between 8:00 and 9:00 A.M. range from 7 to 18 µg/100 ml, and fall to 2 to 9 µg/100 ml by 11:00 P.M. Because the concentration of corticosteroid-binding globulin is increased by pregnancy, estrogen, or oral contraceptive administration, total plasma cortisol also increases under these conditions; however, free cortisol remains normal. Severe liver disease decreases the metabolic clearance rate of corticosteroids, but because of negative feedback control, plasma concentrations of total and free cortisol remain normal.

Serum Dehydroepiandrosterone Sulfate. This androgen is secreted almost exclusively from the adrenal and becomes the major constituent of 17-ketosteroids (17-KS) in the urine. Measurement of this steroid in serum can be used to assess adrenal androgen production. Normal values in adult males range from 130 to 550 µg/100 ml and in adult females during the reproductive years from 60 to 340 µg/100 ml.

Urinary Free Cortisol. This quantity reflects the non-protein-bound cortisol in plasma and correlates well with cortisol secretion rate. As measured by radioimmunoassay, normal values for adults are up to 100 µg/day.

17-Hydroxycorticosteroids (17-OHCS). As shown in Figure 4–3, cortisol, cortisone, and 11-deoxycortisol (compound S), because of their dihydroxyacetone side chain, react with phenylhydrazine in sulfuric acid to produce a yellow color (Porter-Silber method). Urinary 17-hydroxycorticosteroids, used as an index of secreted cortisol, account for only 30% of the cortisol secreted. Normal values for adults range from 3 to 10 mg/day or less than 10 mg/g creatinine; for children normal values are 3 mg/m^2/day.

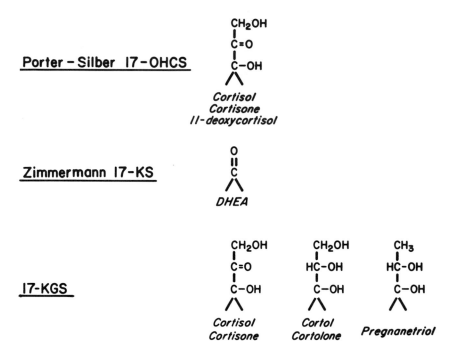

Figure 4–3. Structures of steroids measured in urinary 17-hydroxysteroids (17-OHCS), 17-ketosteroids (17-KS), and 17-ketogenic steroids (17-KGS).

17-Ketogenic Steroids (17-KGS). Urinary 17-ketogenic steroids are the steroids that can be converted into 17-ketosteroids by oxidation with sodium bismuthate. Figure 4–3 illustrates the side-chain groups necessary for this reaction. This test for cortisol secretion is nonspecific but was used in the past because it was a simple laboratory procedure. Normal values in adults are less than 20 mg/day.

17-Ketosteroids (17-KS). Urinary 17-ketosteroids are used to estimate adrenal androgen production. Dehydroepiandrosterone sulfate, dehydroepiandrosterone, androstenedione, testosterone, and to a lesser extent cortisol contribute to urinary 17-KS. Testosterone and cortisol are metabolized to products measured as 17-KS. Normal values in adult males are 10 to 22 mg/day and in adult females, 5 to 15 mg/day.

ADRENOCORTICAL INSUFFICIENCY

Adrenocortical insufficiency results primarily from deficient cortisol and in some cases deficient aldosterone and androgen production by the adrenal. Since the adrenal cortex is normally stimulated by pituitary ACTH, cortisol deficiency may result from adrenal disease (primary adrenal insufficiency) or from pituitary or hypothalamic disease (secondary adrenal insufficiency).

Primary

Primary adrenocortical failure was described by Addison in 1855 and included cases of idiopathic adrenal atrophy, tuberculosis, and metastatic tumor; most commonly adrenal insufficiency is caused by idiopathic adrenal atrophy and less frequently by tuberculosis. Rare causes include bacterial or mycotic infection, sarcoidosis, amyloidosis, hemochromatosis, bilateral adrenalectomy, abdominal irradiation, adrenal vein thrombosis, adrenal artery embolus, metastatic carcinoma, anticoagulant therapy, and adrenolytic drugs.

Secondary

This disease entity is most commonly caused by iatrogenic corticosteroid administration, which suppresses CRH and ACTH secretion resulting in adrenal atrophy. Other causes include pituitary tumors, tumors of the third ventricle, trauma, encephalitis, optic glioma, craniopharyngioma, basilar meningitis, stalk section, postpartum pituitary necrosis, and hypophysectomy for pituitary tumors.

Symptoms and Signs

Acute adrenal insufficiency is a potentially fatal medical emergency. Clinical features include nausea, fever, and shock, progressing to diarrhea, muscular weakness, increased and then decreased temperature, hypoglycemia, hyponatremia, and hyperkalemia.

Cardinal signs of *chronic adrenal insufficiency* are weakness and weight loss, hyperpigmentation, hypotension, nausea, vomiting, diarrhea, and vitiligo. Other symptoms are salt craving, muscle cramps, flank tenderness, and loss of body hair especially in females. The ear cartilage may calcify in longstanding adrenal insufficiency.

Pathophysiology

The clinical features are due to deficient cortisol, aldosterone, and androgen effects in steroid target tissues. In addition to abnormal function of the brain and gastrointestinal cells, cortisol deficiency impairs gluconeogenesis in liver and kidney, and impairs the muscular arteriolar constrictor response to catecholamines.

In primary adrenal insufficiency lack of the inhibitory feedback effect of cortisol on ACTH and LPH secretion by the pituitary results in increased melanin in the skin. Increased pigmentation occurs in areas exposed to light or pressure such as the face, neck, knuckles, elbows, knees, mucous membranes, skin creases in the palms, and scars acquired after the onset of adrenal failure.

Aldosterone deficiency results in renal sodium loss from decreased sodium reabsorption at the distal tubule. This loss causes a decrease in total body sodium, plasma volume, pressor response to catecholamines, cardiac output, and renal blood flow. Lack of aldosterone also impairs renal secretion of potassium and hydrogen ions resulting in hyperkalemia and metabolic acidosis.

The adrenal androgens, dehydroepiandrosterone, dehydroepiandrosterone sulfate, and androstenedione, have weak biologic activity and are converted to testosterone, which has potent bioactivity. In the female these androgens are mainly responsible for the growth of pubic and axillary hair. Deficiency of adrenal androgen results in loss of body hair.

Secondary adrenocortical failure is usually associated with deficiency of gonadotropins, GH and TSH. The isolated lack of ACTH from pituitary or hypothalamic lesions is rare. Suppression of ACTH secretion due to prolonged use of supraphysiologic doses of glucocorticoids is common. When the steroids are discontinued, the pituitary gland secretes little ACTH even though corticosteroid levels are low. Recovery of the hypothalamic-pituitary-adrenal axis may take months. The patient is consequently vulnerable to adrenal failure in times of stress during this period. The hypothalamus and pituitary must recover first; then the trophic effect of ACTH on the adrenal restores adrenal responsiveness to normal.

Diagnosis

ACTH Stimulation Test

The diagnosis of adrenocortical insufficiency is primarily based on the plasma cortisol determination during the *ACTH stimulation test*. For this 1-hour test, 250 μg cosyntropin (the 1 to 24 amino acid sequence of ACTH) is given intravenously. Peak cortisol values occur at 30 to 60 minutes. A normal test consists of a baseline cortisol greater than 5 μg/100 ml, an increment between baseline and stimulated cortisol greater than 7 μg/100 ml, and a stimulated cortisol level greater than 18 μg/100 ml. An inadequate cortisol response to this test indicates adrenal insufficiency, and further tests are required to distinguish primary from secondary adrenal insufficiency.

The *prolonged ACTH stimulation test* may be used to differentiate between primary and secondary adrenal insufficiency. In response to successive injections of long-acting ACTH (1 mg cosyntropin gel) or an 8-hour infusion of ACTH (250 μg cosyntropin), the diagnosis of primary adrenal insufficiency is made if the plasma cortisol fails to rise above 18 μg/100 ml. In secondary adrenal insufficiency, the cortisol response to this test is normal.

Plasma ACTH

Baseline plasma ACTH is elevated in primary adrenal insufficiency but maintains a circadian rhythm. A significantly elevated plasma ACTH is useful in diagnosing primary adrenocortical insufficiency.

Tests of Immunity

Once the diagnosis of primary adrenal insufficiency is made, a positive tuberculin skin test implicates tuberculosis as the cause. If adrenal microsomal and mitochrondrial antibodies are detected in serum, idiopathic, probably autoimmune, adrenal atrophy can be diagnosed with certainty.

Insulin Tolerance Test

To document secondary adrenal insufficiency, the insulin hypoglycemia and metyrapone stimulation tests are useful. In order to interpret these tests, the adrenal cortex must be fully responsive to ACTH. In performing an insulin tolerance test in patients suspected of having hypopituitarism, the dose should not exceed 0.1 U soluble insulin/kg body weight. Blood samples are drawn at 0, 15, 30, 45, 60, and 90 minutes. The blood glucose should fall to less than 40 mg/100 ml and to less than 50% of the basal level to be an adequate stimulus for ACTH release. A normal response is a cortisol level at 45 to 90 minutes equal to or greater than 20 μg/100 ml, with an increment of at least 8 μg/100 ml. If the response to insulin-induced hypoglycemia is normal, one can assume all components of the hypothalamic-pituitary-adrenal axis are normal.

Metyrapone Test

The metyrapone test is also useful to assess pituitary ACTH reserve. Metyrapone inhibits the enzyme 11β-hydroxylase, which is the final step in cortisol synthesis. The decrease in cortisol following 2 to 3 g metyrapone orally at 11:00 P.M. results in increased ACTH secretion; the adrenal responds by secreting 11-deoxycortisol (compound S). A normal response consists of a compound S value at 8:00 A.M. greater than 7 μg/100 ml. Abnormal responses to metyrapone and hypoglycemia with a normal response to ACTH confirm the diagnosis of secondary adrenocortical insufficiency.

Associated Conditions

Patients with idiopathic Addison's disease are prone to other autoimmune disorders, which may develop before or years after the diagnosis of adrenal disease. These disorders include Hashimoto's thyroiditis, hyperthyroidism of Graves' disease, pernicious anemia, diabetes, hypoparathyroidism, primary hypogonadism, vitiligo, and moniliasis.

Treatment

Acute Adrenal Insufficiency

Cortisol (hydrocortisone) is the drug of choice for initial treatment because it does not require metabolism for its biologic action. Acute adrenal insufficiency is treated by intravenous hydrocortisone: 100 mg injected as a bolus initially and then every 6 hours for 24 to 48 hours. Fluid replacement is given as 5% glucose in saline solution, 4 L over 4 hours; saline solution is administered to treat shock. Sympathomimetic agents and blood transfusions are rarely indicated. From 20 to 40 mEq potassium may be added to the second and third liter to replace the total body deficit. As soon as the patient can tolerate oral fluids, glucocorticoids may be administered orally. Although hydrocortisone (cortisol) is the glucocorticoid secreted by the normal adrenal, prednisone is frequently given for chronic replacement therapy because the cost is less. For example, on day 2, oral prednisone, 10 mg every 8 hours, may be given. On day 3, 5 mg every 6 hours may be given and on day 4, 5 mg every 8 hours. On days 5 and 6, reduce the prednisone dosage to 7.5 mg daily and maintain this dose.

In addition to glucocorticoid therapy, a mineralocorticoid is usually required in the therapy of primary adrenal insufficiency. For example, 0.05 to 0.10 mg fluorocortisol acetate (Florinef) may be added daily when oral prednisone is begun. Mineralocorticoid replacement is not usually necessary in secondary adrenal insufficiency.

Chronic Adrenal Insufficiency

Prednisone (7.5 mg orally per day) and fluorocortisol (0.05 to 0.1 mg orally per day) are maintenance therapy. A normal diet is prescribed, with additional salt for excessive heat or humidity. The patient should carry extra prednisone for oral use, hydrocortisone hemisuccinate for intramuscular use in an emergency, and medical identification—a card or bracelet stating diagnosis, medication and dosage, and physician's name and telephone number.

During stress glucocorticoid dosage is increased to mimic normal function. For a "flu" syndrome with fever or a dental extraction, double the normal maintenance dosage for 2 to 3 days. For gastroenteritis, patients should receive parenteral hydrocortisone.

For glucocorticoid coverage during surgical procedures, 100 mg hydrocortisone is given with preoperative medication, 100 mg intravenously during the surgical procedure, then 75 mg every 8 hours. Rapidly taper hydrocortisone to the normal dosage once the acute stress ends.

ADRENOGENITAL SYNDROME (CONGENITAL ADRENAL HYPERPLASIA)

Definition

Adrenogenital syndrome comprises a group of genetically transmitted inborn errors of the enzyme systems involved in cortisol synthesis by the adrenals. The defect is transmitted as an autosomal recessive, and the frequency of the abnormal gene is between 1:100 and 1:150 in North America. Deficient cortisol synthesis leads to increased pituitary ACTH release, with hyperplasia of the adrenal glands and increased production of a number of steroids, including testosterone, in the virilizing syndrome. Other steroids are converted to testosterone in extra-adrenal tissues.

Pathophysiology

Increased elaboration of testosterone in this syndrome exposes the fetus to excessive quantities of circulating testosterone and continued virilization after birth. In the female fetus this condition leads to fusion of the labia and clitoral hypertrophy giving an appearance at birth of ambiguous external genitals (Fig. 4–4). The degree of fusion varies; in extreme cases a male-like phallus develops and the urethra opens at the tip. The male fetus also undergoes virilization although abnormalities at birth are more difficult to detect. Untreated infants and children continue to show effects of virilization postnatally; manifestations are increased somatic growth; advancement of epiphyseal maturation; premature development of pubic, axillary, and facial hair; acne; lowering of the voice pitch; and increased growth of the phallus. In spite of growth of the penis in boys, the testes generally do not grow in size to a concomitant degree, and spermatogenesis is diminished or absent. In the female, signs of puberty, such as breast development and menstruation, do not occur. Although virilization nearly always occurs, in rare forms of the syndrome testosterone cannot be produced and absence of fusion of the scrotal folds occurs, leading to feminization of the male fetus.

In addition to virilization (or rarely, feminization), other symptoms and signs develop because of excessive production of other steroids. Signs and symptoms of cortisol deficiency are rare because the enzymatic block is rarely complete, and under excessive ACTH stimulation, the adrenal cortex can produce adequate resting levels of cortisol. However, the adrenals are unable

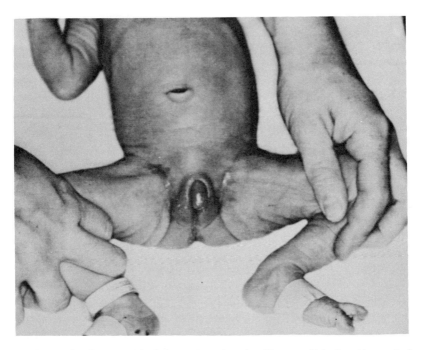

Figure 4–4. Ambiguous genitalia in newborn female with congenital adrenal hyperplasia. Note enlargement of the clitoris and partial labial fusion.

to produce the increased amounts of cortisol usually secreted under conditions of stress.

About half these patients have aldosterone deficiency and develop life-threatening salt-losing crises, marked by increasing lethargy, vomiting, dehydration, hyponatremia, and hyperkalemia. In another group of patients hypertension develops as a result of excessive production of 11-deoxycorticosterone.

Diagnosis (Figs. 4–5, 4–6, and 4–7).

21-Hydroxylase Deficiency

This most common type of deficiency is characterized by production of 21-deoxysteroids. The steroid nucleus can be hydroxylated at the 11 and 17 positions but not at the 21 position. As a result, progesterone, 17-hydroxyprogesterone, and 11,17-dihydroxyprogesterone accumulate in the blood and, after appropriate reduction, undergo excretion in the urine as follows: Progesterone is converted to pregnanediol, 17-hydroxyprogesterone to pregnanetriol, and 11,17-dihydroxyprogesterone to 11-keto or 11-hydroxypregnanetriol. Presence of the 17,20-desmolase in the adrenal results in conversion of some of these substances to 17-ketosteroids such as androstenedione and dehydroepiandrosterone, and these are excreted in the urine. Reduction of these 17-ketosteroids by a 17-reductase in the adrenals and in peripheral organs leads to formation of testosterone. Plasma levels of estradiol are also increased although feminization does not occur.

In about half the subjects, salt-losing crises may occur because of deficiency in aldosterone synthesis. Aldosterone is a 21-hydroxylated compound, and deficiency of 21-hydroxylase might naturally be expected to lead to aldosterone deficiency. Surprisingly, the non-salt-losers with 21-hydroxylase deficiency actually have an increased production of aldosterone. They do not develop signs of hyperaldosteronism because of the antagonistic effects exerted by progesterone and 17-hydroxyprogesterone on the renal response to aldosterone.

A clear explanation of why some patients with 21-hydroxylase deficiency have aldosterone deficiency and others aldosterone excess is not available. The diagnosis of 21-hydroxylase deficiency is based on increased 17-ketosteroids and pregnanetriol in the urine and increased 17-hydroxyprogesterone in the blood.

11 β-Hydroxylase Deficiency

In the second most frequent enzymatic defect, absence of 11-hydroxylation leads to formation of 11-deoxycortisol (compound S), which is physiologically inert, and 11-deoxycorticosterone, which is a potent retainer of sodium and may cause hypertension. Patients with this form of the disorder are virilized because of the production of testosterone. Some are hypertensive but none are salt losers. The diagnosis in these patients is made by increased amounts

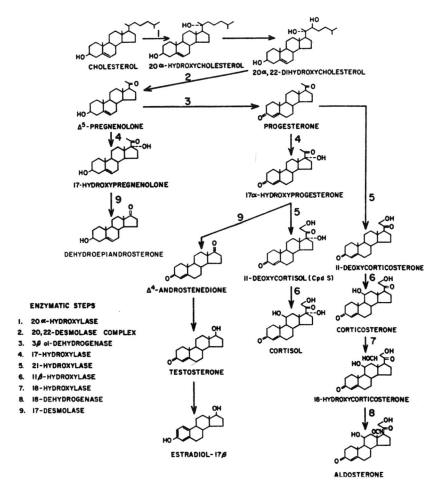

Figure 4–5. The major biosynthetic pathways for adrenal steroids. (From Temple, T.E., and Liddle, G.W.: Annu. Rev. Pharmacol., *10*:199, 1970.)

of 17-ketosteroids and tetrahydro-S in the urine with normal urinary pregnanetriol. Compound S is increased in the plasma.

17 α-Hydroxylase Deficiency

Patients with this syndrome exhibit hypogonadism because the inability to hydroxylate at the 17 position exists in both adrenals and gonads, and they cannot elaborate adequate quantities of either testosterone or estradiol. Excessive quantities of 11-deoxycorticosterone are formed and lead to hypertension. 17-ketosteroid excretion is low, pregnanetriol is normal, and the diagnosis is made by finding excessive quantities of 11-deoxycorticosterone and corticosterone in the blood or urine.

3 β-Dehydrogenase Deficiency

In this syndrome pregnenolone cannot be converted to progesterone; therefore cortisol, aldosterone, and testosterone cannot be formed. Scrotal fusion does not occur in male fetuses, and because of impairment of aldosterone synthesis, salt-losing crises occur. Also present are 17-hydroxylation, 17,20-desmolase activity, and increased excretion of 17-ketosteroids but not pregnanetriol.

20,22-Desmolase Deficiency

Deficiency of the enzyme catalyzing the conversion of cholesterol to pregnenolone leads to severe adrenal insufficiency characterized by marked deposition of lipids in the adrenals and is referred to as a lipoid adrenal hyperplasia. Symptoms of aldosterone deficiency occur with hyponatremia and dehydration. Excretion of 17-ketosteroids and other adrenal steroids is within normal limits. Virilization does not occur.

Treatment

Treatment is with glucocorticoid in amounts sufficient to suppress ACTH production. Generally the amounts must be equivalent to between 2 and 3 times the normal secretory rate, which is about 12 mg cortisol/m^2/day. These amounts are considerably in excess of those used for treatment of primary adrenal failure. Adequacy of therapy is checked by monitoring for signs of virilization, measurement of appropriate steroids in plasma or urine (e.g., 17-ketosteroids and pregnanetriol), and bone age roentgenograms. For aldosterone deficiency, 9-fluorocortisol is administered orally in a dosage of 0.05 to 0.1 mg daily. For crises intravenous sodium chloride solutions and intramuscular deoxycorticosterone injections are used.

CUSHING'S SYNDROME

Definition

Cushing's syndrome is a symptom complex due to excess glucocorticoid production by the adrenal cortex or sustained administration of glucocorticoids. Spontaneous Cushing's syndrome occurs with a female:male ratio of 3:1.

Cushing's syndrome may be classified as ACTH-dependent or ACTH-independent. Table 4–2 lists the frequency of occurrence of spontaneous Cushing's syndrome; however, the most common cause is therapy with exogenous glucocorticoids or ACTH.

Pathophysiology

Cushing's Disease

Pituitary-dependent bilateral adrenocortical hyperplasia (Cushing's disease) comprises 68% of the cases of Cushing's syndrome. In this disease, abnormal pituitary corticotrophs secrete excessive amounts of ACTH and LPH. This results in increased 24-hour production of cortisol and increased adrenal growth. X-ray evidence of a pituitary tumor is present initially in approximately 7% of patients and may develop following bilateral adrenalectomy. Small pituitary adenomas are present in most patients at the time of diagnosis. These pituitary tumors are usually chromophobe adenomas, rarely basophilic adenomas or eosinophilic adenomas. Plasma ACTH is normal or slightly elevated in the presence of elevated plasma cortisol levels indicating decreased sensitivity to cortisol feedback suppression of ACTH. The episodic secretion of ACTH and cortisol, which normally is maximal in the early morning hours and minimal during the first part of sleep, is exaggerated in Cushing's disease so that, although secretory episodes are still more frequent in the early morning hours, the minimum level of cortisol during the night is much higher than normal.

Ectopic ACTH Syndrome

The clinical ectopic ACTH syndrome is excessive production of biologically active ACTH (and in some cases CRH) by nonendocrine tumors arising from lung, thymus, pancreas, or other organs. Pigmentation and hypokalemic alkalosis are presenting features. The pigmentation is due to ACTH and LPH secreted by the tumor. Hypokalemic alkalosis is due to the mineralocorticoid effects of excessive cortisol and 11-deoxycorticosterone (DOC). Other common physical findings of Cushing's syndrome are minimal or absent.

Tumors of the Adrenal Cortex

Adrenal tumors account for 8% of patients with Cushing's syndrome; fewer than 50% of these patients have adrenocortical carcinoma. However, in children Cushing's syndrome is usually due to adrenal carcinoma. Plasma ACTH is suppressed because of negative cortisol feedback at the hypothalamus and pituitary, and the normal adrenal tissue is atrophic. Adrenal carcinomas may secrete large amounts of many steroids including estrogens. Increased estrogens cause feminization, primarily in males.

Nodular Adrenal Hyperplasia

In nodular adrenocortical hyperplasia, both adrenal glands are involved. Plasma ACTH is usually undetectable and cannot be stimulated, but after adrenalectomy, ACTH often rises to high levels similar to those in Cushing's disease.

Symptoms and Signs

Table 4–3 lists the frequency of symptoms and signs in patients with Cushing's syndrome. Obesity is the most common symptom and is predominantly in the face, trunk, cervicodorsal and supraclavicular regions. The limbs are relatively thin due to muscle wasting. Typically there is a round "moon" face and dorsal "buffalo" hump.

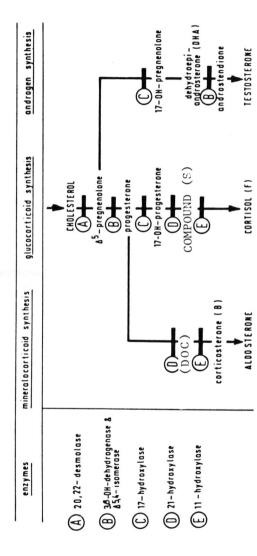

Figure 4–6. The inborn errors in steroid synthesis. (From Zurbrügg, R.P.: Endocrine and Genetic Diseases of Childhood. 2nd Ed. Edited by L.I. Gardner. Philadelphia, W.B. Saunders, 1975.)

URINARY EXCRETORY PRODUCTS OF ADRENAL STEROIDS

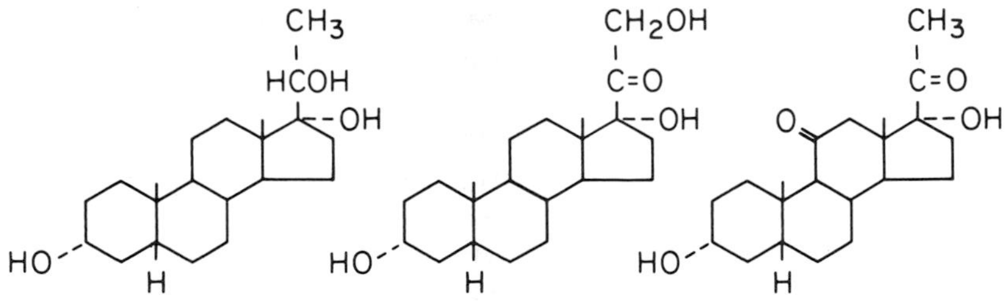

Pregnanetriol   Tetrahydro-S   11 Keto-pregnanetriol

Figure 4–7. Structure of three steroids found in the urine in various forms of congenital adrenal hyperplasia.

Table 4–2.   Classification of Spontaneous Cushing's Syndrome

	Incidence (%)
ACTH dependent	
Cushing's disease	68
Ectopic ACTH-secreting tumor	15
ACTH independent	
Adenoma	5
Carcinoma	3
Nodular adrenal hyperplasia	9
Adrenocortical rest tumor	<1

Table 4–3.   Incidence of Clinical Manifestations

	Incidence (%)
Obesity	90
Hypertension	85
Glucosuria and decreased glucose tolerance	80
Menstrual and sexual dysfunction	76
Hirsutism, acne, plethora	72
Stria, atrophic skin	67
Weakness, proximal myopathy	65
Osteoporosis	55
Easy bruisability	55
Psychiatric disturbances	50
Edema	46
Polyuria, polyphagia	16
Ocular changes and exophthalmos	8

Hypertension is in the range of 150 to 180 systolic and 90 to 110 diastolic. It may be due to increased mineralocorticoid secretion, primarily 11-deoxy-corticosterone, or the weak mineralocorticoid activity of large amounts of cortisol.

Decreased glucose tolerance is common but overt diabetes and ketosis are uncommon. The actions of cortisol to stimulate gluconeogenesis and lipolysis are antagonistic to the actions of insulin and cause secondary hyperinsulinism.

Amenorrhea or oligomenorrhea is secondary to increased adrenal androgens and, in some cases, increased estrogens, which suppress the LH surge and ovulation. Males may have decreased libido, testicular softening, and gynecomastia.

Hirsuitism is of two types. Cortisol excess produces lanugo-like hair over the face and body. Androgen excess results in acne, seborrhea, temporal recession, deep voice, coarse hairs on the upper lip and chin, and a male escutcheon.

Purple stria over the abdomen and breasts develop secondary to the catabolic effects of cortisol on the skin and the coloring of erythrocytosis. Capillary fragility results in easy bruisability although the clotting mechanism is normal. Proximal muscle weakness results from decreased muscle mass due to the protein catabolic effects of cortisol and from hypokalemia.

Osteoporosis and kyphosis occur in adults; retardation of growth occurs in children. These changes are due to the protein catabolic effect and negative calcium balance (vitamin D antagonism) induced by glucocorticoids. Excess glucocorticoid also suppresses secretion of growth hormone (GH) and inhibits the action of somatomedins on bone and cartilage.

Psychiatric disturbances are common in Cushing's syndrome and may not remit following treatment. Up to 70% of patients with Cushing's disease have emotional disorders, primarily depression.

Diagnosis

The presence of Cushing's syndrome is established by:
1. Loss of circadian rhythm of plasma cortisol.
2. Lack of suppression of cortisol secretion by low dose dexamethasone (1 mg overnight or 2 mg over 24 hours).
3. Increased urinary excretion of cortisol and its metabolites.
4. Lack of cortisol response to hypoglycemia.

Circadian Rhythm

Circadian rhythm can be estimated by plasma cortisols drawn at 8:00 A.M. and midnight. Plasma cortisol levels at midnight normally are less than 8 µg/100 ml. In Cushing's syndrome, conditions of stress, and severe depression, all values throughout the day are similar. Plasma cortisol levels are increased throughout the day during pregnancy and estrogen therapy due to increased cortisol binding globulin.

Low Dose Dexamethasone Suppression

The overnight dexamethasone suppression test uses 1 mg dexamethasone given at 11:00 P.M. In Cushing's syndrome, plasma cortisol at 8:00 the next morning is greater than 4 μg/100 ml. The standard low-dose dexamethasone suppression test consists of administration of 0.5 mg dexamethasone every 6 hours for 2 days; this procedure results in urinary 17-hydroxysteroids of less than 5 mg/day after 24 hours and less than 3.5 mg/day after 48 hours in normal subjects; greater values are seen in Cushing's syndrome.

Twenty-four Hour Urinary Steroids

Baseline 24-hour 17-hydroxysteroids are usually greater than 20 mg in males and greater than 15 mg in females with Cushing's syndrome; urinary excretion in excess of 10 mg/g creatinine is usually seen. In Cushing's syndrome, 17-ketosteroid excretion is usually greater than 22 mg/24 hours in males or 15 mg/24 hours in females. However, in Cushing's disease (bilateral adrenal hyperplasia), 17-ketosteroids may be normal. Values for 17-ketosteroid greater than 40 mg/24 hours suggest adrenal carcinoma. Urinary free cortisol excretion is greater than 100 μg/24 hours in Cushing's syndrome.

Insulin Tolerance Test

The cortisol response to insulin-induced hypoglycemia is useful in differentiating Cushing's syndrome from obesity and severe depression. Patients with Cushing's syndrome fail to respond to a blood glucose less than 40 mg/100 ml with an increase in cortisol of at least 8 μg/100 ml. In addition, patients with Cushing's syndrome fail to have a GH rise in response to insulin-induced hypoglycemia.

Tests useful in diagnosing the pathogenesis of Cushing's syndrome include:
1. High-dose dexamethasone suppression (8 mg).
2. Metyrapone test.
3. Plasma ACTH.
4. ACTH stimulation test.
5. Radiologic tests.

High Dose Dexamethasone Suppression

The high dose dexamethasone suppression test consists of 2 mg dexamethasone administered every 6 hours for 48 hours. In Cushing's disease urinary 17-hydroxysteroids are suppressed at least 50%. In Cushing's syndrome due to other causes, no suppression usually occurs. Rarely, there is periodic secretion of ACTH and cortisol with a cycle of 10 days or more; this secretion may result in spontaneous increase or decrease in urinary steroids during the dexamethasone suppression test and invalidate the test.

Metyrapone Test

Following 3 g metyrapone at 11:00 P.M., plasma 11-deoxycortisol (compound S) at 8 the next morning is normally 7 to 18 μg/100 ml. In Cushing's disease, the compound S response to metyrapone is greater than normal. In adrenal tumors the compound S response usually equals the pretreatment baseline cortisol consistent with autonomous ACTH-independent production of steroids by the tumor.

Plasma ACTH

Plasma ACTH in Cushing's disease may be normal (less than 100 pg/ml) or slightly elevated. In clinically evident ectopic ACTH syndrome, plasma ACTH is greater than 200 pg/ml. In patients with adrenal tumors plasma ACTH is usually undetectable.

ACTH Stimulation Test

The administration of 25 U (250 μg) cosyntropin (Cortrosyn) given intravenously results in more than a twofold increase in plasma cortisol in patients with bilateral adrenal hyperplasia. Patients with adrenal adenoma may or may not have a normal increase in plasma cortisol. Over 90% of patients with adrenal carcinoma are unresponsive to ACTH.

Radiologic Tests

In Cushing's disease polytomography of the sella turcica may reveal sellar enlargement and erosion of the sellar floor if the pituitary adenoma is a macroadenoma (greater than 1 cm in diameter). Computerized tomography (CT) scanning of the sellar area may reveal suprasellar or lateral extension of the pituitary tumor. Most patients with Cushing's disease have normal sella polytomograms and CT scans; however, on pituitary exploration a microadenoma is usually found.

An adrenal scan with radioiodinated cholesterol, adrenal CT, or arteriography may be useful to differentiate unilateral adrenal adenoma from bilateral adrenal hyperplasia. Other tests useful in localizing an adrenal tumor include intravenous pyelogram with tomography, and venography with selective venous sampling from the inferior vena cava and each adrenal vein for cortisol measurements. This testing localizes the site of excess cortisol secretion.

Treatment

The treatment of choice for Cushing's disease is transsphenoidal microsurgery to selectively remove the pituitary microadenoma, which is the source of excess ACTH secretion.

Mild or moderate Cushing's disease may be treated initially with pituitary irradiation. The remission rate is about 30%.

Adrenal adenomas or carcinomas are most effectively treated by surgical removal. Inoperable patients may be treated with o,p'-DDD (Mitotane), which is specifically toxic to the adrenal cortex and inhibits adrenal hormone synthesis. Ectopic ACTH syndrome is preferably treated by removal of the tumor. Inoperable patients may be treated with o,p'-DDD, aminoglutethimide or metyrapone to block cortisol synthesis. Bilateral nodular hyperplasia is usually treated by subtotal or total adrenalectomy.

Postoperatively, replacement therapy with cortisol and mineralocorticoid is necessary. This therapy is detailed in the section on adrenal insufficiency.

PRIMARY ALDOSTERONISM

Definition

Primary aldosteronism refers to the adrenal gland's excessive and autonomous production of aldosterone, the major adrenal mineralocorticoid. The term primary signifies that hypersecretion of aldosterone has its origin within the adrenal gland, whereas in various forms of secondary aldosteronism the stimulus is extra-adrenal in origin. There are two major pathologic forms of primary aldosteronism. Most cases of primary aldosteronism are due to a single or, infrequently, multiple aldosterone-producing adrenal adenomas. Between 15 and 30% of all cases have bilateral adrenocortical hyperplasia as the source of excessive aldosterone production. In rare cases, primary aldosteronism is caused by an adrenal carcinoma.

Primary aldosteronism is an uncommon disease involving, at the most, 1% of all hypertensive patients. Yet, when considered in light of the estimated 23 million hypertensives in the United States, this form of curable hypertension demands careful consideration in any patient with elevated blood pressure.

Pathophysiology

Almost all the pathophysiologic events in primary aldosteronism can be explained in terms of the effects of aldosterone on sodium and potassium transport. Aldosterone excess results in increased sodium reabsorption, increased total body sodium, and hypervolemia; however, at a certain point, no further sodium retention occurs because proximal tubular sodium reabsorption decreases and sodium excretion increases. This mineralocorticoid "escape" phenomenon explains why patients with primary aldosteronism rarely exhibit progressive volume expansion or edema. Excessive aldosterone production in primary aldosteronism causes arterial hypertension in all patients, which can be explained by volume expansion, arteriolar sodium content, vascular and sympathetic reactivity. All degrees of blood pressure elevation from mild and labile to severe and sustained hypertension occur in primary aldosteronism, although malignant hypertension is rare. Many patients with primary aldosteronism have hypertension only; they lack any other discernible signs or symptoms. Thus, differentiation of this disease from the larger essential hypertensive population on a clinical basis may be difficult.

The second major event of aldosterone excess is increased renal tubular secretion of potassium eventuating in both intracellular and extracellular depletion of this electrolyte. When symptoms do occur in primary aldosteronism, most of them can be attributed to potassium depletion. A major function of potassium is to maintain excitability of nerve and muscle by contributing to the electrical potential difference across the cell membrane. Potassium depletion in primary aldosteronism results in muscle weakness and fatigue, which is usually more pronounced in the lower extremities and, on rare occasion, progresses to complete, transient paralysis. Another consequence of potassium depletion, particularly if severe, is a defect in urinary concentration. Thus, patients frequently have nocturnal polyuria sometimes associated with polydipsia. The exact pathophysiology of kaliopenic nephropathy is poorly understood but may be due to alterations of distal tubule and collecting duct permeability to water. Although polyuria and polydipsia are frequently resistant to vasopressin administration, potassium repletion can completely reverse these symptoms and the renal lesion. Chronic hypokalemia also alters the electrical potential of myocardial cells, leading to the electrocardiographic findings of U waves and widened Q-T interval. Another frequent association most likely related to hypokalemia is diminished glucose tolerance or clinical diabetes mellitus in about 50% of patients with primary aldosteronism. Hypokalemia directly impairs insulin release from the pancreatic β cell and may also influence the peripheral action of insulin. Aldosterone excess also increases hydrogen ion secretion, and not uncommonly metabolic alkalosis is noted in primary aldosteronism. The alkalosis is not due to a direct aldosterone effect but seems best correlated with the degree of hypokalemia.

Symptoms and Signs

The common symptoms of primary aldosteronism include muscle weakness, fatigue, and nocturia. There are few typical physical stigmata of this disease. Arterial hypertension is a constant finding. Accompanying prolonged blood pressure elevation, there may be mild to moderate hypertensive retinopathy and left ventricular hypertrophy. Edema is almost always absent. Prolonged hypokalemia can blunt certain circulatory reflex responses so that postural hypotension with bradycardia can occur. In a minority of patients, tetanic findings such as the Chvostek and Trousseau signs can be elicited.

Diagnosis

The major diagnostic criteria for primary aldosteronism include:
1. Arterial hypertension.
2. Hypokalemia with excessive urine potassium excretion that is augmented by salt loading.
3. Suppressed plasma renin activity.
4. Elevated aldosterone levels that fail to be suppressed during volume expansion.

In the untreated hypertensive patient, a serum potassium of less than 3.5 mEq/L is suggestive of primary aldosteronism. A major diagnostic problem is the significant number of hypertensives with diuretic-induced hypokalemia. In distinguishing diuretic-induced hypokalemia, several days after stopping the diuretic, a 24-hour *urine potassium* excretion should be less than 40 mEq.

In patients with mineralocorticoid-induced hypokalemia, potassium excretion persists at greater than 40 mEq/24 hours. Second, in borderline hypokalemia with suspicion of primary aldosteronism, salt loading (sodium chloride tablets 2 g thrice daily) for 5 days induces further hypokalemia in patients with primary aldosteronism. This condition is due to increased delivery of filtered sodium to the distal sodium-potassium exchange site, resulting in increased potassium excretion. The dependence of potassium excretion on sodium intake explains why some patients with hyperaldosteronism are normokalemic. An additional outpatient procedure that can help confirm a suspected case of primary aldosteronism is administration of spironolactone, a specific mineralocorticoid antagonist. Administration of large doses (400 to 600 mg/day) should normalize serum potassium and blood pressure over a 4- to 6-wk period in most cases of primary aldosteronism.

The next diagnostic step is to demonstrate suppression of *plasma renin activity*. In normal man, plasma renin activity increases with any form of volume depletion, such as sodium restriction, hemorrhage, upright posture, or diuretic administration. Likewise, volume expansion suppresses plasma renin activity, and the chronic hypervolemia of primary aldosteronism accounts for the suppressed levels seen in this disease. Several methods of volume depletion have been used to evaluate renin responsiveness, the most physiologic being 5 days of dietary sodium restriction (10 mEq sodium daily) combined with 4 hours of upright posture. A more practical method of testing renin response is administration of a potent diuretic agent, such as furosemide (60 mg orally) with measurements of renin after 5 hours of upright posture. Although suppressed renin activity is found in all cases of primary aldosteronism, it is also present in 25% of the essential hypertensive population.

The final diagnostic confirmation of primary aldosteronism rests on demonstrating elevated levels of *plasma* or *urine aldosterone*. The majority of patients with primary aldosteronism demonstrate elevated baseline aldosterone levels, but some patients overlap into the normal range. Chronic hypokalemia may itself reduce aldosterone production by the adrenal tumor. To circumvent this problem, volume expansion is performed to test the suppressibility of aldosterone. Immediate or prolonged volume expansion by most methods does not suppress aldosterone levels in primary aldosteronism based on the relative autonomy of the adrenal tumor. In contrast, in normal subjects or in other forms of hypertension, adequate volume expansion results in a 50 to 80% fall in aldosterone from baseline. Volume expansion may be performed by oral salt loading (200 to 300 mEq sodium intake for 5 days), infusion of normal saline solution (2 L for 4 hours), or administration of a potent mineralocorticoid (10 mg deoxycorticosterone acetate twice daily or 200 μg fluorocortisol thrice daily) for 3 days. Lack of aldosterone suppression in a hypertensive patient with hypokalemia and low renin is the final confirmation of the diagnosis of primary aldosteronism.

The differential diagnosis of primary aldosteronism is given in Table 4–4. These disorders include those that biochemically mimic primary aldosteron-

Table 4—4.   Differential Diagnosis of Primary Aldosteronism

	Plasma renin	Plasma aldosterone	Blood pressure	Serum potassium
Primary aldosteronism	low	high	high	low
Edematous disorders	high	high	normal	low
Malignant hypertension	high	high	high	low
Renovascular hypertension	normal or high	normal or high	high	normal or low
Congenital adrenal hyperplasia (11- and 17-hydroxylase deficiency)	low	low	high	low
Cushing's syndrome	low or normal	normal or low	high	low
Liddle's syndrome	low	low	high	low
Barter's syndrome	high	high	normal or low	low
Licorice ingestion	low	low	high	low
Low-renin essential hypertension	low	normal or low	high	normal

ism. Secondary aldosteronism is an elevation of aldosterone due to increases in the renin-angiotensin system. Secondary aldosteronism is most conveniently divided into diseases with or without hypertension. The edematous disorders without hypertension make up most cases of secondary aldosteronism and include the nephrotic syndrome, cirrhosis with ascites, and congestive heart failure. These underlying diseases lead to disturbances in circulating blood volume, which stimulate the renin-angiotensin-aldosterone axis. Secondary aldosteronism with hypertension is most commonly due to malignant or accelerated hypertension. This disorder has been associated with high levels of renin and aldosterone due to decreased renal perfusion and is frequently accompanied by marked hypokalemia and metabolic alkalosis. Renal vascular hypertension can produce secondary aldosteronism, but hyperaldosteronism and hypokalemia are uncommon in this disorder. Cushing's syndrome, especially the ectopic ACTH syndrome, can occur with hypertension and hypokalemia. In most cases, the classic physical stigmata of Cushing's syndrome direct attention toward the proper diagnosis. Certain forms of congenital adrenal hyperplasia, including the 11β-hydroxylase and 17α-hydroxylase deficiency syndromes, result in hypertension and hypokalemia, which respond to glucocorticoid therapy. Liddle's syndrome, which is a familial disorder of increased sodium retention, results in hypertension and hypokalemia. This abnormality is attributed to an increased activity of the nonaldosterone-dependent site for distal tubular sodium and potassium exchange. Other rare causes of hypertension and hypokalemia are tumors producing either renin or a mineralocorticoid. A rare familial form of primary aldosteronism in children with hypertension and hypokalemia responds to glucocorticoid therapy. Excessive ingestion of licorice can mimic primary aldosteronism by causing hypertension, hypokalemia, and renin suppression. Licorice contains glycyrrhizin, which in excess acts as a mineralocorticoid by binding to aldosterone receptor sites. Finally, approximately one-fourth of patients with essential hypertension may demonstrate low levels of plasma renin activity. However, the differential diagnosis rests on the fact that most of this group are normokalemic and have aldosterone levels in the normal to low range.

Adrenal Adenoma versus Hyperplasia

The final diagnostic consideration is preoperative distinction between adrenal adenoma and bilateral hyperplasia. The importance of this distinction is that the majority of patients with hyperaldosteronism due to bilateral hyperplasia do not have normal blood pressure following bilateral total adrenalectomy. This result is in marked contrast to patients with aldosterone-producing adenomas, where surgical correction of hypertension is the rule. Recent work has shown that plasma aldosterone increases in response to upright posture in the hyperplasia group and remains unchanged or falls in patients with adenoma. This simple clinical procedure may be useful preoperatively to separate the two groups.

Intravenous urography, retroperitoneal pneumography, and adrenal arteriography have not been successful in distinguishing adrenal adenoma from hyperplasia. Adrenal venography with venous sampling for aldosterone determination and adrenal scintigraphy employing ^{131}I-19-iodocholesterol have an accuracy of 95% for diagnosing unilateral adrenal adenoma and 90% for diagnosing bilateral hyperplasia.

Treatment

Surgical procedure is recommended for patients with aldosterone-producing adenomas and medical therapy for bilateral adrenal hyperplasia. At operation, most adenomas are small, often less than 1 cm in diameter; however, the entire adrenal gland containing the tumor is usually excised. Sometimes no tumor tissue is located, and a subtotal or total adrenalectomy is necessary. Surgical outcomes in the adenoma group result in 70% correction of hypertension and significant improvement in the remainder. Since ACTH and cortisol remain intact in primary aldosteronism, pre- and postoperative steroid replacement is usually not needed. It is important preoperatively to replenish body potassium, usually accomplished with oral potassium supplementation. Alternatively preoperative treatment with spironolactone (400 to 600 mg daily) has been advocated to normalize potassium preoperatively.

Medical therapy with spironolactone is the treatment of choice in patients with bilateral hyperplasia, but the results have been variable, and long-term evaluation of this therapy is not available. In addition, long-term spironolactone treatment is frequently accompanied by impotence and gynecomastia in males and menstrual abnormalities in females. The antiserotonergic drug cyproheptadine has been useful in some cases. Improved understanding of the pathophysiology of bilateral hyperplasia is needed to permit more rational therapy.

HYPORENINEMIC HYPOALDOSTERONISM

Pathophysiology

Hyporeninemic hypoaldosteronism occurs primarily in patients with renal disease, commonly interstitial nephritis or nephropathy. Hyperkalemia and metabolic acidosis result from aldosterone deficiency. Renal secretion of potassium and hydrogen ions is impaired; the resulting hyperkalemia further increases the acidosis by reducing renal ammonia production. The hypoaldosteronism appears to be due to decreased renin release by the kidney. Plasma concentrations of renin and aldosterone are low and do not increase normally in response to sodium restriction and upright posture. Aldosterone release does occur in response to ACTH or angiotensin II infusion.

Diagnosis

In a patient with chronic hyperkalemia, hyperchloremic acidosis, and modest renal insufficiency, the diagnosis of hyporeninemic hypoaldosteronism is based on low plasma renin and aldosterone levels in response to sodium restriction and upright posture. Adrenal insufficiency should be excluded by demonstrating that the cortisol response to ACTH is normal.

Treatment

Hypokalemia and acidosis respond to mineralocorticoid therapy with fluorocortisol. Higher doses (usually 0.2 mg/day) are required to treat this disorder than are needed in adrenal insufficiency, perhaps because the diseased kidney is resistant to the steroid. Some patients, especially those with hypertension and increased fluid volume, may require therapy with a diuretic such as furosemide instead of or in addition to mineralocorticoid therapy to correct hyperkalemia and acidosis.

ADRENAL MEDULLA

Physiology

The adrenal medulla is derived embryonically from primitive neural crest tissue. The major secretory products of the adrenal medulla and the sympathetic nerve endings are the catecholamines, epinephrine and norepinephrine. A third member of this group, dopamine, appears to be most important within the central nervous system. These dihydroxylated phenolic compounds have diverse functions, including regulation of the neural and cardiovascular systems.

The following biotransformations are involved in the syntheses of catecholamines:

1. Tyrosine	tyrosine hydroxylase →	Dihydroxyphenylalanine(dopa)
2. Dopa	dopa decarboxylase →	Dopamine
3. Dopamine	dopamine β-oxidase →	Norepinephrine
4. Norepinephrine	N-methyl transferase →	Epinephrine

The postganglionic sympathetic nerves and adrenal medulla contain all the enzymes to synthesize catecholamines from the amino acid, tyrosine. The first step requires the microsomal enzyme, tyrosine hydroxylase, which is rate limiting for the entire biosynthetic sequence. The second reaction involves the cytoplasmic enzyme, dopa decarboxylase, to produce dopamine, which is taken up by active transport into cytoplasmic storage granules. Within these granules, dopamine is oxidized to norepinephrine by dopamine β-oxidase. The last transformation, yielding epinephrine, involves the enzyme phenylethylamine N-methyl transferase, present only in the adrenal medulla and the organ of Zuckerkandl. Thus, in the adrenal medulla, epinephrine constitutes about 75% of the end product, whereas norepinephrine is the major extraadrenal product. Evidence suggests that the last enzyme is regulated by glucocorticoids. Because of the close anatomic relationship between the adrenal cortex and medulla, drainage through the adrenal portal system results in high medullary steroid concentrations.

Catecholamine release involves migration of the cytoplasmic storage granules to the cell surface where they are discharged by exocytosis. Upon stimulation and membrane depolarization, the granules discharge not only catecholamines but also ATP and the enzyme, dopamine β-oxidase. The fate of released catecholamines appears to be complex. Some are bound to the specific α- and β-adrenergic receptors in various target tissues to initiate their diverse physiologic effects. However, a major portion of released catecholamines is taken up again by the neuron for storage in new cytoplasmic granules. This reuptake transport pathway serves as an efficient, economical process to reutilize these amines. The third fate of these compounds is metabolic inactivation and excretion in the urine. Two primary enzyme systems are responsible for inactivation of catecholamines (Fig. 4–8). The primary enzyme is catechol-O-methyl transferase, present in most tissues, especially liver and kidney. The resulting inactive methylated amines, metanephrine and normetanephrine, are either excreted in the urine or further metabolized by oxidative deamination by the enzyme, monoamine oxidase. The final metabolic product is vanillylmandelic acid. Under normal conditions, vanillylmandelic acid comprises about 75% of total urinary catecholamines, and metanephrines about 10%. Finally, about 1% consists of free catecholamines, which are excreted unaltered in the urine.

PHEOCHROMOCYTOMA

The most common tumor of sympathetic origin in adults is pheochromocytoma, which derives from chromaffin cells of the adrenal medulla or extraadrenal ganglia. Other rare neoplasms of sympathetic origin include neuroblastoma, ganglioneuroma, and chemodectoma. Although the incidence of pheochromocytoma is less than 0.5% of all patients with hypertension, this disorder is of major importance because it represents a curable form of hypertension.

The tumor occurs with equal frequency in both sexes and has been found at all ages from infancy to the eighth decade. Pheochromocytomas occurring in childhood are frequently bilateral, more often malignant, and associated with increased familial incidence. Being of neural crest origin, these tumors can occur at any location along the primitive chromaffin system. Most commonly, they arise in the adrenal medulla or sympathetic ganglia along the abdominal aorta. Less than 5% of tumors are extra-abdominal, usually occurring in the thoracic sympathetic chain. About 15% of tumors are multiple and 10% are malignant.

Pathophysiology

Most findings in pheochromocytoma can be attributed to the pharmacologic action of the major catecholamines, epinephrine and norepinephrine. The effects of these sympathomimetic amines are partially determined by their receptor-binding affinity to various target tissues. The adrenergic nervous system has two types of receptors, α and β. The α-adrenergic receptors are predominantly involved in maintenance of peripheral circulation, with additional effects on gastrointestinal sphincter constriction, pupil dilatation, and sweating. The β-receptors increase cardiac rate and inotropism, and also cause peripheral vasodilation, bronchodilation, and decreased gastrointestinal motility. Norepinephrine has predominantly α effects, whereas epinephrine acts on both α and β receptors. Catecholamine action is effected when receptor binding activates the cell membrane enyzme, adenylate cyclase, to form intracellular cyclic AMP from ATP.

Hypertension in those with pheochromocytoma is an α effect related to excess norepinephrine. Blood pressure elevation may be sustained or paroxysmal, depending on the nature of catecholamine release. Sustained hypertension is seen in approximately half of the cases and, if other symptoms are mild or nonspecific, can mimic essential hypertension. Orthostatic hypotension is an important finding occurring in over 60% of patients with pheochromocytoma. This postural fall in blood pressure may be volume-related, but more likely reflects attenuation of normal circulatory reflexes. In addition, a few patients can have severe hypotension and shock, presumably related to a high production of epinephrine relative to norepinephrine.

Table 4–5 outlines the various modes of presentation of pheochromocytoma, emphasizing the propensity of these tumors to mimic several common illnesses. Erroneous initial diagnosis is common. Classic findings with pheochromocytoma, in order of decreasing frequency, are hypertension, headache, sweating, palpitations, pallor, nausea, tremor, weakness, flushing with heat intolerance, epigastric and chest pains, and paresthesias. Paroxysmal attacks are often precipitated by postural changes, smoking, palpation of the abdomen, overeating, induction of anesthesia, urination, exercise, and certain drugs. Attacks may occur a number of times per day or several months apart. These episodes are often followed by extreme prostration.

The hypermetabolic features of pheochromocytoma, which can resemble hyperthyroidism, include tremor, weight loss, heat intolerance, and increased basal metabolic rate. One important differential finding is that constipation, not hyperdefecation, characterizes pheochromocytoma. In fact, the catecholamines drastically reduce gastrointestinal motility and increase sphincter tone, leading to other common findings, e.g., nausea, abdominal pain, and, at times, symptoms of intestinal obstruction. Catecholamines block insulin release and increase gluconeogenesis and fatty acid mobilization, accounting for the high incidence of abnormal glucose tolerance, fasting hyperglycemia, and glycosuria in this disease. If other findings of hypermetabolism are minimal, an initial diagnosis of diabetes mellitus may be made. Similarly, because certain symptoms, including sweating, headache, hypermetabolism, and emotional lability, are common to pregnancy, the onset of hypertension in pregnancy often leads to the diagnosis of toxemia. Some believe that pheochromocytoma has an increased incidence in pregnancy and, if unrecognized, leads to increased morbidity and mortality in both mother and fetus. Autonomic nervous system abnormalities, such as postural hypotension, sweating, palpitations, and chest pains, in a nervous individual may suggest psychoneurosis. The corollary is that many patients with essential hypertension have one or more features suggesting pheochromocytoma; but only few of this group turn out to have the disease. A rare patient with pheochromocytoma has a large abdominal mass without symptoms of catecholamine excess; these large tumors degrade catecholamines within the tumor, yielding low or normal catecholamine levels but high levels of inactive metabolites. Catecholamine excess can also produce a specific myocarditis and myocardial necrosis. In this setting, the patient may manifest signs of severe, refractory congestive heart failure masking the more common findings in this disease. Myocardial damage may reflect a direct inflammatory effect of catecholamines on cardiac tissue. Pheochromocytoma can lead to malignant hypertension. Occasionally, these patients have a stroke.

Associated Familial Disorders

Although the majority of pheochromocytomas occur sporadically, they also show a familial occurrence with autosomal dominant inheritance. Pheochromocytoma can be associated with medullary carcinoma of the thyroid. The relationship of these two diseases is based on their common embryonic origin from neural crest cells. This association, termed multiple endocrine adenomatosis, type II (type IIa), has a high incidence of bilateral pheochromocytoma and production of calcitonin by the malignant "C" cells, which comprise the thyroid carcinoma. There may be associated parathyroid gland hyperplasia or adenomas. The high prostaglandin and serotonin content of the thyroid tumor may account for the flushing and diarrhea seen in this syndrome. Familial multiple endocrine adenomatosis type III (type IIb) is

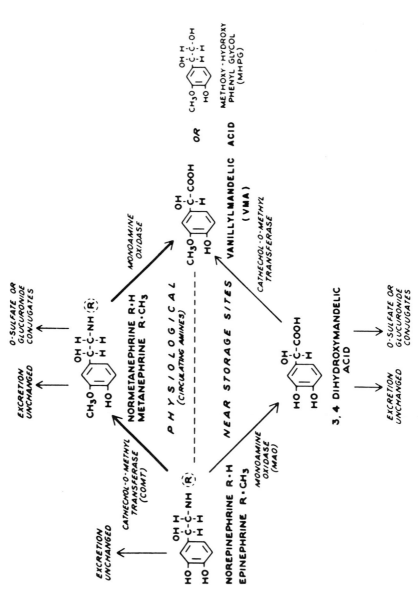

Figure 4–8. Pathways for metabolic degradation of catecholamines. (From Williams, R.: Textbook of Endocrinology, 5th Ed. Philadelphia, W.B. Saunders, 1974.)

Table 4–5. Modes of Presentation in Pheochromocytoma

Disorder	*Symptoms*
Paroxysmal attack	Hypertension, headache, sweating, pallor, palpitation, nausea, chest and abdominal pain, tremor
Sustained hypertension	Symptoms mild or nonspecific, suggesting essential hypertension
Hypermetabolism	Tremor, sweating, weight loss, increased basal metabolic rate, suggesting hyperthyroidism
Increased blood glucose	Suggesting diabetes mellitus
Decreased gastrointestinal motility	Suggesting abdominal obstruction or Hirschsprung's disease
Hypertension in pregnancy	Mimics toxemia of pregnancy with hypermetabolism and psychic changes
Anxiety syndromes	Orthostatic dizziness, palpitations, paresthesias, and tremor, suggesting psychoneurosis or hyperventilation syndrome
Abdominal mass	Patient may be relatively free of symptoms if large tumor rapidly metabolizes catecholamines
Hypotension	May mimic any of the more common forms of shock
Congestive heart failure	Catecholamine induced myocardiopathy may mimic more common causes of congestive heart failure

associated with mucosal neuromas and marfanoid habitus in addition to bilateral pheochromocytomas and medullary thyroid carcinoma.

Pheochromocytoma is frequently associated with other neuroectodermal syndromes, particularly neurofibromatosis, in 5 to 10% of patients. Other common neurocutaneous findings in pheochromocytoma include café-au-lait spots, hyperpigmentation, and axillary freckling. A higher incidence of other neuroectodermal disorders such as Lindau's disease, Sturge-Weber syndrome, and tuberous sclerosis has also been noted.

Symptoms and Signs

Despite the striking symptoms of pheochromocytoma (see Table 4–5), findings on physical examination often are nonspecific. Although weight loss is commonly described, as many as 30% of patients may be overweight, dispelling the adage that one never sees a "fat pheo." Examination of the skin may reveal café-au-lait spots, other dermatologic abnormalities, and diaphoresis. The thyroid gland may be nodular. The veins of the dorsum of the hand may not be apparent due to intense venoconstriction. Catecholamine-induced myocarditis may manifest itself as arrhythmias, gallop rhythms, and signs of congestive heart failure. A palpable abdominal tumor is found in 10 to 15% of cases, and palpation may elicit an attack. Frequently, however,

Table 4–6.   Normal Values

Plasma Concentrations	
Catecholamines: Epinephrine (supine)	≤75 ng/l
Norepinephrine (supine)	50–440 ng/l
Urinary Excretion Rates	
Catecholamines	≤100 μg/24 hr
Metanephrines	≤1.2 mg/24 hr
Vanillylmandelic acid	≤6.5 mg/24 hr

the patient has hypertension and an otherwise negative physical examination, so specific laboratory testing is needed.

Diagnosis

Screening hypertensive patients for pheochromocytoma can be accomplished with urinary assays for total free catecholamines, metanephrine, normetanephrine, and vanillylmandelic acid (VMA) or by assay of plasma catecholamines (Table 4–6).

Total Free Catecholamines

This assay measures the sum of norepinephrine and epinephrine excreted unaltered in the urine and is best quantified by the trihydroxyindole fluorometric method. Various separatory procedures make it possible to fractionate norepinephine and epinephrine for purposes of localizing adrenal and extraadrenal tumor sites. Several pharmacologic compounds produce a false-positive elevation of catecholamines, the most common being the antihypertensive agent, α-methyldopa. Other interfering compounds include isoproterenol, theophylline, and sympathomimetic agents present in several commonly used drugs. Since this sensitive procedure is expensive and technically more difficult than the other assays, it should not be used for routine screening. The normal adult secretion of free catecholamines is less than 100 μg/day.

Metanephrines and Normetanephrines

These 3-methoxy metabolites can be measured by a relatively simple photometric method, usually expressed as total metanephrines. Many consider this the most reliable assay because it is virtually free from major interfering substances and is specific and sensitive. Monoamine oxidase inhibitors and α- methyldopa will falsely elevate urinary metanephrines. Normal values are less than 1.2 mg/day.

Vanillylmandelic Acid (VMA)

This acid is the final product of catecholamine metabolism. It is measured by organic extraction, conversion to vanillin, and spectrophotometric assay. This procedure is specific; however, the VMA screening tests are nonspecific since they measure phenolic acids in such foods as bananas, coffee, nuts, and chocolate. In addition, the monoamine oxidase inhibitors and α-methyldopa result in a misleading decrease in VMA excretion. Normal values are less than 6.5 mg/day.

If these assays are done by correct methods, most persons with pheochromocytoma show an elevation of free catecholamines (99%), total metanephrines (97%), and VMA (90%). Therefore, in routine screening of hypertensive patients, the best recommendation is a single measurement of either total metanephrines or VMA and confirmation of abnormal levels by assay of total free catecholamines. Traditionally, most measurements have been done on 24-hour urine specimens, a procedure that is plagued by the problem of inaccurate collection. To circumvent this problem, either a timed 2- to 3-hour single-voided specimen or a random urine sample expressed per milligram of creatinine is useful if collected during or immediately after a severe attack.

Plasma Catecholamines

Levels of total resting supine plasma catecholamines are elevated in most cases of pheochromocytoma (≥2000 ng/L), but there is overlap with the levels in essential hypertensive patients in the range of 1000 to 2000 ng/L. In patients whose total plasma catecholamines fall within this range, the rise in blood pressure and plasma catecholamines in response to 2 mg intravenous glucagon distinguishes patients with pheochromocytoma from those with essential hypertension. The greatest value of plasma catecholamines has been to help localize tumors by frequent sampling along the course of the vena cava.

Pharmacologic Tests

Before the availability of accurate urinary tests for pheochromocytoma, the monitoring of blood pressure during administration of pharmacologic agents that stimulated or blocked catecholamine release was utilized to diagnose this disease. Today, with accurate tests of catecholamine levels, these potentially hazardous and inaccurate procedures are rarely employed. However, an occasional patient may have normal or equivocal catecholamine levels; then these provocative tests, using tyramine, histamine, or glucagon, may be carried out in conjunction with obtaining plasma samples or a timed urine specimen for catecholamines. The α-adrenergic blocking agent phentolamine should be available to counteract a hypertensive crisis. Histamine and tyramine tests should not be performed in a severely hypertensive patient.

Tumor Localization

The studies most helpful for tumor localization include abdominal computerized axial tomography scan, selective angiography, and adrenal venous sampling for catecholamine levels. Certain simple preoperative procedures, such as roentgenograms of the chest and thoracic spine, are done to locate the rare extra-abdominal tumors. Angiography may be accompanied by severe, often fatal reactions, which may be prevented by premedication (for 4 to 5 days) with the α-blocking agent phenoxybenzamine.

Treatment. Proper preoperative management has dramatically reduced the morbidity and mortality of surgical procedures. Phenoxybenzamine (10 mg orally twice daily) is administered preoperatively and increased to 40 to 100 mg daily until symptoms are controlled. One may administer α-methyltyrosine (1 to 4 g/day), to reduce catecholamine biosynthesis by competitive inhibition of tyrosine hydroxylase. Phentolamine, a shorter-acting α-blocker, is used to control more severe paroxysms. A high-sodium diet may be given preoperatively to counteract volume depletion. Usually, β-blockade with propranolol is not necessary preoperatively unless cardiac arrhythmias occur.

Therapy during surgical procedure should include monitoring of pulse, arterial and venous pressure, and electrocardiogram throughout the procedure. Anesthetic agents should not release catecholamines or sensitize the myocardium; most modern anesthetic agents appear acceptable. If a hypertensive attack occurs during induction of anesthesia or at operation, phentolamine (1 to 5 mg intravenously) should be given. Ventricular arrhythmias are best treated with propranolol (1 to 3 mg intravenously). During the operation when the tumor is localized, it is important to ligate the venous drainage before excision to prevent excessive catecholamine release. Immediately after removal of the tumor, the blood pressure may fall precipitously; administration of a plasma expander before tumor removal usually prevents this complication. Surgical results are extremely rewarding; in fact, normotension resumes in the early postoperative period. A check of urinary catecholamines should be made the week after the operation to document complete tumor removal.

For inoperable pheochromocytoma, chronic medical therapy is necessary; the drug of choice is the inhibitor of tyrosine hydroxylase, α-methyltyrosine. Unfortunately, for most cases of malignant pheochromocytoma, medical therapy is the only choice since these tumors respond poorly to antitumor therapy such as radiation or cytotoxic agents.

CLINICAL PROBLEMS

Patient 1. This 37-year-old white woman was admitted to the hospital with severe weakness. Her history dates back 10 years, when she noted that her fingers had areas of loss of pigmentation. Over the past year, she developed total body alopecia, including loss of head, axillary, and pubic hair. She also noted increased pigmentation and freckling of the face, back, hands, elbows, and knees. Four months before admission she became severely fatigued, nauseated, and weak. She was diagnosed as having the "flu" and placed on bed rest for 3 weeks without improvement. During this time she had a 15-pound weight loss, extreme weakness, abdominal pain, and anorexia. She was only able to retain liquids; solid foods caused epigastric pain, vomiting, and left lower quadrant cramping. Upon standing she had light-headedness, palpitations, dyspnea, and fullness in her ears. There was no history of fever, chills, sweats, cough, or exposure to tuberculosis. She had a past history of goiter and had complaints of cold intolerance, dry skin, somnolence, and constipation. There was no family history of endocrine disorders, tuberculosis, or alopecia.

PHYSICAL EXAMINATION. This examination revealed a thin, pale, chronically ill woman. Blood pressure (BP) supine was 100/60; on standing no BP could be auscultated, only a systolic pressure by palpation. Pulse rate went from 84 to 120 upon standing. Total alopecia of the scalp accompanied increased pigmentation along her wig line. Increased freckling and vitiligo were apparent around the eyes. No mucosal pigmentation was noted. The thyroid was slightly enlarged, firm, and irregular without discrete nodules. The lungs were clear to percussion and auscultation. There was no costovertebral angle tenderness. She had dark pigmentation around the nipples. There was no axillary or pubic hair. Heart examination revealed tachycardia without abnormal sounds or murmurs. The abdomen was soft with minimal tenderness in the left lower quadrant and no rebound tenderness. There were no masses; liver and spleen were not palpable. Vitiligo covered the hands. Neurologic examination was normal except for generalized muscle weakness. Deep tendon reflexes were symmetrical with normal relaxation phase.

LABORATORY DATA. Hematocrit (HCT), 39%; white blood count (WBC), 6900 with 87 segs, 9 lymphocytes, 3 monocytes, and 1 undifferentiated cell. Platelets were adequate. Serum Na, 135 mEq/L; K, 6.7 mEq/L; Cl, 99 mEq/L; CO_2, 24.8 mEq/L; glucose, 118 mg/100 ml; creatinine, 1.0 mg/100 ml; blood urea nitrogen (BUN), 18 mg/100 ml. Serum, calcium, magnesium, and liver function tests were normal. Electrocardiogram showed peaked T waves suggestive of hyperkalemia. Chest roentgenogram was normal.

Serum cortisol, 1.0 μg/100 ml; after ACTH stimulation, cortisol remained 1.0 μg/100 ml. Serum aldosterone, 1.7 ng/100 ml (normal, 6 to 30 ng/100 ml in upright position). Urinary 17-OH steroids, less than 1.0 mg/24 hours. Urinary 17-ketosteroids, 5.0 mg/24 hours. Plasma ACTH, 310 pg/ml (normal, 8:00 A.M. 30 to 120 pg/ml). Serum vitamin B_{12}, 993 pg/ml (normal, 330 to 1025 pg/ml); T_4, RIA, 7.2 μg/100 ml; T_3, 103 ng/100 ml (normal, 80 to 180 ng/100 ml); TSH, 2 μU/ml (normal, 0.5 to 5 μU/ml).

QUESTIONS
1. What is the pathophysiology of the patient's symptoms?
2. What is your diagnosis, and what is the cause of the disease?
3. What other diseases are associated with this disorder?
4. What therapy would you initiate at the time of diagnosis?
5. If the patient were hypothyroid, what would be the danger in treating her with thyroxine only?

Patient 2. This 5-year-old boy was first seen with complaints of excessive growth, pubic hair, and acne (Fig. 4–9). At 3 weeks of age he was admitted to the hospital with complaints of poor feeding, failure to gain weight, and vomiting. Physical examination revealed evidence of dehydration; serum sodium, 110 mEq/L; serum potassium, 9.5 mEq/L; urine sodium, 72 mEq/L; urine potassium, 15 mEq/L; 17-ketosteroids, 4.2 mg/24 hours (normal, less than 0.5 mg/24 hours); pregnanetriol, 3.2 mg/24 hours (normal, less than 0.5 mg/24 hours). He was treated with intravenous fluid, deoxycorticosterone acetate, 1 mg/24 hours, and cortisone, 10 mg/day. One week later he was discharged with serum Na, 142 mEq/L; K, 4.8 mEq/L; urine 17-ketosteroids, 0.5 mg/24 hours; and pregnanetriol, 0.3 mg/24 hours.

At the age of 11 months he was readmitted to the hospital with recurrence of vomiting, dehydration, and evidence of pneumonia. Serum Na, 115 mEq/L; K, 9.4 mEq/L; urine 17-ketosteroids, 5.8 mg/24 hours, and pregnanetriol, 2.4 mg/24 hours. Bone age was 1 year. Cortisone dosage was increased to 15 mg/day. Florinef (9α-fluorocortisol), 0.1 mg daily, was substituted for deoxycorticosterone. Cortisone was given only intermittently because parents thought it was responsible for hyperpigmentation.

At the age of 3 years he had an upper respiratory infection and was seen at the hospital. Dehydration was no longer evident; 17-ketosteroids, 10.1 mg/24 hours (normal, less than 2.0 mg/24 hours); pregnanetriol, 12.5 mg/24 hours; serum Na, 130 mEq/L; K, 5.8 mEq/L. Cortisone dosage was increased to 20 mg/day. Parents were unable to understand the need for cortisone and Florinef. They were skeptical of the need for cortisone and one day took him to a physician who told them nothing was wrong with the boy's adrenals.

At age 5, he was referred to UCLA's clinic at the insistence of the school nurse who had noted his large size, hoarse voice, increased muscularity, acne, pubic hair, enlarged penis, and hair growth on the upper lip. Physical examination confirmed these findings. His height was 131 cm (about 6 SD above the mean), and his weight was 31 kg (also 6 SD above the mean). Serum sodium was 140 mEq/L; serum K was 4.6 mEq/L. Although the penis was greatly enlarged, the testes were normal in size for his age. Bone age was 12 years.

Over the next few years, his height continued well above the ninety-fifth percentile. He continued to take his medications sporadically. At age 9½, serum testosterone was 440 ng/100 ml, FSH and LH were unmeasurable. 17-ketosteroids were 84.8, and pregnanetriol was 18 mg/24 hours. Serum 17α-hydroxyprogesterone was 64 ng/ml (normal, less than 0.2 ng/ml). At age 9, he had developed testicular enlargement on the right side. This testicle was explored and a mass removed. The cells of this mass resembled Leydig cells. At this time, his bone age was 15 years.

QUESTIONS
1. Which tests support the diagnosis of congenital adrenal hyperplasia?

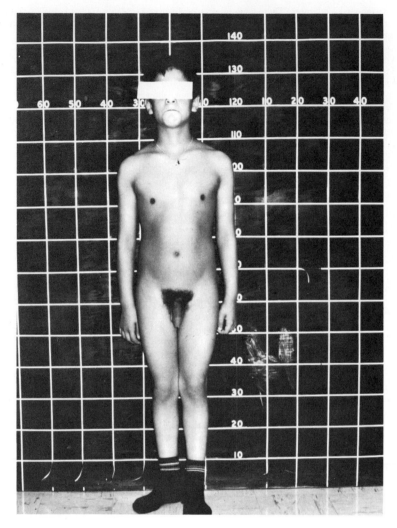

Figure 4–9.   Patient at 5 years.

2. What are the reasons for his salt loss? What enzymatic defects are associated with salt retention?
3. How does the urinary pregnanetriol establish the enzymatic defect? Does measurement of pregnanediol in the urine assist in this diagnosis?
4. Why is this boy tall? What will his adult height be—normal, short, or tall?
5. What is the nature of the testicular tumor?

Patient 3. This 10-year-old child was admitted to the hospital because of ambiguous external genitalia. The patient's mother had had a normal pregnancy. Because of the appearance of the external genitalia, the child was considered to be a boy and raised as such. Pubic and axillary hair appeared at the age of 2 years and acne at 4 years. The voice became low-pitched, and precocious development of the phallus was evident. The patient had been treated intermittently with 25 mg cortisone by mouth daily, but steroid treatment had ceased 4 or 5 years prior to admission. The patient had been in apparent good health throughout childhood and was the star of his school baseball team.

PHYSICAL EXAMINATION. The examination on admission revealed an elevated BP of 179/130 in an apparently precocious boy with well-developed musculature. Facial and body hair was of the normal adult male distribution, and acne of the face and trunk was present. There was grade II hypertensive retinopathy. Urologic examination revealed a hypertrophic clitoris and hypospadias, which was actually a urogenital sinus, and large rudimentary labial-scrotal folds. An organ thought to be a prostate gland was palpable on rectal examination, but the uterus could not be palpated. A smear of the buccal epithelium was chromatin positive. Karyotyping of a leukocyte culture revealed 46 chromosomes and an XX sex chromatin pattern. Skeletal roentgenograms showed advanced bone age with closure of all epiphyses. At that time, the height age was 8 years. Multiple views of the chest revealed cardiomegaly involving predominantly the left ventricle. The electrocardiogram showed a pattern of left ventricular hypertrophy. The intravenous pyelogram (IVP) was normal. A urethrogram and vaginogram showed a slit-like opening into the verumontanum, which was considered to be the vagina. An infantile uterus was also noted.

LABORATORY DATA. Pertinent laboratory data on admission included hematocrit, 42%; white blood cell count, 9000/mm with 67% neutrophils and 32% lymphocytes; blood urea nitrogen, 20 mg/100 ml; serum Na, 146; K, 4.1; Cl, 100 mEq/L.

The patient's steroid values are shown in the following table.

	Patient's Values	*Normal Values*
Compound S in serum (11-deoxycortisol)	13–25 µg/100 ml	<0.1 µg/100 ml
17-ketosteroids in urine	22–32 mg/24 hr	0.5–3.0 mg/24 hr
Pregnanetriol in urine	1.1 mg/24 hr	<0.5 mg/24 hr
Tetrahydro compound S in urine	25 mg/24 hr	<0.5 mg/24 hr
Tetrahydrocortisol and tetrahydrocortisone in urine	<4 mg/24 hr	4–10 mg/24 hr

Treatment with 25 mg cortisone/day was started, and the BP gradually declined to levels of about 110/70. Urinary excretion of 17-ketosteroids fell to between 5 and 8 mg/24 hours. Under anesthesia, the "hypospadias" was found to be a urogenital sinus with the urethra opening into a vaginal pouch. On laparotomy, enlarged cystic ovaries, fallopian tubes, and a uterus were found. The female internal genitalia were removed, and plastic reconstruction of the external genitalia was performed so the urethra opened at the tip of the phallus. Testosterone was administered by monthly injection.

QUESTIONS

1. What enzyme defect is responsible for this patient's problem?
2. What is the differential diagnosis of progressive virilization in a female?
3. What types of congenital adrenal hyperplasia are characterized by hypertension?

Patient 4. A 33-year-old woman described development of protruding abdomen, rounded face, increased facial hair, calf cramps, weakness, and recent leg ulcers that would not heal. She gave a history of hypertension recently diagnosed, menstrual irregularity, and swelling of her hands and feet for 2 years. Friends had commented that she looked older and had round rosy cheeks. She denied visual symptoms, acne, stria, and increased thirst or urination.

PHYSICAL EXAMINATION. BP, 155/100; P, 80 reg.; R, 15; T, 98.0. She was a well-developed white woman, with plethoric round face and protuberant abdomen. Skin was dry and thin, with bruises over her lower extremities. Soft downy hair was heavy over mustache area and chin. Visual fields were normal. Supraclavicular and dorsal fat pads were not enlarged. Examination of the chest and heart was normal. The abdomen had increased fat centrally. Extremities had no pitting edema. Neurologic examination was normal.

LABORATORY DATA. Complete blood count, urinalysis, and electrolytes were normal. Oral glucose tolerance test was mildly diabetic, with fasting glucose of 100, 1 hour of 200, 2 hours of 150, and 3 hours of 120 mg/100 ml.

| | Plasma cortisol (μg/100 ml) | | 17-hydroxycorticosteroids |
	A.M.	P.M.	mg/24 hr
Basal	22	18	18.3
	25		17.9
2 mg dexamethasone/day	24		12.7
	21		15.5
8 mg dexamethasone/day	15		6.3
	10		4.5

Plasma ACTH, 80 to 120 pg/ml.
IVP, skull and sella films were normal.
Chest roentgenogram: mild demineralization of ribs with 2 old fractures.

QUESTIONS

1. What physical findings indicate glucocorticoid excess?
2. What laboratory data help diagnose Cushing's syndrome and its cause in this case?
3. What is the expected adrenal disorder?
4. What additional laboratory tests would aid in diagnosing a macroadenoma of the pituitary?

Patient 5. This 55-year-old white male was admitted for progressive, generalized weakness of 3-year duration. He had been hypertensive for 9 years and was treated with thiazide diuretics. For the past 2 years, he had experienced nocturia 3 or 4 times nightly but did not have increased thirst. Recently, the weakness had progressed from intermittent to constant and was associated with muscle cramps. He also described frontal headaches occurring daily in the morning for the past year. He denied anorexia, weight loss, chest pain, dyspnea, and edema. There was no family history of hypertension, diabetes, renal or muscular disease. He was taking no medication except the diuretic. He denied excessive licorice ingestion or use of steroids.

PHYSICAL EXAMINATION. The examination revealed a well-developed man. BP, 190/110 supine, 176/96 upright; pulse, 80/minute supine, 92/minute upright; respiration (R), 20/minute; temperature (T), 99.4°. Funduscopic examination disclosed mild arteriolar attenuation. Cardiac exam revealed no cardiomegaly or murmurs but an S4 gallop at the apex. Abdomen was soft without organomegaly, masses, tenderness, or bruits. Pulses were all palpably present and equal; extremities had no edema. Muscle atrophy or fasciculations were not evident, but generalized weakness to muscle testing was noted. Cranial nerves, deep tendon reflexes, and sensory system were intact.

LABORATORY DATA. Hematocrit is 44% and WBC is 8700 with normal differential.

Results of urinalysis are specific gravity, 1.007; pH, 6.0, negative for glucose and protein. The serum creatinine is 1.2 mg/100 ml; BUN, 18 mg/100 ml; creatinine clearance, 80 cc/min.

| Electrolytes | Serum (mEq/L) | | | | Urine (mEq/24 hr) | |
	Na	K	Cl	CO₂	Na	K
120 mEq	144	2.6	104	33	62	69
Na intake	144	2.8	110	34	84	72
10 mEq Na intake	143	3.4	107	32	12	56
After saline infusion						
(2 L normal saline solution in 4 hours)	144	2.4	108	33	108	92

17 hydroxysteroids—3.8 mg/24 hours (normal, 3 to 10 mg/24 hours)
17-ketosteroids—8 mg/24 hours (normal, 10 to 22 mg/24 hours)
Serum thyroxine and T₃ uptake—normal
Urine VMA—5.9 mg/24 hours (normal, less than 6.5 mg/24 hours)
Glucose tolerance test: Fasting, 90 mg/100 ml; 1 hour, 160 mg/100 ml; 2 hours, 140 mg/100 ml; 3 hours, 120 mg/100 ml

Plasma renin activity		Patient (ng/ml/hr)	Normal Range (ng/ml/hr)
120 mEq Na intake:	Supine	0.3	1.0–2.2
	Upright	0.5	1.8–5.8
10 mEq Na intake:	Supine	0.5	1.8–8.2
	Upright	0.9	2.2–12.3
4 hours postdiuretic:	Upright	0.8	1.8–6.4
(60 mg furosemide)			

Urine aldosterone excretion—33 μg/24 hours (normal, 10 to 15 μg/24 hours)

Plasma aldosterone (ng/100 ml)		Patient	Normal Range
120 mEq Na intake:	Supine	22	2–10
	Upright	36	3–16
200 mEq Na intake:	Upright	32	1–5
Saline infusion	pre	20	50–80% suppression
(2 L normal	post	17	from baseline
saline/4 hours)			

ECG—suggests left ventricular hypertrophy, prolonged QT interval, flattening of T waves
Chest roentgenogram—mild left ventricular hypertrophy
Rapid sequence IVP—normal

QUESTIONS

1. What symptoms suggest aldosteronoma?
2. What is the pathophysiology of these symptoms?
3. How would serum and urine potassium determinations in the basal state and after saline infusion aid in the diagnosis of the patient?
4. What further diagnostic procedures would aid in clarification of the disorder and in the decision for surgical procedure versus medical therapy in this case?

Patient 6. This 32-year-old white male electrician was in excellent health until 6 months ago. At that time, he noted sudden onset of an intense frontal headache with sweating and tightness in the chest, coming on usually at work after sudden movements and changes in position. Afterwards, he felt "washed out" but continued to work. These episodes continued, and the patient ascribed the symptoms to "nerves," as he had recently separated from his wife. During this time, he also noted some postural dizziness and a nauseated feeling, which he related to recent obstipation. On one occasion, he sought medical help and was told that his BP was high. He was given a sedative, but did not return for follow-up as instructed. Two weeks prior to admission, he began to experience mild exertional dyspnea and noted ankle swelling. At this time, he had one episode of rapid heart rate diagnosed in a local emergency room as atrial tachycardia, which responded to digitalis and propranolol therapy. Because of a BP of 220/130 noted on that visit, the patient was referred for further evaluation. A family history of hypertension included his mother and one brother. The patient's past medical history revealed excellent health, and he was taking no medication.

PHYSICAL EXAMINATION. The examination revealed a well-developed, thin man who appeared nervous and tremulous. BP, 185/125 supine, 145/112 upright; R, 16/minute; T, 98°; pulse, 96 supine, 108 upright. Examination of the fundi showed grade I arteriolar narrowing. The thyroid gland was normal in size. Carotid pulses were equal and strong. His skin was moist and his hair was matted. The lungs had bilateral rales. Cardiac exam revealed normal rhythm; point of maximal impulse (PMI) was forceful and sustained; a third heart sound was heard at the apex. Pulses were all strong and equal, with no bruits. Abdominal exam revealed no tenderness, masses, or organomegaly. Extremities had 1+ pitting edema.

LABORATORY DATA
Hgb, 15.2; HCT, 44%; WBC, 8500 with normal differential.
Na, 142; K, 4.1; HCO₃, 28; Cl, 96 mEq/L; creatinine, 1.2 mg/100 ml; BUN, 18 mg/100 ml; FBS, 125 mg/100 ml; Ca, 9.6 mg/100 ml: P, 3.3 mg/100 ml; cholesterol, 256 mg/100 ml.
Liver function tests normal.
Oral glucose tolerance test mildly diabetic.
Serum thyroxine, 6.4 μg/100 ml.

Chest roentgenogram, moderate left ventricular hypertrophy and increased vascular marking in upper lung fields.

ECG, normal sinus rhythm.

Rapid sequence IVP with nephrotomograms suggested a mass on the medial side of the left kidney in the paraspinal area.

Urine VMA, 14.6 mg/24 hours

Urine metanephrine, 3.1 mg/24 hours

Total free catecholamines, 280 μg/24 hours; urine norepinephrine 196 μg/24 hours.

Transfemoral venogram, mass in the left adrenal area.

Catecholamine levels by selective venous catheterization:

Site	Catecholamine (μg/L)
Inferior vena cava (IVC) at diaphragm	8
Left adrenal vein	22
Right adrenal vein	6
IVC low	12

QUESTIONS

1. What is the pathophysiology of the patient's symptoms?
2. What is the significance of a 30% ratio of epinephrine to total catecholamines?
3. What further diagnostic studies would rule out endocrine disorders associated with pheochromocytoma in this patient?
4. What effect would propranolol have on the patient's blood pressure?

Patient 7. This 45-year-old Mexican-American woman was admitted to hospital in July, 1980, for evaluation of bizarre behavior and confusion. She had been well until 3 months before, when she was hospitalized for renal failure secondary to bilateral ureteral obstruction. Cervical biopsy revealed undifferentiated cervical carcinoma. A laparotomy was performed and revealed the uterus entirely infiltrated with tumor, as well as multiple positive para-aortic nodes. A left nephrostomy was placed, and the patient's BUN fell to the low 20's. The patient was discharged and treated by radiation therapy with 7000 rads to the pelvis and 5000 rads to the para-aortic chain.

She did well until May, 1981, when she was readmitted for bizarre behavior and confusion. The patient had no focal findings and had a normal computed tomographic brain scan, EEG, and lumbar puncture. A serum potassium of 2.8 was noted and treated with potassium supplementation. She was discharged on potassium and thorazine without change in her mental status. In July, 1981, she was readmitted for hypokalemia (potassium, 2.1).

PHYSICAL EXAMINATION. The examination revealed an obese, plethoric white woman with a full face. The skin showed multiple ecchymoses, and she had facial hirsutism. No acne, buffalo hump, or pigmented striae were present. Extremities showed 4 + edema. Neurologic examination revealed a confused disoriented female, with no focal findings.

LABORATORY DATA

Date	Blood						Urine		
	Na⁻	Cl⁻	HCO₃⁻	K+	BUN	FBS	Na+	K+	OSM
3/05/81	140	103	25	3.1	12	104	5.5	19	172
7/27/81	147	92	36	2.1	24	255	17	65	701

Serum cortisol—baseline, greater than 50 μg/100 ml
　　　　　　　after 1 mg dexamethasone, greater than 50 μg/100 ml
　　　　　　　after 8 mg dexamethasone for 3 days, greater than 50 μg/100 ml

QUESTIONS

1. What is the pathophysiology of sodium retention, edema, and hypokalemia in this patient?

2. What medication could you use to decrease cortisol production?
3. What would be this patient's compound S response to metyrapone?

SUGGESTED READING

Adrenal Insufficiency
Baxter, J.D., and Tyrrell, J.B.: The adrenal cortex. *In* Endocrinology and Metabolism. Edited by P. Felig, J.D. Baxter, A.E. Broadus, and L.A. Frohman. New York, McGraw-Hill, 1981.
Irvine, W.J., and Toft, A.D.: Diagnosing adrenocortical insufficiency. Practitioner, *218*:539, 1977.
Nelson, D.H.: Addison's disease (primary adrenal insufficiency). *In* The Adrenal Cortex: Physiological Function and Disease. Philadelphia, W.B. Saunders, 1980.
Nerup, J.: Addison's disease—clinical studies. A report of 108 cases. Acta Endocrinol., *76*:127, 1974.

Adrenogenital Syndrome
Hamilton, W.: Congenital adrenal hyperplasia. Clin. Endocrinol. Metab., *1*:503, 1972.
Korth-Schutz, S., et al.: Serum androgens as a continuing index of adequacy of treatment of congenital adrenal hyperplasia. J. Clin. Endocrinol. Metab., *46*:452, 1978.
Lippe, B.M., et al.: Serum 17-alpha-hydroxyprogesterone, estradiol and testosterone in the diagnosis and management of congenital adrenal hyperplasia. J. Pediatr., *85*:782, 1974.
Nelson, D.H.: Congenital adrenal hyperplasia and defects in biosynthesis of the corticosteroids. *In* The Adrenal Cortex: Physiological Function and Disease. Philadelphia, W.B. Saunders, 1980.

Cushing's Syndrome
Aron, D.C., et al.: Cushing's syndrome: problems in diagnosis. Medicine, *60*:25, 1981.
Baxter, J.D., and Tyrrell, J.B.: The adrenal cortex. *In* Endocrinology and Metabolism. Edited by P. Felig, J.D. Baxter, A.E. Broadus, and L.A. Frohman. New York, McGraw-Hill, 1981.
Findling, J.W., et al.: Selective venous sampling for ACTH in Cushing's syndrome. Differentiation between Cushing's disease and the ectopic ACTH syndrome. Ann. Intern. Med., *94*:647, 1981.
Gold, E.M.: The Cushing syndromes: changing views of diagnosis and treatment. Ann. Intern. Med., *90*:829, 1979.
Wolfsen, A.R., and Odell, W.D.: The dose-response relationship to ACTH and cortisol in Cushing's disease. Clin. Endocrinol., *12*:557, 1980.

Primary Aldosteronism
Biglieri, E.G., and Baxter, J.D.: The endocrinology of hypertension. *In* Endocrinology and Metabolism. Edited by P. Felig, J.D. Baxter, A.E. Broadus, and L.A. Frohman. New York, McGraw-Hill, 1981.
Ganguly, A., et al.: Control of plasma aldosterone in primary aldosteronism: distinction between adenoma and hyperplasia. J. Clin. Endocrinol. Metab., *37*:765, 1973.
Hogan, M.J., et al.: Location of aldosterone-producing adenomas with [131]I-19-iodocholesterol. N. Engl. J. Med., *294*:410, 1976.
Oparill, S., and Haber, E.: The renin-angiotensin system. N. Engl. J. Med., *291*:389, and *291*:446, 1974.
Weinberger, M.H., et al.: Primary aldosteronism. Diagnosis, localization, and treatment. Ann. Intern. Med., *90*:386, 1979.

Hypoaldosteronism
Nelson, D.H.: Clinical disturbances of aldosterone secretion. *In* The Adrenal Cortex: Physiological Function and Disease. Philadelphia, W.B. Saunders, 1980.
Schambelan, M., and Sebastian, A.: Hyporeninemic hypoaldosteronism. Adv. Intern. Med., *25*:385, 1979.

Pheochromocytoma
Bravo, E.L., et al.: Circulating and urinary catecholamines in pheochromocytoma. Diagnostic and pathophysiologic implications. N. Engl. J. Med., *301*:682, 1979.
Cryer, P.E.: Diseases of the adrenal medullae and sympathetic nervous system. *In* Endocrinology and Metabolism. Edited by P. Felig, J.D. Baxter, A.E. Broadus, and L.A. Frohman. New York, McGraw-Hill, 1981.
Engelman, K.: Phaeochromocytoma. Clin. Endocrinol. Metab., *6*:769, 1977.

CHAPTER 5

Sexual Differentiation and Development

Barbara Lippe

SEXUAL DEVELOPMENT AND DIFFERENTIATION OF THE FETUS

The events in the sequence of embryonic and physiologic changes controlling sexual differentiation of the fetus begin with fertilization. The genotype of the zygote, normally 46 XX or 46 XY, confers so-called genetic sex to the fetus. The successive events of internal and external "sexual" organogenesis and differentiation are initiated primarily by the somatic and germ cell components of the fetal gonads and the subsequent development of normal hormonal and biochemical mechanisms.

Gonadal Development

The first step in sexual differentiation occurs during the fourth week of fetal gestation (fertilization age) when the gonadal ridges differentiate. They are paired proliferations of the coelomic epithelium and underlying mesenchyme arising on either side of the midline. The epithelium proliferates, penetrates the underlying mesenchyme of the so-called indifferent gonad, and forms a number of irregularly shaped "sex cords." At this time, primordial germ cells, located in the yolk sac, migrate by amoeboid movement (control mechanism unknown) along the dorsal mesentery and by the sixth week have invaded the genital ridges. The interaction between the differentiating somatic cells of the gonad and the germ cells determines the second step in sexual differentiation. Three events occur:

1. Germ cells must reach each genital ridge for a fertile gonad to develop. (At this point the concept of laterality becomes important because subsequent embryonic events are dependent on processes occurring in each gonad, independently, and may or may not be the same on each side.)

2. The chromosomal component that the germ cell confers must be the same on each side if the same type of gonad is to be induced on each side.
3. The somatic components of the gonad must be "induced" to form a testis, or else an ovary will form.

In the normal male, a specific testicular inducer called H-Y antigen is synthesized, secreted, and bound to cell surface membranes early in embryogenesis. The regulatory genes for the synthesis of this material are on the short arm of the Y chromosome, whereas other regulator genes for its expression may be on the X chromosome and/or an autosome. The H-Y antigen is believed to be responsible for the primary differentiation of the genital somatic cells into a testis. Because it is present prior to gonadal differentiation and then binds to the differentiating cells, it can induce a testis even if the karyotype of the gonadal ridge cells is XX (gonadal sex-reversal). If the H-Y antigen is produced in less than "normal" quantity (presumably from a developing embryo in whom all cells do not bear the appropriate genetic message to synthesize the material), only part of a genital ridge, or one but not both ridges, may be induced to become a testis. In the normal female, H-Y antigen is not present, and somatic components of both genital ridges differentiate into ovaries.

As germ cells penetrate the differentiating gonad, a second regulatory step may occur. If the karyotype of the germ cell is different from the phenotype of the gonad (i.e., an XX germ cell in a developing testis), the germ cell will usually not survive. However, in some cases evidence suggests that the germ cell can induce somatic sex-reversal at that time; XY germ cells may act as a second inducer and may direct an XX genital ridge into testicular differentiation. Finally, there may be other regulators of induction, including receptors of the H-Y antigen inducer, which also affect differentiation.

The process of testicular development is so rapid that it is complete by the ninth fetal week, whereupon the testicle begins to function. Ovarian organogenesis occurs at a slower rate than the testicular counterpart. It involves continued development of cortical cords from the germinal epithelium and continued invasion by primordial germ cells, so that the maximum number of germ cells is present before the ovarian structure becomes evident. The medulla then begins to take on a cord-like appearance, germ cells group around the cords and enter the first meiosis, and follicles and stroma develop. This recognizable ovarian structure may not be present until 17 to 20 weeks of fetal gestation. Unlike the testis, which retains its structure whether or not its germ cells are viable, if the germ cells of the ovary fail to develop and to maintain normal follicles, the ovarian structure may lose its integrity and may become fibrotic. This postulated mechanism may explain the streak ovary in patients with X chromosome monosomy or deletions (Turner's syndrome (45 XO) and its variants). A normal karyotype is not necessary for induction of the ovary, but normal germ cells are necessary for its continued preservation. Thus, the ultimate potential of the gonad is a result of multiple directors of differentiation and function.

Internal Genital Duct Development

During the earliest stage of fetal development, series of paired mesodermal ducts appear. The first, the pronephric ducts, are present by 3 weeks (and degenerate soon thereafter). By 4 weeks the mesonephric ducts are present bilaterally and develop in close proximity to the genital ridge. If a testicle is developing, its close apposition to the mesonephros results in the organization of this duct (then called wolffian duct) into the duct of the epididymis, the ductus deferens, seminal vesicle, and the common ejaculatory duct at the level of the bladder trigone. Jost showed that a small amount of locally secreted testosterone, from each testicle, is responsible for this organization (on each side). However, the amount of testosterone is not sufficient (or does not cross-over) to influence ductal development on the contralateral side. This process of male internal genital ductal development is obvious by 9 weeks and may be complete by 14 weeks. In the absence of the developing testis, the meso-nephric duct degenerates by 10 weeks.

At 5 weeks the paramesonephric ducts develop lateral to the developing genital ridges (not as close as the mesonephric duct). If a testis is developing, müllerian regression substance is secreted by this testis (again locally, af-fecting development on one side), and the paramesonephric duct (müllerian duct) will regress. Müllerian regression substance is a glycoprotein of about 20,000 daltons, and is secreted by testicular Sertoli cells. It acts only on one side, and must therefore be secreted bilaterally for müllerian regression to occur bilaterally. This substance is the only known fetal regressor.

When a testicle is not present (or there is a failure of production or action of müllerian regression substance), the paramesonephric duct develops into a fallopian tube, a hemiuterus (on each side), and the upper two-thirds of the vagina. An ovary does not directly influence this process. Because of the more lateral development of the müllerian duct in relation to the developing gonad, no direct connection exists between the gonad and this potential ex-cretory unit. Thus, excreted ova must pass free into the peritoneum to reach the fimbriated end of the fallopian tube, whereas the testicle has a closely incorporated excretory system. These steps for internal genital development are summarized in the center of Figure 5–1.

External Genital Development

This final step in fetal sexual differentiation involves two complex embry-onic mechanisms: (1) the development of the excretory system, both urogenital and alimentary (many of the steps of which are under embryonic controls that are unknown and unrelated to the "sex" of the fetus) and (2) the development of that part of the external genitalia that is associated with sex assignment and that is under the influence of circulating androgen.

At three weeks, cloacal folds develop around the cloacal membrane and unite cephalad to form the genital tubercle. At the sixth week, the cloacal membrane is subdivided into the urogenital and anal membranes, and the

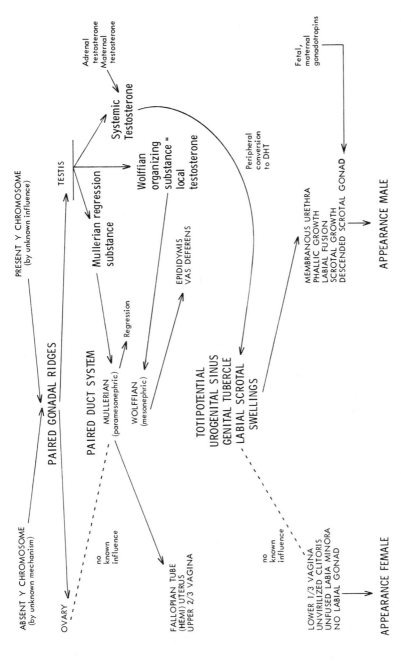

Figure 5–1. Development of the genital tract. This diagram outlines the factors that influence the development of each level of sexual differentiation.

cloacal folds into the urethral folds and the anal folds. Concomitantly, a second set of paired structures, the genital swellings, develops on either side of the urethral folds. These events occur in the fetus of either "sex" and result in common indifferent primordia for external genital development. By the eighth week, the cloaca is divided into an anterior urogenital groove (sinus) and posterior anorectal canal, and this step, too, is independent of hormonal ("sex") control (although subject to congenital anomalies) (Fig. 5–2*A*). It is only after eight weeks' gestation, when the fetal testis is functioning, that the development of the external genitalia diverges.

In the normal male, the genital tubercle rapidly elongates, pulls the urethral folds forward to form a deep urogenital or urethral groove, and by 12 weeks forms the penile urethra (Fig. 5–2*B*). This process is under the influence of

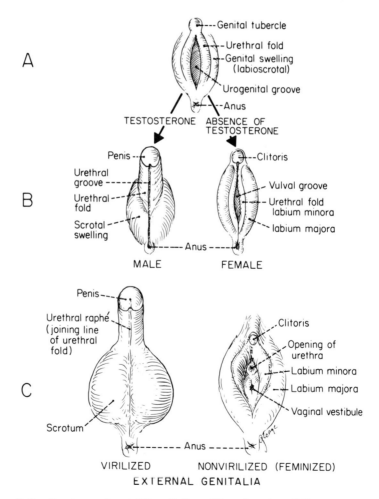

Figure 5–2. Development and differentiation of the external genitalia.

circulating testosterone (and its peripheral conversion of dihydrotestosterone (DHT) by 5-α reductase, with subsequent normal "reception" by the tissues). The final formation of the glandular urethra (to the tip of the phallus) is not under the influence of testosterone and does not occur in this process, but later (fourth month), as an invagination of penile ectoderm to reach the urethral lumen. This process explains the frequent occurrence of hypospadias independent of disorders of adequate testosterone production. The genital swellings move caudally to make up the halves of the scrotum (Fig. 5–2C).

In the female, in whom the levels of circulating androgen are normally lower, the indifferent primordium develops more slowly into the female genitalia. This development can be considered the unmodified embryonic pathway of the fetal genitoexcretory system. The genital tubercle elongates only slightly to form the clitoris (although this organ always has the potential to elongate under the influence of androgen, and may do so at any time during prenatal or postnatal development if circulating androgen increases). The urethral folds are not pulled anteriorly and therefore do not fuse. Instead they remain as the labia minora (Fig. 5–2B). By 14 weeks' gestation the relative position of the urethral orifice is fixed, and exposure to androgen will no longer pull the urethral folds or labia minora anteriorly. Therefore, while later exposure to androgen may enlarge the clitoris, it will not fuse the labia in the female or result in a phallic urethra. The time limit of this embryonic event may help date prenatal exposure to androgen; a virilized female exposed after 14 weeks may have clitoromegaly but does have unfused labia and a normally positioned urethra. Finally, the genital swellings do not migrate, but enlarge to form the labia majora, and the urogenital groove remains open to form the vaginal vestibule (Fig. 5–2C).

PATHOGENESIS AND DIFFERENTIAL DIAGNOSIS OF AMBIGUOUS GENITALIA

Ambiguity of the external genitalia at birth is a consequence of a sporadic developmental anomaly or is secondary to a derangement in the hormonal environment of the fetus or its ability to respond to hormonal stimuli. Since the ambiguity is the obvious clinical feature, an approach to the differential diagnosis and the definition of pathogenesis proceeds from what the clinician first sees.

The presence or absence of a palpable lower inguinal or scrotal gonad is an important clinical feature, since a gonad in this position, almost always testicular or partly testicular histologically, usually rules out simple virilization of a female baby. A normal ovary can herniate but, if so, appears just outside the inguinal ring. Only the rare condition of ovarian ectopia results in an ovary positioned well into the labial fold. Conversely, the absence of external gonads most often signifies a virilizing syndrome in a female infant.

The buccal smear cannot be used in the initial design of the work-up or as a significant aid in the explanation of pathogenesis because: (1) it is unreliable; e.g., it results in many false-negative chromatin determinations in genotypically XX infants, and (2) even appropriately identified chromatin positivity tells nothing about the presence or absence of a Y in the karyotype, nor can mosaic cell lines be easily defined. A complete chromosomal karyotype is therefore essential, but is only one part of the evaluation. The karyotype of the infant is not the ultimate determinant in the gender assignment of the child and may help only in classifying some of the unusual disorders associated with ambiguity. A normal blood "female karyotype" (46 XX) may be found in an infant with testes, as may a normal "male karyotype" (46 XY) be found in an infant with a vagina and uterus. The evaluation requires that the internal and external anatomy of the infant be completely defined and that the biochemical cause for either incomplete masculinization or excessive virilization be identified.

In the ambiguous infant without a palpable scrotal gonad the following five conditions are most often found:

1. Female with congenital adrenal hyperplasia: salt-losing form.
2. Female with congenital adrenal hyperplasia: non-salt-losing form.
3. Female who has been iatrogenically virilized by maternal ingestion of virilizing substances.
4. Female who has been virilized by maternal overproduction of androgen.
5. Female in whom the source of intrauterine virilization is never found ("idiopathic") and the internal anatomy is normal for a female.

In the ambiguous infant with a palpable scrotal gonad, as many as nine different mechanisms may be identified:

1. Asymmetric or mixed gonadal dysgenesis—secondary to a mosaic karyotype at the gonadal level (45 XO/46 XY or some variant), which is usually identified in the blood karyotype but may have to be inferred.
2. True hermaphrodite—secondary to mosaic karyotypes or Y-derived genetic material at the gonadal level, which may or may not be identified in the blood karyotype.
3. Male pseudohermaphroditism, type I—X-linked recessive; found in an XY male with testes. This is a form of partial peripheral insensitivity to dihydrotestosterone.
4. Male pseudohermaphroditism, type II—autosomal recessive; found in an XY male with testes. This is secondary to an enzymatic deficiency of 5-α-reductase and results in failure to synthesize dihydrotestosterone.
5. Male with inability to make müllerian regression substance—autosomal recessive or X-linked defect.
6. Male with an error in pathway of testosterone synthesis—these enzymatic defects are autosomal recessive: (1) 20,22-desmolase deficiency, (2) 3-hydroxysteroid dehydrogenase deficiency, (3) 17-hydroxylase deficiency, (4) 17,20-desmolase deficiency, and (5) 17-ketosteroid reductase deficiency.
7. Male with congenital malformations—congenital anomalies that are developmental and not secondary to known hormonal or genetic mechanisms.

8. Male with as yet undetermined defects in androgen action—has testes, XY karyotype, and normal enzymes but fails to virilize adequately.
9. Male with hypopituitarism—the key clinical feature is a microphallus associated with other features of hypopituitarism.

A flow sheet for the clinical evaluation leading to the differential diagnosis of these 14 conditions is found in Figure 5–3. The karyotype, not included in the flow sheet, is supplemental information.

GONADAL FUNCTION FROM BIRTH TO PUBERTY

The mechanisms that control gonadal function actually begin in the fetus. Fetal hypothalamic-pituitary activity can be demonstrated in the second trimester and good evidence suggests that a component of fetal gonadal activity is directly stimulated by fetal pituitary gonadotropin. Toward the end of gestation, fetal gonadotropin secretion decreases. This decrease is a consequence of negative feedback inhibition from increasing circulating levels of sex steroids on the fetal hypothalamic-pituitary axis. At birth, the rapid decline in these circulating steroids following placental separation results in a surge of gonadotropin and an increase in gonadally derived hormones. In the male infant during the first three months of life, plasma testosterone concentrations may rise to levels as high as those detected in midpuberty. In the female infant, the rise in estradiol is less striking, but it does occur. These increased concentrations of gonadal steroids are believed to be responsible for negative hypothalamic-pituitary feedback, resulting in a second decline in gonadotropins in the first year of life. In the infant without gonads in whom steroids cannot be secreted in response to the gonadotropin surge in the neonatal period, the gonadotropins do not decline during the first year.

Following this phase of gonadal control, a second control mechanism becomes operative. This mechanism appears to be central neural inhibition of hypothalamic release of gonadotropin releasing hormone (GnRH). Studies in higher primates indicate that the normal pubertal cyclic release of pituitary FSH and LH is a consequence of pulsatile GnRH secretion. These pulses occur at 60- to 90-minute intervals. In the prepubertal state, neural inhibitory mechanisms appear to suppress or to modulate either the amplitude or the frequency of the GnRH release and thereby to prevent the pubertal pattern of FSH and LH release. This central inhibition is largely independent of gonadal feedback inhibition because even the agonadal child experiences a decline in gonadotropins between the ages of about 2 and 10 years. Neither mechanism results in total inhibition because low but fluctuating concentrations of both FSH and LH can be detected in both the plasma and urine of males and females throughout childhood. As the child matures, a gradual lessening of the inhibitory mechanisms appears to occur. The mechanisms responsible for this central shift are unknown. In early puberty, higher amplitude gonadotropin surges are detected first during sleep. In association with these pulses (presumably the consequence of a change in the pulsatile nature of GnRH secretion), gonadal steroids rise. This rise is most easily demonstrated in the male,

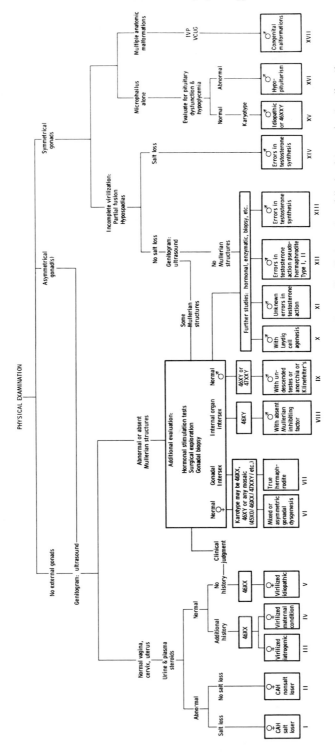

Figure 5–3. Newborn with ambiguous genitalia. This diagram outlines the studies that most rapidly lead to understanding the pathogenesis and determining the sex assignment of the newborn with sexual ambiguity.

in whom the nocturnal plasma testosterone concentration may reach levels well into the pubertal range, while the daytime concentration may still be a prepubertal value. The lessening of inhibition appears to be both at the central control of GnRH release and at the level of response of the hypothalamic-pituitary axis to the gonadal steroid feedback. This process shifts from negative inhibition to positive feedback, so that response to GnRH then becomes augmented despite increased production of sex steroids.

The clinical implications of the gradual changes that occur in the hypothalamic-pituitary-gonadal axis in the prepubertal and early pubertal child are as follows:

1. Hormonal concentrations vary with age and range over an overlapping spectrum of "normal" (see Table 5–1). Therefore, single hormonal determinations are often not helpful in assessing, describing, or diagnosing a clinical state.

2. Many of the static and dynamic tests of hypothalamic-pituitary-gonadal axis used in adults are of little value prior to puberty.

   a. Clomiphene does not stimulate an LH surge in the prepubertal child and in fact may add to the negative feedback system already present.

Table 5–1. Plasma Hormones in Females and Males

Plasma Hormones in Females				
Age // Tanner Stage	Testosterone (ng/100 ml)	Estradiol (pg/ml)	FSH (mIU/ml)	LH (mIU/ml)
Neonate	<50	25	3	
0–3 mo	—	20	3	<2
1 yr	—	<20	2	<2
2–8 yr	7–20	<20	3	<3
9–10 // 2	<30	<30	3	3
11–12 // 3–4	<40	40	5	4
13–14 // 3–5	<50	50	11	8
15 // 5	<56	>50	12	9
16 and over // adult	<56	>50	4–20	4–20
Plasma Hormones in Males				
Age // Tanner Stage	Testosterone (ng/100 ml)	Estradiol (pg/ml)	FSH (mIU/ml)	LH (mIU/ml)
Neonate	50	20		
0–3 mo	up to 200	<20	<2	—
1 yr	15	<30	2	2
2–9 yr	10–15	<30	4	2
10–11 // 2	25–100	<30	4	6
12–13 // 3–4	50–300	<40	6	9
14–15 // 4–5	100–500	<40	8	14
16–21 // adult	300–1100	14–36	2–15*	2–15 *

*Occasional normal subjects have lower values.

b. GnRH administration as an infusion or single bolus may not stimulate FSH or LH release since pulses of the appropriate amplitude and frequency appear to be necessary, especially in the unstimulated state.

c. Basal serum FSH and LH determinations from children between the ages of two and ten years may be normally low in both the normal and agonadal child. Only later do FSH and LH concentrations rise to castrate concentrations in the agonadal child and become clearly helpful in this diagnosis. In the child with delayed puberty, low concentrations of FSH and LH do not distinguish between a hypothalamic defect, a pituitary defect, or a simple delay in maturation.

d. Major increases in basal estradiol and testosterone determinations often lag behind clinical features of puberty and are frequently more helpful in confirming a clinical impression of "delayed" puberty than in making an etiologic diagnosis. Sleep-related surges of hormone might be helpful in characterizing the developing pattern of puberty but are clinically difficult to obtain.

SECONDARY SEXUAL DEVELOPMENT

The physical changes that occur during puberty in the female and male have been arbitrarily divided into stages of sequential development in order to demonstrate that the age of onset of earliest pubertal changes is variable, but the rate or progression of change thereafter is less variable and may be anticipated. Therefore, a standard nomenclature for describing each stage allows the observer to evaluate the rate and degree of progression.

Female Pubertal Development

The physical standards and the associated mean ages most commonly applied are those of Tanner and Marshall, but these standards are limited to breast development and pubic hair growth (Table 5–2).

The ovaries and uterus are difficult to assess by physical examination, but radiographic and pathologic evidence suggests that enlargement of the ovary is the first physical change during puberty. Uterine enlargement can be documented by pelvic examination (or more recently by ultrasonography). When these changes have occurred, more than 90% of girls show breast development, followed in some months by growth of pubic hair, with subsequent progression to adult characteristics in 3 years. From 5 to 10% of girls have pubic hair first, with breast development following within a year. If more than a year separates the two, the sequence is abnormal and suggests failure of adequate estrogen production (a pattern often seen in Turner's syndrome).

Menarche

The first menstrual period is a consequence of ovarian estrogen production and uterine growth and endometrial proliferation. It occurs at a mean interval of 2.3 years after breast development is first noted. In American girls the most recent mean age reported was 12.8 years. This figure would place

Table 5–2. Female Secondary Sexual Development

Tanner Stage	Description	Age (yr) (mean ± 2 SD)
Breast		
1	Prepubertal	
2	Subareolar breast budding (often begins unilaterally and with tenderness)	10.5 ± 2
3	Widening of breast tissue and areola without separation of contours	12 ± 1
4	Areola and papilla project above the plane of enlarging breast	13 ± 2
5	Mature breast—areola and breast in same plane— papilla erect	15 ± 3
Pubic Hair		
1	Absence of pubic hair (downy fine body hairs may be present on mons at any age)	
2	A few long pigmented hairs develop over mons or on labia majora	11.7 ± 2.5
3	Hair curls and spreads over mons	12.4 ± 2.2
4	Abundant hair limited to mons	13 ± 2
5	Adult escutcheon with spread of hair to medial thighs	14.4 ± 2.2

menarche at a point close to breast and pubic hair stage 4. Menarche is best correlated with skeletal maturation, and the highest correlation is with a bone age of 13. Some data suggest that body weight (and perhaps more precisely, percentage of body fat) may have a direct relation to initiation of puberty and time of menarche in females. This "critical weight" hypothesis (mean 48 kg) is being investigated.

Growth

The rate of growth in height accelerates significantly during puberty and reaches its peak in most girls during breast and pubic hair stages 2 and 3 (preceding menarche). The intensity of the "spurt" seems related to the time of occurrence; i.e., in the year preceding menarche, early developers gain more height than do late developers. This theory accounts for the lack of a significant difference in the adult heights of "early and late growers" (as opposed to the anecdotal impression that early developers "end-up" shorter). Among American girls, menarche is achieved at a mean height of 158 cm.

Male Pubertal Development

In contrast to female pubertal stages, those described for the male cover a greater number of physical variables. There are at least four measures of genital development (testicular enlargement, scrotal changes, phallic enlargement, and prostatic enlargement) as well as pubic hair changes and other somatic changes such as axillary hair, facial hair and hairline, laryngeal development, and body habitus. This development has been summarized in Figure 5–4, in which stage 1 is prepubertal, stage 5 is fully pubertal, and stage 6 represents further changes, which may not occur until the middle of the third decade.

The key to male pubertal staging is testicular size. Because the testis is an ellipsoid organ, accurate length and diameter measurements are difficult to obtain. Significant changes in volume occur with small changes in any one dimension. Volume itself is a more accurate means to assess testicular growth, and standards have been developed by Prader, using ellipsoids of known volume (milliliters). The most significant changes occur between 1 and 2 ml (onset of puberty), 5 and 8 ml (progression beyond size of testis of a patient with Klinefelter's syndrome), and 15 + ml (adult size). Since phallic enlargement may not be present until the testis has enlarged to 5 ml or greater, boys at this stage are often erroneously misdiagnosed as being prepubertal.

Pubic Hair

Staging is similar to that in girls, with early stages characterized by long, straight, downy hairs, followed by coarsening of the hair, then darker pigmentation, and finally development of a male escutcheon with extension of

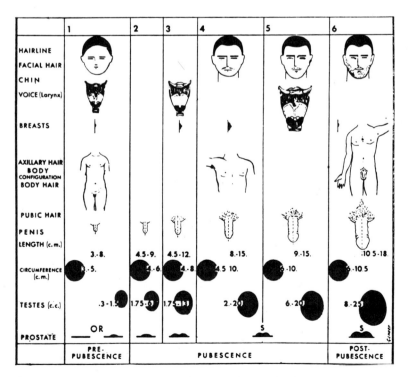

Figure 5–4. Male pubertal development. (From Schonfeld, W.A.: Am. J. Dis. Child., 65:535, 1943.)

hair upward onto the linea alba. Since changes of testicular volume and phallic enlargement can both be easily quantitated and described, precise pubic hair staging is less important in the male.

Gynecomastia

Enlargement of the male breast, either unilateral or bilateral, is a normal response in the pubertal male, occurring in as many as 70% of males at some time during puberty. It is usually transitory in nature, lasting 1 to 2 years. The development of breast tissue appears to be secondary to a high ratio of estradiol to testosterone, which may occur during the early stages of puberty, and resolution may occur as that ratio reverses with increasing testosterone production. Excessive size of the breasts or persistence of breast tissue beyond the adolescent years may necessitate surgical removal, but again, the tissue is not usually pathologic. However, postpubertal development of gyneco-mastia signals an abnormality in hormonal secretion or milieu and needs evaluation. A few pathologic conditions are characterized by pubertal gy-necomastia. These conditions may be chromosomal in origin (i.e., Klinefel-ter's (47 XXY) syndrome, with testicular hyalinization and failure of pro-gression in volume beyond 4 to 5 ml), or they may represent a primary abnormality in testosterone metabolism or action, such as failure of dihydro-testosterone (DHT) synthesis or partial end-organ resistance to DHT due to "receptor abnormalities." These latter conditions almost invariably have some degree of structural genital abnormality associated with them.

Growth

The pubertal growth spurt period in the male is longer than in the female, with a tendency to reach its peak velocity at a mean age of 15.5 years. The peak velocity is less intense than the female's, but the extended time period leads to ultimate taller stature. Since the onset of the growth spurt and puberty are related and correlate with skeletal maturation (bone age), assessment of puberty and its consequent hormonal changes is a requisite for the evaluation of growth during this time interval.

CLINICAL CONDITIONS OF ABERRANT GROWTH AND PUBERTAL DEVELOPMENT

The interrelationship between the maturation of the hypothalamic-pituitary axis, gonadal responses, and pubertal growth and development makes it nec-essary to consider disorders of growth and pubertal development together in the adolescent.

Delayed Growth and Puberty

Based on the mean age ± 2 standard deviations (SD) for the onset of pubertal changes, 2% of girls fail to exhibit breast development by age 13 years, and 2% of boys fail to have testicular enlargement by 13.5 years. The majority of these children progress into puberty within 1 to 2 more years and have no demonstrable somatic or hormonal abnormalities. Bone age and height age are usually concordant in these children, their prior growth rates are usually normal, and the first signs of puberty are usually seen when the bone age reaches 11 years in girls and 11 to 12 years in boys. Uncharacterized genetic factors may be responsible for the time of initiation of puberty, and the term *constitutional growth delay* is applied. There is often a family history of a similar pattern in one parent, a first-degree parental relative, or a sibling. The condition appears to be more common in boys.

Following is a list of the conditions that can be responsible for the small fraction of children with pubertal delays (with or without growth delay) that are not "constitutional."

Systemic Disorders
    1. Generalized—infectious, inflammatory, neoplastic
    2. Specific Organ System—cardiovascular, respiratory, gastrointestinal, renal, neuromuscular
    3. Endocrine—undiagnosed or poorly controlled conditions
Hypothalamic Dysfunction
    1. Generalized—postinfectious, inflammatory, or traumatic dysfunction
    2. Specific—lesion or process causing dysfunction
        a. Congenital malformation—midline defect or cleft syndrome associated with failure to produce releasing hormone
        b. Craniopharyngioma with suprasellar extension
        c. Infiltrative lesion—histiocytosis X
        d. Hypothalamic tumor
    3. Syndromes—associated with dysfunction
        a. Kallmann's—anosmia and hypogonadotropic hypogonadism
        b. Prader-Willi (mental retardation, hypogonadism, hypotonia, and obesity)
        c. Laurence-Moon-Bardet-Biedl (mental retardation, hypogonadism, retinitis pigmentosa, and hand anomalies)
        d. Anorexia nervosa
    4. Idiopathic or familial—failure to produce or secrete hypothalamic releasing substances
Pituitary Dysfunction
    1. Generalized—infectious, granulomatous, vascular (insufficiency or infarct), autoimmune insufficiency
    2. Specific—lesion or process causing dysfunction
        a. Congenital malformation—pituitary aplasia or hypoplasia
        b. Craniopharyngioma—with pituitary destruction
        c. Adenoma
        d. Histiocytosis X
    3. Syndromes—associated with primary pituitary gonadotropin deficiency (postulated but not proved)
Gonadal Dysfunction
    1. Generalized—gonadal failure as a consequence of systemic condition such as cystic fibrosis, or secondary to autoimmune destructive process
    2. Specific—lesion or process
        a. Congenital
        Ovarian or pure gonadal dysgenesis in the female
        Uterine—congenital absence; appears with primary amenorrhea
        Testicular—anorchia or "vanishing testis"
        b. Chromosomal
        Ovarian—gonadal dysgenesis
        Testicular—Klinefelter's syndrome
        c. Infectious, inflammatory traumatic
        Ovarian—secondary to pelvic inflammatory disease, torsion, or therapeutic radiation
        Uterine—secondary to pelvic inflammatory disease; mimics primary or secondary amenorrhea

Testicular—secondary to orchitis, torsion, or vascular insufficiency (after orchiopexy or herniorrhaphy); following radiation or chemotherapy (especially cyclophosphamide)
d. Enzymatic syndromes—autosomal dominant and recessive forms of male pseudohermaphroditism; degrees of pubertal delay with or without ambiguous genitalia
e. Miscellaneous
Ovarian—insensitivity to gonadotropin syndrome
Testicular—associated with neuromuscular disorders such as myotonic dystrophy; disorders associated with cryptorchidism and pubertal delay (such as Noonan's syndrome)

Systemic disorders causing delay (see preceding list) vary from overt generalized or organ system disease with clinical debilitation (such as cystic fibrosis) to occult conditions in which the growth and pubertal delay may precede all clinical symptoms (such as early inflammatory bowel disease). In most conditions the mechanism appears to be centrally mediated, with diminished gonadotropin release. The condition of anorexia nervosa in females combines elements of a systemic disorder (weight loss) with those of a primary hypothalamic dysfunction (reversion of the pattern of gonadotropin secretion to an early pubertal or prepubertal pattern). The complex relationship between body weight and hypothalamic control of gonadotropins remains unclear.

As one evaluates the other levels at which dysfunction can affect puberty, the concentration and pattern of gonadotropin are key determinants in the differential diagnosis. In most hypothalamic and pituitary disorders, delay is associated with hypogonadotropic hypogonadism, whereas gonadal, chromosomal, and enzymatic disorders usually have associated hypergonadotropism (see preceding list).

CONDITIONS OF PRECOCIOUS SEXUAL DEVELOPMENT

Precocious puberty is defined as the progressive development of secondary sexual characteristics in a female prior to the age of seven years and in a male prior to the age of nine years. Isosexual precocity denotes characteristics appropriate for the gender of the child (feminization of the female and virilization of the male). Heterosexual precocity implies major characteristics at variance with gender (i.e., feminization of the male or virilization of the female). Isosexual precocity can then be subdivided depending on the pathogenesis of the process.

1. True Isosexual Precocity—due to early activation of the hypothalamic-pituitary axis
   a. Idiopathic—80% in females; 50% in males.
   b. Secondary to a CNS lesion or malformation.
   c. Associated with a systemic condition or syndrome, such as McCune-Albright's polyostotic fibrous dysplasia.
   d. Part of the "overlap syndrome" of primary hypothyroidism.
2. Isosexual Precocity—independent of the hypothalamic-pituitary axis
   a. Secondary to ectopic gonadotropin secretion.
   b. Gonadal autonomy—ovarian or testicular tumor.
   c. Extragonadal hormone production—usually adrenal.
   d. Exogenous hormonal exposure.

e. Factitious—local vaginal bleeding that is nonhormonal in origin.
3. Heterosexual Precocity—usually results from the abnormal production or exposure to androgen or estrogen independent of the hypothalamic-pituitary axis, as in 2 a-d.

When precocious secondary sexual characteristics are present but do not progress, the following conditions may be defined:

1. Female with Precocious Thelarche—The cause is unclear, but the natural history is usually of stabilization at Tanner stage II or III. True puberty begins appropriately.
2. Male with Prepubertal Gynecomastia—A search for a feminizing lesion must be made, but in its absence this rare condition is benign and nonprogressive.
3. Precocious Adrenarche—The females have pubic and/or axillary hair prior to age seven, and males have such hair prior to age nine. This condition is more common in females. Recent hormonal studies suggest adrenal overproduction of weak androgens. The condition tends to be nonprogressive and benign.

CLINICAL PROBLEMS

Patient 1. You are called to the delivery room to consult on the gender identification of a 7-pound, 2-ounce baby born with ambiguous genitalia.

PHYSICAL EXAMINATION. The baby is vigorous, and the physical examination apart from the genitalia appears normal. The external genitalia are as diagrammed (Fig. 5–5). A midline organ looks like an enlarged clitoris or a phallus with hypospadias. There is no obvious urethral orifice.

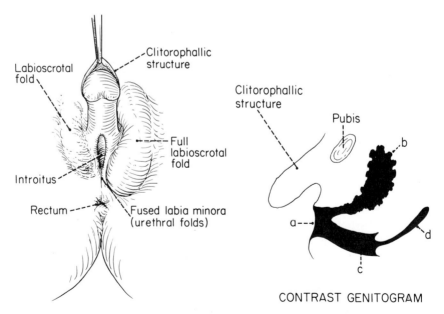

Figure 5–5. Patient 1. *A*, Diagram of external genitalia of this newborn; *B*, Lateral view of her contrast genitogram.

The labial folds are somewhat scrotalized and can be described as a bifid scrotum. The folds are asymmetric with a fullness on one side (the left). Midline fusion from the rectum anteriorly is incomplete. A small vault-like orifice is present, and urine appears to emanate from within it.

Having talked with the parents and the grandparents, you transfer the baby to the nursery.

LABORATORY DATA. The following laboratory studies are ordered:

1. Contrast genitogram.
2. Pelvic ultrasonography.
3. 24-hour urine collections for steroids.
4. Plasma steroid determinations.
5. Blood karyotype.

The first results you get are those from the radiologic studies, followed on day 3 by a preliminary karyotype. Two cell lines, 45 XO and 46 XY, are described. On day 4 the fullness in the left fold increases in size, the baby becomes irritable and seems ill, and surgical intervention appears necessary to correct the "incarcerated" hernia.

QUESTIONS

1. What did you tell the parents initially?
2. Was the baby named?
3. Was a birth certificate filed?

The genitogram contrast study showed the following structure in the lateral film. Label the structures (Fig. 5–5*B*):

4. a.
5. b.
6. c.
7. d.
8. The ultrasound study of the pelvis does not show any gonadal structures, but some structure appears to the right of the midline deep in the pelvis. It is most likely _____
9. Describe the clinical condition that the baby's physical examination, contrast studies, and subsequent karyotype best fit.
10. What was found at operation?
11. What gender assignment was made, and what future surgical procedures could be contemplated?

Patient 2. A 3-year-old girl is referred for evaluation of swelling of the breasts for 4 months. She has otherwise been healthy and had normal motor and intellectual development.

PHYSICAL EXAMINATION. She is 98 cm tall (1 SD above the mean) and weighs 17 kg (1 SD above the mean). Her fundi are benign and her skin is unremarkable. A complete neurologic examination is normal.

She has stage III breast development. Although there is no axillary hair, several long strands of pubic hair are noted. The clitoris is not enlarged, but the labia minora are thickened. On rectal examination there are no adnexal masses.

LABORATORY DATA. The following laboratory data are obtained. Plasma FSH—8 mIU/ml, LH—5 mIU/ml, estradiol—48 pg/ml, bone age— 5 yr, and skull series normal. A pelvic ultrasound study shows enlargement of the uterus with symmetrical enlargement of the ovaries.

QUESTIONS

1. What information from her past history would be helpful in evaluating her height and weight?
2. What dermatologic findings, if present, would have been significant in the evaluation of the breast development?
3. In what way does the neurologic examination influence the further work-up of this patient?
4. What diagnosis do the laboratory studies suggest?

Patient 3. A 13-year-old girl is brought by her adoptive parents for evaluation of short stature and primary amenorrhea. They had been told that her natural mother's pregnancy was "normal," but gestation time was unknown. She was 3.5 kg and 51 cm at birth and spent the first 2½ years at home with her natural mother. At the time of her adoption at 3 years, she was 88 cm tall and weighed 10 kg. The reasons for her adoption are unclear, and the heights of her natural parents are unknown.

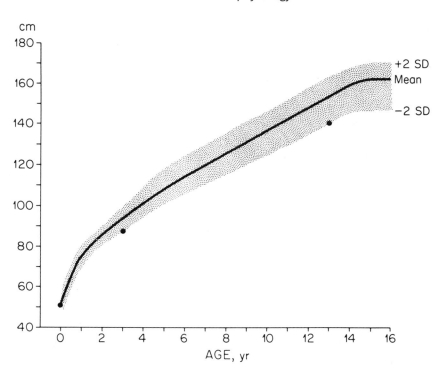

Figure 5–6. Growth chart for patient 3 (see text for details).

PHYSICAL EXAMINATION. She was 140 cm tall and weighed 30 kg (Fig. 5–6). She was shy but of normal intelligence. Her physical examination was positive in that she had a slightly low hairline and one observer felt she had a high-arched palate. She had a prepubertal but otherwise normal physical examination.

LABORATORY DATA. This evaluation revealed a normal blood count and urinalysis and normal serum creatinine. Her T_4 was "lost" by the laboratory. The girl's bone age was reported as 10 years and a skull roentgenogram was normal, although special views of the sella were suggested for better resolution. Her plasma FSH was 3 mIU/ml and LH was 2 mIU/ml.

QUESTIONS

1. Based on the growth data, how likely is it that this girl has hypothyroidism?
2. Based on the growth data and bone age, how likely is it that she is developing a craniopharyngioma; should cone-down sella films and computed tomography be performed?
3. Based on the gonadotropins, how likely is it that she has Turner's syndrome and should chromosome studies be ordered?
4. What is the most likely diagnosis? How do you test this endocrinologic problem?

SUGGESTED READING

Sexual Development and Differentiation of the Fetus
Blanchard, M.G., and Josso, N.: Source of the anti-müllerian hormone synthesized by the fetal testis: müllerian-inhibiting activity of fetal bovine Sertoli cells in tissue culture. Pediatr. Res., *8*:968, 1974.
Donahoe, P.K., et al.: The range of activity of müllerian inhibiting substance. Pediatr. Res., *9*:289, 1975.
Gordon, J.W., and Ruddle, F.H.: Mammalian gonadal determination and gametogenesis. Science, *211*:1265, 1981.

Haseltine, F.P., and Ohno, S.: Mechanisms of gonadal differentiation. Science, *211*:1272, 1981.

Jost, A.: A new look at the mechanisms controlling sex differentiation in mammals. Johns Hopkins Med. J., *130*:38, 1972.

Lippe, B.M.: Ambiguous genitalia and pseudohermaphroditism. Pediatr. Clin. North Am., *26*:91, 1979.

Wachtel, S.S., et al.: Serologic detection of a Y-linked gene in XX males and XX true hermaphrodites. N. Engl. J. Med., *295*:750, 1976.

Walsh, P.C., et al.: Familial incomplete male pseudohermaphroditism, type II. N. Engl. J. Med., *291*:944, 1974.

Wilson, J.D., et al.: Familial incomplete male pseudohermaphroditism, type 1. N. Engl. J. Med., *290*:1097, 1974.

Gonadal Function from Birth to Puberty

Boyar, R.M., et al.: Synchronization of augmented luteinizing hormone secretion with sleep during puberty. N. Engl. J. Med., *287*:582, 1972.

Grumbach, M.M.: The neuroendocrinology of puberty. *In Neuroendocrinology.* Edited by D.T. Krieger and J.C. Hughes. Sunderland, Mass., Sinauer Associates, 1980.

Knobil, E., and Plant, T.M.: Hypothalamic regulation of LH and FSH secretion in the rhesus monkey. *In* The Hypothalamus. Edited by S. Reichlin, R.J. Baldessarini, and J.B. Martin. New York, Raven Press, 1978.

Kulin, H.E., and Reiter, E.O.: Gonadotropin and testosterone measurements after estrogen administration to adult men, prepubertal and pubertal boys, and men with hypogonadotropism: evidence for maturation of positive feedback in the male. Pediatr. Res., *10*:46, 1976.

Parker, D.C., et al.: Pubertal sleep-wake patterns of episodic LH, FSH and testosterone release in twin boys. J. Clin. Endocrinol. Metab., *40*:1099, 1975.

Prader, A.: Testicular size, assessment and clinical importance. Triangle, *7*:240, 1966.

Disorders of Puberty

Boyar, R.M., et al.: Anorexia nervosa: immaturity of the 24-hour luteinizing hormone secretory pattern. N. Engl. J. Med., *291*:861, 1974.

Crawford, J.D., and Osler, D.C.: Body composition at menarche: The Frisch-Revelle hypothesis revisited. Pediatrics, *56*:449, 1975.

CHAPTER **6**

Female Reproductive Disorders

Glenn D. Braunstein

NORMAL MENSTRUAL CYCLE

Between menarche and menopause, the reproductive organs of most women undergo a series of closely coordinated changes at approximately monthly intervals; together these actions comprise the normal menstrual cycle. A menstrual cycle begins with the first day of genital bleeding (day 1) and ends just prior to the next menstrual period. The following discussion describes the individual changes that take place in the hypothalamus, pituitary, ovaries, and sexual accessory organs during the normal cycle. Figures 6–1, 6–2, and 6–3 depict these events; for illustrative purposes, the depicted menstrual cycles are 28 days long, although normal cycle length varies from 25 to 34 days.

Hypothalamus

The area of the central nervous system above the pituitary and surrounding the third ventricle contains numerous nuclei that control a variety of bodily processes. Experimental studies in lower mammals have indicated that three nuclei are especially concerned with reproduction in the female. The preoptic anterior hypothalamic nucleus is sensitive to the feedback effects of gonadal steroids and appears primarily responsible for the cyclic discharge of the decapeptide, gonadotropin-releasing hormone (LRH or GnRH), while the ventromedial and arcuate nuclei in the median eminence control the tonic and presumably the microsecretory bursts of LRH. Discharge of LRH into the hypothalamo-hyophyseal portal system results from stimulation of dopaminergic neurons in the basal hypothalamus and by the norepinephrine released from neurons whose axons terminate in this area, but whose cell bodies are located outside the hypothalamus.

During the first half of the menstrual cycle (follicular or proliferative phase), and during the latter half (luteal or secretory phase), estradiol (E_2) alone or

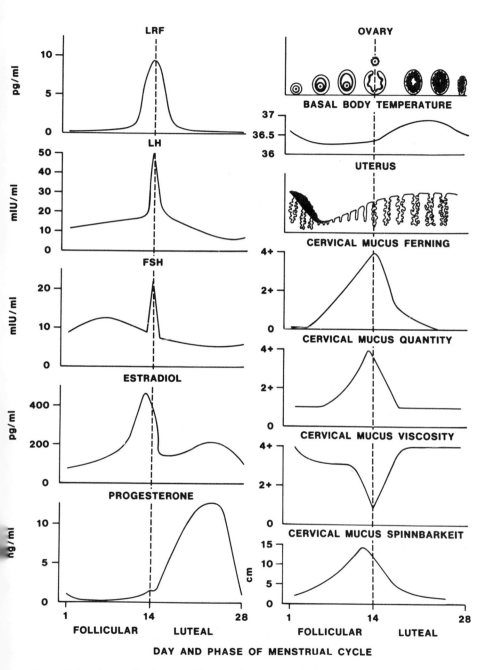

Figure 6–1. Composite diagram of hormonal and morphologic changes during the normal menstrual cycle.

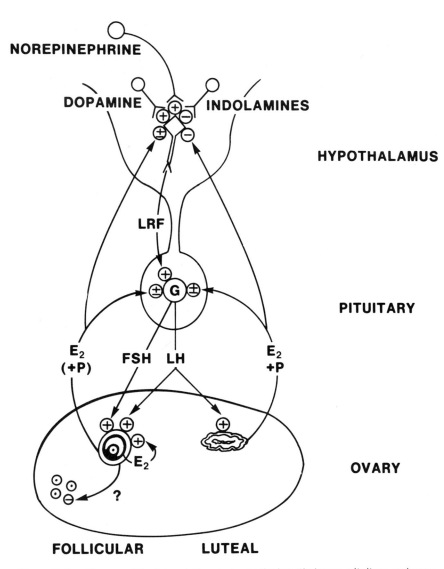

Figure 6–2. Diagram of the interrelations between the hypothalamus, pituitary, and ovary during the normal menstrual cycle. See text for discussion. (G: gonadotrope, LRF: gonadotropin-releasing hormone, E_2: estradiol, P: progesterone, +: positive feedback or stimulation, and −: negative feedback or inhibition.)

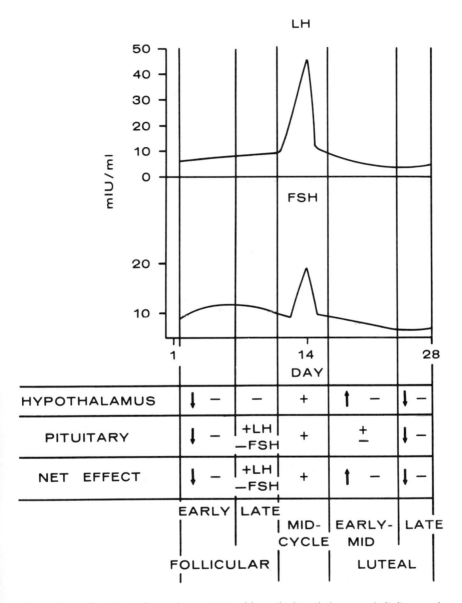

Figure 6–3. Feedback effects of gonadal steroids on the hypothalamus and pituitary, and the net result during the normal menstrual cycle. See text for description. (+: positive feedback or stimulation, −: negative feedback or inhibition, ↑: increasing, and ↓: decreasing.)

in conjunction with progesterone (P) acts in a negative feedback fashion to suppress secretion of LRH. However, at midcycle (approximately day 14), there is a secretory surge of LRH release, which appears to be related to the rapid rise in E_2, or to the peak levels of this steroid achieved just prior to the LRH surge, or to synergism between E_2 and P. Therefore, a positive feedback situation appears to be present at midcycle, with E_2 (and possibly P) stimulating the release of LRH.

Pituitary

The gonadotropic hormones, luteinizing hormone (LH) and follicle-stimulating hormone (FSH), are synthesized in the same basophilic cells, the gonadotropes. Under the influence of LRH, both LH and FSH are synthesized and secreted by these cells in a continuous and episodic pattern with a midcycle surge. The amplitude and frequency of secretion are modulated by the gonadal steroid concentrations.

During the first half of the follicular phase, when the E_2 levels are low, FSH gradually rises owing to decreased negative feedback. The FSH levels decrease during the second half of the follicular phase under the influence of increased negative feedback by E_2. At midcycle, there is a surge of FSH that results both from the midcycle surge of LRH and from enhanced sensitivity of the gonadotropes to the effects of LRH. This enhanced sensitivity is probably due to a positive feedback effect of gonadal steroids. The negative feedback suppression by the high levels of E_2 plus P during the luteal phase results in the suppression of FSH release until a few days before menstruation begins, when the FSH levels begin to rise owing to a fall in the E_2 and P concentrations.

The LH levels during the follicular phase gradually rise, initially through decreased negative feedback by the low E_2 levels and then by apparent positive E_2 feedback. As with FSH, a midcycle surge of LH occurs secondary to LRH stimulation and enhanced sensitivity of the gonadotropes to LRH. A progressive decline of LH during the first two-thirds of the luteal phase is due to the negative feedback effects of the gonadal steroids, primarily on LRH release and to a lesser extent on gonadotrope sensitivity to LRH. Just prior to the beginning of the next menstrual cycle, the LH levels begin to rise, coinciding with the fall in E_2 and P.

Ovaries

The morphologic events that take place in the ovaries are the result of both gonadotropin stimulation and intraovarian "short-loop" feedback control mechanisms. During the late luteal phase of the preceding cycle and during the early part of the follicular phase, FSH stimulates 10 to 15 primary follicles, composed of oogonia surrounded by a single layer of granulosa cells, to develop into secondary follicles with several layers of granulosa cells. By an unknown intraovarian mechanism (possibly due to ovarian androgen secretion by the largest follicle), all but one of the follicles become atretic. Proliferation of the granulosa cells of the remaining follicle under the influence of FSH and the formation of E_2 and antral fluid, stimulated by both FSH and LH, take place during the remainder of the follicular phase. Between 12 and 30 hours following the midcycle LH peak, follicular rupture takes place with the extrusion of the egg. The mechanism responsible for ovulation is unknown, but may be related to the rapid increase in intrafollicular fluid accumulation and progesterone-induced synthesis of enzymes, which weaken the follicular wall. After ovulation, LH induces the transformation of the follicle into a corpus luteum.

During the last few days of the luteal phase of the preceding menstrual cycle, the levels of E_2 rapidly decrease and remain low during the early part of the follicular phase. Under the influence of FSH and LH, the levels of E_2 rise slowly during the first half of the follicular phase and more rapidly during the second half, peaking approximately 24 hours before the LH peak. Just before ovulation, the E_2 levels decrease, only to rise again when corpus luteum steroidogenesis begins. Progesterone levels continue to decline during the first half of the follicular phase and then rise gradually, reaching a peak during the middle of the luteal phase. The thermogenic effect of P leads to a parallel rise in the basal body temperature. Luteal phase E_2 and P secretion are primarily controlled by LH, modulated by intrinsic changes in the sensitivity of the corpus luteum to LH stimulation.

Uterus

The uterine endometrium is composed of three layers. The basal layer is not lost during menses and serves to regenerate the other two layers during the cycle. A superficial layer of compact columnar epithelial cells lines the endometrial cavity, with an intermediate layer of spongiosum. These two layers show the principal endometrial changes during the menstrual cycle. Approximately five days after the start of the menses under the influence of rising levels of E_2, the denuded endometrium begins to be regenerated from the basal layer. At that time, the surface epithelium is cuboidal with a compact stroma and straight glands. During the proliferative phase the endometrial lining increases in width, the epithelium becomes more columnar and the glands elongated. After ovulation, the E_2 secreted by the corpus luteum maintains the growth of the endometrium, while P induces the glands to become coiled, sawtoothed, and secretory. As the levels of E_2 and P decline during the late luteal phase, the stroma becomes edematous, endometrial and blood vessel necrosis occurs, and menstrual bleeding ensues. Because the histologic changes during the menstrual cycle are so characteristic, endometrial biopsies may be used to accurately date the stage of the cycle and assess the tissue response to gonadal steroids.

Endocervix

The endocervical glands also undergo cyclic changes in morphology and function. The product of these glands—the cervical mucus— demonstrates a series of characteristic changes. Under the influence of E_2, the quantity, elasticity, water content, and sperm penetrability of the mucus increases, peaking at midcycle, while the viscosity and cell count decrease. The changes in viscosity and elasticity, spinnbarkeit, are easily quantitated by measurement of the length that the cervical mucus can be stretched. Ferning, the ability of the sodium chloride present in the cervical mucus to crystallize in an arborized pattern as the mucus dries, is also a manifestation of the estrogen effect and reaches a peak at midcycle. During the luteal phase, P induces a decrease in the quantity, pH, spinnbarkeit, sperm penetrability, and ferning ability of the mucus, with a concomitant increase in the viscosity and cellular content.

Vagina

Four well-defined layers of cells make up the stratified squamous epithelium of the vagina. The basal germinal layer is not desquamated and is responsible for regeneration of the epithelium. The other three layers—the parabasal, the intermediate or precornified squamous, and the cornified squamous epithelium—change during the cycle. In the proliferative phase, the estrogens induce thickening of the vaginal epithelial cell layers and increase the number of cornified cells. After ovulation, stimulation by P results in more precornified cells, an increased number of polymorphonuclear leucocytes, cellular debris, and clumping of the desquamated cells. These changes may be quantitated by a variety of histologic methods and are useful qualitative indices of estrogen stimulation.

Summary of Hormonal Events During the Menstrual Cycle

The low levels of E_2 and P at the end of the preceding cycle induce a rise in the FSH and LH concentrations, which in turn stimulate follicular growth and E_2 production during the early follicular phase. The rise in E_2 suppresses FSH, but not LH, during the last half of the follicular phase. Because of the rapid rate of rise of E_2, the absolute amount of E_2, or synergism of P and E_2, LRH secretion increases and the sensitivity of the gonadotrope to LRH increases, resulting in a midcycle LH and FSH secretory discharge. The rapid elevation of gonadotropin concentrations results in further growth of the follicle and secretion of antral fluid, which together with possible weakening of the follicular wall due to enzymes brings about ovulation. The LH-stimulated secretion of E_2 and P by the corpus luteum results in LRH suppression and, therefore, LH and FSH suppression. The decreased LH levels, together with the inherent decreasing sensitivity of the corpus luteum to LH, leads to a decrement in E_2 and P secretion, which through decreased negative feedback inhibition results in rising levels of FSH and LH and a new cycle.

VARIATIONS OF THE MENSTRUAL CYCLE

The preceding discussion describes the typical, normal, ovulatory menstrual cycle observed in the majority of women between the ages of 25 and 40 years. However, approximately 20% of the cycles in apparently normal women may be abnormal. This percentage of abnormal cycles increases at both ends of the reproductive years. A brief discussion of the hormonal and clinical findings in several varieties of such cycles follows.

Short Luteal Phase

This abnormality is characterized by cycle lengths that are usually short because of a decreased duration of the luteal phase (10 days or less), with an inadequate rise and duration of rise of the basal body temperature, lower-than-normal serum progesterone levels, and endometrial development that does not correspond with the cycle date. This defect appears to be the result of an inadequate early follicular FSH rise and subsequent incomplete maturation of the follicular steroid-producing cells that become luteinized. If this defect persists, it may lead to infertility.

Inadequate Luteal Phase

These cycles are often found in obese, oligomenorrheic women and during the menopausal transition. The amount of P secreted by the corpus luteum is not great enough to mature the endometrium fully. Hence, the cycle lengths may be short or long, and the endometrial development is always out of phase with the cycle date. The pathogenesis of this defect is similar to that of the short luteal phase.

Long Follicular Phase

Prolonged cycles with delayed, but ultimately normal, follicular maturation and ovulation are commonly found shortly after menarche. The duration of the luteal phase and the hormonal patterns during this phase are completely normal.

Short Follicular Phase

Regularly menstruating, premenopausal women may demonstrate short ovulatory cycles, which are characterized by a short follicular phase, with lower than normal midcycle and luteal E_2 levels. This condition appears to be an age-related decrease in E_2 secretory ability of the follicles and corpus luteum. The endometrial lining and cervical mucus usually do not develop properly during this type of cycle.

Anovulatory Cycle

Although a variety of pathologic processes may lead to anovulatory cycles, the menopausal transition is often characterized by long cycles with irregular bleeding. During the menopause, which usually takes places between 45 and 55 years, the ovaries undergo an obliterative endarteritis that ultimately leads to a reduction in ovarian size and replacement of the parenchyma with connective tissue. As the E_2 production decreases, the gonadotropins rise and the woman may experience a variety of signs and symptoms of the menopause, including hot flushes, sweating, and atrophy of the breasts, vagina, and vulva.

Early during the menopausal transition, the rising gonadotropin levels may be sufficient to stimulate some follicular estrogen synthesis. If ovulation does not occur and P is not secreted, the endometrium continues to proliferate, eventually resulting in irregular, prolonged shedding. These irregular cycles may persist from months to years before the woman becomes amenorrheic.

FEMALE REPRODUCTIVE DISORDERS

Disorders that affect the glands and organs involved in female reproduction are common. Although such topics as the endocrinology of pregnancy, contraception, and infertility fall into this category of gynecologic endocrinology, they are not discussed here. Rather, this section concentrates on two problems, amenorrhea and hirsutism. These topics were chosen because disorders of virtually all the endocrine glands may result in either one or both of these problems. Therefore, they illustrate the close interaction of the endocrine glands in maintaining normal female reproductive homeostasis.

Amenorrhea

Amenorrhea, or the absence of menses, occurs in every woman surviving to the age of 60. Many women have long lapses between menses during the first 1 or 2 years after menarche, with between 40 and 55% of the cycles being anovulatory. During the active reproductive years, pregnancy is the most common physiologic cause of amenorrhea. Between the extremes of menarche and the menopause, a variety of pathologic processes may produce the symptoms of amenorrhea or oligomenorrhea.

Definitions

Primary amenorrhea is the absence of a menses in a phenotypic female by age 17. Older publications often set the age limit between 18 and 20 years. However, the age of menarche has been decreasing at a rate of 4 months per decade from 1830 until 1968 (secular trend). In the United States, the age of menarche at present is approximately 12.8 ± 1.2 (SD) years. Therefore, the age of 17 is $3\frac{1}{2}$ SD from the mean, justifying the previously cited age limit for defining primary amenorrhea. *Secondary amenorrhea* is the absence of a menses for a period equal to or greater than 3 times the length of the usual menstrual cycle in a previously menstruating female. *Oligomenorrhea* refers to infrequent, irregular bleeding episodes, at intervals of more than 45 days.

Causes of Primary Amenorrhea

Primary amenorrhea is a symptom of an underlying disorder that may involve the genital tract, ovaries, adrenal, thyroid, pituitary, or hypothalamus. This section lists the causes of primary amenorrhea and then describes some of the clinical and laboratory features associated with these disorders.

Vaginal Disorders
  Vaginal aplasia
  Imperforate hymen
  Congenital vaginal atresia

Uterine Disorders
  Congenital absence of the uterus
  Endometritis
Ovarian Disorders
  XO gonadal dysgenesis and variants
  XX gonadal dysgenesis
  XY gonadal dysgenesis
  Congenital absence of the gonad
  Testicular feminization syndrome
  17-hydroxylase deficiency of the ovaries and adrenals
  Autoimmune oophoritis
  Resistant ovary syndrome
  Polycystic ovary syndrome
Adrenal Disorders
  Congenital adrenal hyperplasia
Thyroid Disorders
  Hypothyroidism
Pituitary-Hypothalamic Disorders
  Hypopituitarism
  Constitutional delay in the onset of menses
  Nutritional disorders

Vaginal Aplasia. This condition most frequently involves the upper third of the vagina and is often associated with absence of the uterus and fallopian tubes due to defective müllerian duct development. Anomalies of the urinary tract may also be present.

Imperforate Hymen. At menarche, cyclic monthly lower abdominal pain, often with a palpable lower abdominal mass, occurs without visible menstruation. Pelvic examination usually reveals a bluish hymeneal membrane at the lower part of the vagina, which is distended with menstrual secretions (hematocolpos). This condition is a form of cryptomenorrhea in which menstruation occurs but does not appear externally owing to the obstruction. In some individuals distention of uterus (hematometria) and fallopian tubes (hematosalpinx) also occurs. This distention may lead to retrograde menstruation with hemoperitoneum, resulting in endometriosis. Surgical excision of the hymeneal membrane is curative.

Congenital Vaginal Atresia. Membranous or fibrinous obliteration may occur at any level of the vaginal canal, owing to incomplete fusion of the müllerian duct structures with the vaginal plate originating from the urogenital sinus. Symptoms are similar to those occurring with an imperforate hymen.

Congenital Absence of the Uterus. This disorder is usually associated with absent or rudimentary fallopian tubes and absence of the upper third of the vagina due to defective development of the müllerian duct. Congenital anomalies of the urinary tract, vertebral column, and heart may also occur in such patients.

Endometritis. Chronic and acute inflammation and destruction of the endometrium by diseases such as tuberculosis or schistosomiasis may prevent the normal endometrial ripening and shedding during the menstrual cycle.

XO Gonadal Dysgenesis (Turner's Syndrome). This syndrome is thought to result either from the fertilization of a hypoploid (lacking a chromosome) gamete, egg or sperm, by a normal gamete or from the loss of the second sex chromosome when fertilization has established an XX or XY zygote. These patients are characterized by short stature, streaked gonads, and a variety of somatic abnormalities. The prevalence of this syndrome is one in 2000 to 3000 female newborns and accounts for approximately 25 to 40% of patients with primary amenorrhea. The short stature is present at birth, with height and weight below the third percentile. The final adult height is almost uniformly below 5 feet and is related in part to the parental height. Growth hormone (GH) secretion is normal, and the response to exogenous GH is poor. Somatomedin levels have been reported to be elevated, implying an end-organ resistance to its effect. The gonads are replaced with bilateral fibrous streaks, which are characterized by sheets and whorls of fibrous tissue with absence of germinal tissue. The uterus, fallopian tubes, and external genitalia are structurally normal, although often hypoplastic. Multiple somatic anomalies have been noted, including triangularly shaped facies, hypoplastic chin, epicanthal folds, abnormally shaped and low-set ears, high-arched palate, strabismus, short and broad neck (often with webbing), low posterior hairline, multiple pigmented nevi, broad shield-like chest with widely spaced nipples, congenital lymphedema of the hands and feet, clinodactyly, short fourth and fifth metacarpals, cubitus valgus, multiple renal malformations, coarctation of the aorta (25 to 30%), and osteopenia. The frequency of diabetes mellitus, red-green color blindness, hypertension, and chronic lymphocytic thyroiditis is increased in these patients. Ovarian estrogen secretion is decreased, and FSH and LH levels are increased. A buccal smear reveals the absence of the Barr body (inactivated X chromosome), and a karyotype establishes the diagnosis. Postzygotic loss of an X chromosome may result in mosaicism. These patients may present with a few or many of the physical stigmata of Turner's syndrome, depending upon what tissues have the deleted X chromosome.

XX Gonadal Dysgenesis. These patients are phenotypic females with streaked gonads, eunuchoid habitus, decreased secondary sexual characteristics, primary amenorrhea, and normal female karyotype. Their pituitary gonadotropins are high and ovarian estrogen secretion is low. In essence, they have gonads that are identical to those found in Turner's syndrome, but do not have the somatic features of Turner's syndrome. Since the E_2 levels are not sufficient to close the epiphyses of the long bones, these patients continue to grow, under the influence of GH, and they develop eunuchoid proportions.

XY Gonadal Dysgenesis. These phenotypic females are similar to the patients with XX gonadal dysgenesis, except that they have a 46 XY karyotype and often develop postpubertal virilization due to androgen secretion from the dysgenetic gonad. Many of these gonads undergo neoplastic transformation to dysgerminomas or gonadoblastomas and, therefore, should be removed.

Congenital Absence of the Gonad. If a gonad is absent after the fifth week of fetal life, both the internal and external genitalia differentiate in a female fashion owing to the lack of testosterone and müllerian duct inhibitory factor. Many of these patients have an XY karyotype. A few patients have had external female genitalia and absence of the internal genitalia, implying a maldevelopment of the müllerian duct primordia.

Testicular Feminization Syndrome. These phenotypic females appear normal at birth, although occasionally an inguinal hernia is present. The growth and development of the patient are usually normal, and breast development occurs at the expected time. However, both axillary and pubic hair are deficient, and no menses occur. Pelvic examination reveals a blind vaginal pouch and no cervix or uterus. The gonads are often located in the inguinal hernia and resemble cryptorchid testes. They may undergo malignant transformation (10 to 20%). The karyotype is 46 XY, and the disorder is transmitted as either a sex-linked recessive trait or a sex-limited autosomal dominant disorder. Testosterone secretion from the testes is normal, and testicular estrogen production is often increased. The defect appears to result from end-organ insensitivity to testosterone and its active metabolite, dihydrotestosterone, with a normal responsiveness to the estrogen secreted from the testes. Because the fetal testes secrete müllerian duct inhibitory factor, the müllerian ducts regress. The resistance to the biologic effects of testosterone leads to regression of the wolffian duct structures, and formation of external genitalia along female lines.

17-Hydroxylase Deficiency of the Ovaries and Adrenals. These women have primary amenorrhea, hypertension, and hypokalemia; they lack secondary sexual characteristics. Plasma cortisol levels are decreased, as are the urinary 17-ketosteroids and estrogen levels. ACTH and gonadotropins are elevated, and the mineralocorticoid, corticosterone, is overproduced. Plasma renin levels are depressed. Replacement of the glucocorticoids does not correct the amenorrhea.

Autoimmune Oophoritis. This rare disorder may cause primary or secondary amenorrhea and is often associated with autoimmune thyroiditis and adrenalitis. Idiopathic hypoparathyroidism, pernicious anemia, diabetes mellitus, myasthenia gravis, Graves' disease, and vitiligo are also seen in this form of polyhormonal disorder. The ovarian steroid production is low, and gonadotropin levels are elevated. This disorder appears to involve cellular immunity, with round cell infiltration of the affected organs and secondary production of autoantibodies directed toward the involved glands. This syndrome may be familial and has been associated with the HLA-B8 histocompatibility antigen.

Resistant Ovary Syndrome. When first seen, patients with this unusual syndrome may have primary or secondary amenorrhea. The ovaries contain normal-appearing, but unstimulated, primordial follicles. Low or low-normal estrogen and elevated levels of gonadotropins are present in the blood. The ovaries are hyporeactive to exogenous stimulation with human menopausal or pituitary gonadotropins. This syndrome is another example of end-organ refractoriness to a hormone, in this instance both LH and FSH.

Polycystic Ovary Syndrome. This condition is most commonly associated with secondary amenorrhea. However, it may occasionally cause primary amenorrhea. It is more fully discussed later in this chapter.

Congenital Adrenal Hyperplasia. Deficiencies of the 21-hydroxylase or 11-hydroxylase enzymes of the adrenal glands, with resultant overproduction of the adrenal androgens, are manifested clinically by primary amenorrhea, virilization, short stature, and hyperpigmentation in the affected females (see Chap. 4). When adequate glucocorticoid replacement therapy is instituted, adrenal androgen levels fall, and ovulatory menstrual cycles may ensue.

Hypothyroidism. Although hypothyroidism in childhood may be associated with isosexual precocious puberty, its occurrence during early adolescence is often accompanied by delayed sexual maturation with low gonadotropin secretion. Growth retardation and other findings of hypothyroidism are usually present.

Hypopituitarism. Partial or panhypopituitarism because of genetic or congenital defects or acquired disorders such as tumors, infiltrative diseases, and infection often results in primary amenorrhea due to deficiency of gonadotropins. Some of the inherited and sporadic forms of hypogonadotropic hypogonadism are caused by a hypothalamic disorder with inadequate stimulation of the pituitary by LRH. When hypopituitarism occurs prepubertally, it results in primary amenorrhea, infertility, lack of secondary sexual development, and a eunuchoid habitus if growth hormone secretion is intact. Agenesis of the olfactory nerves with anosmia or hyposmia may be associated with isolated deficiency of the gonadotropins (Kallmann's syndrome).

Constitutional Delay in the Onset of Menses. Approximately 2% of the women begin menstruating after the age of 17 years. These patients often give a history of late onset of menses in their mothers and other female relatives. They can be distinguished from most women with other causes of hypogonadism by the presence of pubertal changes, such as breast buds, pubic hair, and peak height velocity. This condition is considered to be a delay in the normal maturation of the pituitary-hypothalamic feedback responsiveness to levels of circulating gonadal steroid hormone.

Nutritional Disorders. See discussion later in this chapter.

Diagnostic Evaluation of Primary Amenorrhea

The most important aspects of the evaluation are the history and physical examination. Important background information includes the age of onset of menarche in the patient's mother, grandmothers, and siblings, family history concerning congenital adrenal hyperplasia or congenital hypopituitarism in siblings, symptoms of organic hypothalamic-pituitary disorders, hypothyroidism, and cyclic lower abdominal pain. On physical examination, special attention should be directed toward determining whether the primary amenorrhea is associated with a general lack of secondary sexual maturation or with normal secondary sexual maturation. The former is found with hypothyroidism, organic pituitary-hypothalamic disorders, and all the gonadal disorders except testicular feminization, whereas the latter is characteristic of constitutional delay in the onset of menses and local vaginal or endometrial disorders. Pelvic examination is usually sufficient to diagnose the vaginal causes of primary amenorrhea. The presence of a uterus eliminates testicular feminization and congenital absence of the uterus from consideration. The patient's ability to smell should be formally tested in order to determine whether she has Kallmann's syndrome. Both congenital adrenal hyperplasia and Turner's syndrome have sufficiently distinctive clinical features to allow an accurate preliminary diagnosis.

Laboratory tests should include serum FSH, LH, and E_2 levels, thyroid function tests, and a buccal smear with staining for the inactivated X chromosome (Barr body) and Y chromosome. Elevated gonadotropins with low E_2 levels (hypergonadotropic hypogonadism) point to a primary ovarian cause of the primary amenorrhea, and further evaluation should include chromosome analysis with banding and, if necessary, laparoscopy with gonadal biopsy. Persistently low gonadotropins and E_2 levels (hypogonadotropic hypogonadism) in a patient with primary amenorrhea and lack of secondary sexual maturation require a full hypothalamic-pituitary evaluation in order to eliminate serious organic problems in this area. Endometrial biopsy, hystosalpingography, and laparoscopy may be needed to diagnose primary endometrial problems accurately.

Causes of Secondary Amenorrhea

Of the disorders causing secondary amenorrhea (see list), many may also result in oligomenorrhea. Following the list of causes, the prominent clinical pathologic and endocrinologic features of these disorders are discussed. A few have been discussed in the section dealing with primary amenorrhea and are not described further.

Uterine Disorders
  Pregnancy
  Post-traumatic uterine synechia
  Progestational agents
Ovarian Disorders
  Polycystic ovary syndrome
  Ovarian tumors
  Precocious menopause
  Antimetabolite therapy
Adrenal Disorders
  Cushing's syndrome
  Virilizing adrenal tumors
  Adrenocorticoid insufficiency
Thyroid Disorders
  Hypothyroidism
  Hyperthyroidism
Pituitary Disorders
  Acquired hypopituitarism
  Physiologic or pathologic prolactin secretion

Hypothalamic Disorders
  Tumor and infiltrative diseases
  Drug suppression
  Nutritional disorders
Extrahypothalamic Nervous System Disorders

Pregnancy. The most frequent cause of secondary amenorrhea is pregnancy, which should be considered despite the most vehement protestations of virginity.

Post-traumatic Uterine Synechia (Asherman's Syndrome). Secondary amenorrhea may occur after a uterine curettage, especially in the postpartum or postabortive state, because of formation of adhesions and damage to the basal layer of the endometrium.

Progestational Agents. Prolonged use of progestational agents for contraceptive purposes or for the treatment of endometriosis may induce an irreversible endometrial atrophy.

Polycystic Ovary (Stein-Leventhal) Syndrome. As originally described in 1935, this syndrome is composed of secondary amenorrhea or oligomenorrhea, involuntary infertility, obesity, hirsutism, and enlarged, polycystic ovaries. Since the initial description, the criteria for this entity have been reduced. It now includes any clinical picture associated with enlarged ovaries that have a thickened tunica albuginea and numerous cystic and atretic follicles in the cortex. These patients tend to have high-normal or mildly elevated urinary 17-ketosteroid and serum dehydroepiandrosterone sulfate (DHEA-S) levels, mildly elevated plasma testosterone levels, low or normal FSH levels, and elevated LH levels. Catheterization of the adrenal and ovarian veins has demonstrated that the elevated androgen levels may arise from either or both of these organs. Ovulation and subsequent pregnancies have been achieved by a variety of techniques including unilateral or bilateral ovarian wedge resection, adrenocortical steroid therapy, clomiphene therapy, or human menopausal gonadotropin therapy. The origin of this syndrome has not been established, and some authorities consider it to be a primary hypothalamic disease. This syndrome can occur sporadically or in a familial setting.

Ovarian Tumors. Ovarian tumors that produce excessive androgens or estrogens cause amenorrhea by suppression of the pituitary-hypothalamic axis. The various types include hilus cell tumors, lipoid cell tumors, arrhenoblastomas, dysgerminomas, gonadoblastomas, and granulosa cell tumors.

Precocious Menopause. These patients develop secondary amenorrhea under the age of 40, often preceded by an interval of gradually increasing menstrual irregularities accompanied by menopausal symptoms. The ovaries appear atrophic, with a thickened cortex, interstitial fibrosis, and absent primordial follicles. The E_2 levels are low, and the serum LH and FSH levels elevated. It is presumed that the original primordial ovarian follicles were deficient in quantity.

Antimetabolite Therapy. Antimetabolite drugs, such as cyclophosphamide, and irradiation may result in destruction of the primordial follicles and secondary amenorrhea.

Cushing's Syndrome. Cushing's syndrome due to bilateral adrenocortical hyperplasia from excessive pituitary secretion of ACTH or ectopic ACTH production, or due to adrenocortical carcinoma, may be associated with amenorrhea when adrenal androgen secretion is sufficiently elevated to suppress the pituitary-hypothalamic axis. The excessive steroids may also directly interfere with ovarian steroidogenesis.

Virilizing Adrenal Tumors. These uncommon tumors may produce large amounts of adrenal androgens, resulting in rapid virilization with acne, hirsutism, clitoral enlargement, deepening of the voice, and amenorrhea due to androgen suppression of the pituitary and hypothalamus, and possibly ovarian steroidogenesis.

Adrenocortical Insufficiency. Amenorrhea occurs with chronic adrenal insufficiency at a time when weight loss is a prominent feature. The amenorrhea may be due to hypothalamic abnormalities induced by the malnutrition.

Hypothyroidism and Hyperthyroidism. Oligomenorrhea, amenorrhea, and polymenorrhea (frequent menses) may occur with either of these disorders, irrespective of the underlying thyroid pathologic process. Menstrual irregularities may result from changes in the metabolic clearance rate of the gonadal steroids, as well as pituitary-hypothalamic dysfunction.

Acquired Hypopituitarism. Secondary amenorrhea occurs frequently with partial or complete hypopituitarism, whether due to tumors, vascular problems (aneurysms, postpartum necrosis), trauma (stalk section), infection, or infiltrative disorders. Evidence of other trophic hormone deficiency or prolactin hypersecretion may also be present.

Physiologic Prolactin Secretion. Postpartum amenorrhea in lactating mothers may extend to 10 or more months compared to a mean duration of 2 to 3 months for non-nursing postpartum women. Pregnancy rate in the nursing group is approximately 10%, whereas in the non-nursing group the rate is approximately 75%. Recent studies have suggested that the elevated concentrations of prolactin may inhibit the normal secretion of LRH from the hypothalamus. In addition, hyperprolactinemia inhibits the ovarian response to gonadotropins. Patients with elevated prolactin levels from pathologic processes may also have amenorrhea.

Tumors and Infiltrative Diseases of the Hypothalamus. Craniopharyngiomas, third ventricular ependymomas, optic gliomas, and metastatic tumors to the hypothalamus may lead to deficient LRH production or release. Through similar mechanisms, infiltrative disorders of the hypothalamus, such as sarcoidosis or histiocytosis X, may lead to secondary amenorrhea.

Drug Suppression of the Hypothalamus. Both combination and sequential types of oral contraceptive agents may induce prolonged suppression of the hypothalamus. This condition occurs primarily in women whose menstrual cycles were irregular prior to administration of the pills. Although the majority of patients spontaneously regain their menses, a few may remain amenorrheic for several years. An occult pituitary neoplasm must be ruled out in these

patients. Psychotropic drugs such as phenothiazines may also suppress gonadotropin secretion, while concurrently promoting prolactin release.

Nutritional Disorders. Rapid weight loss, through voluntary dieting or
profound psychologic disturbances (anorexia nervosa), may lead to hypothalamic dysfunction. Patients with anorexia nervosa demonstrate low basal LH
and FSH levels, elevated GH levels, partial diabetes insipidus, and thermo-
regulatory deficiencies. Upon refeeding, the patients develop nocturnal LH
spikes similar to those found during puberty. The mechanism for the hypothalamic suppression is unknown. Hypothalamic amenorrhea occurs in ballet
dancers and long-distance runners; changes in weight and alterations in lean
body mass may be responsible. Secondary amenorrhea has also been observed
with rapid weight gain, although the pathophysiology of this problem has not
been elucidated.

Extrahypothalamic Central Nervous System Disorders. The extrahypothalamic central nervous system may profoundly influence the menstrual cycle.
Both emotional and physical stress may suppress gonadotropin release, with
resulting amenorrhea. This disorder is perhaps best exemplified by the "board-
ing house amenorrhea" of college girls, who are away from home and who
develop amenorrhea of varying lengths while under stress. The phenomenon
of pseudocyesis with the symptoms of pregnancy and weight gain associated
with amenorrhea illustrates that higher cortical areas influence the hypothalamic control of ovulation.

Diagnostic Evaluation of Secondary Amenorrhea

As in the case of primary amenorrhea, the history and physical examination
are extremely important in evaluation of patients with secondary amenorrhea.
A history should include inquiries about unprotected sexual intercourse, recent
curettage or therapeutic abortion, use of progestational agents or oral contraceptives, and recent weight loss or weight gain. These topics help in determining whether the patient's condition is related to pregnancy, post-traumatic
uterine synechia, endometrial atrophy, hypothalamic suppression by birth
control pills, or hypothalamic dysfunction due to rapid weight changes. Similarly, a history of a traumatic childbirth raises the possibility of postpartum
necrosis, and a history of galactorrhea suggests ingestion of drugs such as
phenothiazines or the presence of a chromophobe adenoma. A history of rapid
virilization or symptoms of excessive glucocorticoid production should be
sought in order to eliminate the possibility of ovarian tumors, virilizing adrenal
tumors, and Cushing's syndrome. Physical examination is often sufficient to
diagnose pregnancy, polycystic ovary syndrome, ovarian tumors, Cushing's
syndrome, virilizing adrenal tumors, adrenocortical insufficiency, thyroid disorders, and nutritional disorders.

Laboratory studies, which are outlined in Figure 6–4, include an initial
pregnancy test. If the test is negative, a progesterone challenge should be
performed. If the uterine endometrium is intact and has been exposed to a
sufficient amount of estrogen, the administration of progesterone causes

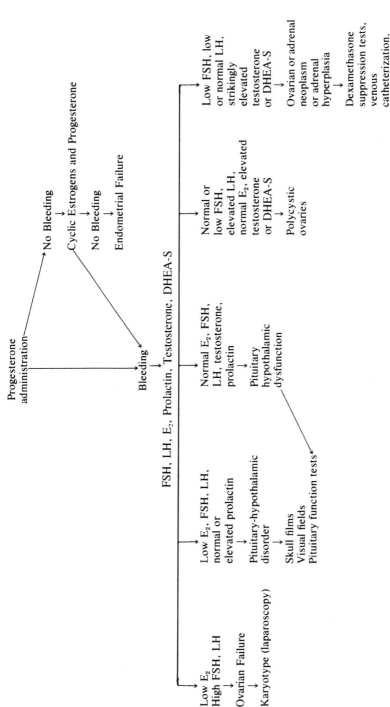

Figure 6–4. Flow sheet for evaluation of secondary amenorrhea.

sloughing of the endometrium. If no sloughing occurs, either the endometrium is atrophic or the estrogen level is not sufficient to have stimulated the endometrium. If the patient fails to menstruate after withdrawal of progesterone, cyclic estrogen and progesterone may be administered for one or two months. If no withdrawal bleeding occurs, endometrial failure is the most likely diagnosis. If withdrawal bleeding occurs, serum FSH, LH, estradiol, testosterone, and serum DHEA-S should be measured. Hypergonadotropic hypogonadism with high FSH, LH, and low E_2 indicates primary ovarian failure and the need for replacement therapy. Hypogonadotropic hypogonadism with low FSH, LH, and E_2 points to a pituitary-hypothalamic dysfunction that needs to be evaluated with skull roentgenograms, visual fields, and pituitary function tests. Low or normal levels of FSH with elevated LH, testosterone, or DHEA-S are most compatible with the polycystic ovary syndrome. Severely elevated serum testosterone levels with normal or slightly elevated DHEA-S levels suggest an ovarian neoplasm, whereas severely elevated DHEA-S levels with mildly or moderately elevated testosterone concentrations suggest an adrenal neoplasm or acquired adrenal hyperplasia. Normal levels of gonadotropins and E_2 are indicative of a mild pituitary-hypothalamic dysfunction, with absence of the LH and FSH midcycle surges required for ovulation.

HIRSUTISM

Hirsutism may be defined as inappropriately heavy hair growth in the androgen-sensitive areas (such as the beard or mustache region) in a woman. Simple hirsutism must be differentiated from virilization, which includes hirsutism and more pronounced evidence of androgen stimulation, with clitoral hypertrophy, deepening of the voice, temporal hair recession, and male-pattern muscular development. Hirsutism is divided into two categories: hirsutism without virilization and hirsutism with virilization.

WITHOUT VIRILIZATION
  Normal Individuals
    Intrinsic Factors
      Familial hirsutism
      Pregnancy
      Menopause
      Idiopathic hirsutism
    Extrinsic Factors
      Trauma
      Drugs
  Pathologic Conditions
    Ovarian Disorders
      Polycystic ovary disease
      Hyperthecosis
    Adrenal Disorders
      Bilateral adrenocortical hyperplasia
    Thyroid Disorders
      Hypothyroidism
    Pituitary Disorders
      Acromegaly
    Congenital Malformation Syndromes
    Porphyria Cutanea Tarda

Without Virilization

Normal women may develop hirsutism due to both intrinsic and extrinsic factors. The amount of hair that grows is related to the potency and concentration of the circulating free androgens, the sensitivity of the hair follicle to these androgens, and the duration of exposure to the androgens. The racial background and familial inheritance of an individual account for the wide range of normalcy in hair growth experienced by females. Women from the Mediterranean area tend to have more hair than those from the northern European countries. When an Italian woman who has a normal amount of hair growth compared to her Italian peers moves to a Scandinavian country, she may be considered to be hirsute by Scandinavian standards. Similarly, Caucasian Americans tend to be more hirsute than American Blacks or Spanish-Americans. Many women who have hirsutism on a familial basis will give a history of mothers and female siblings also having excessive hair when compared to the rest of the population. Of importance with this variety of hirsutism is that the patient's menstrual cycle is usually normal. Physiologic hirsutism may also occur during pregnancy, probably because of androgens secreted by the placenta. During the menopause, preexisting villus hairs may become darkly pigmented, possibly owing to an increase in ovarian androgen secretion under the influence of rising gonadotropin levels. When none of these factors appear to be present in an apparently normal individual, that patient is considered to have idiopathic hirsutism. The pilosebaceous unit (composed of the hair, its follicle, and the sebaceous gland) in these women may have increased sensitivity to normal circulating levels of androgens.

Hirsutism may also occur due to extrinsic factors such as local trauma. Repeated scratching of an area of the skin may increase the blood supply to that area, resulting in increased stimulation to the pilosebaceous unit. Certain drugs such as phenytoin (diphenylhydantoin), diazoxide, glucocorticoids, ACTH, and minoxidil may also cause local stimulation of the pilosebaceous unit and increased hair growth. Pigmented nevi often have hair growing from them.

Multiple pathologic conditions may also give rise to simple hirsutism. The endocrinologic disorders include those of ovarian origin, such as polycystic ovary disease, and hyperthecosis, which is clinically similar to the polycystic ovary syndrome with slightly different ovarian pathologic features. Bilateral adrenocortical hyperplasia from pituitary oversecretion of ACTH (Cushing's disease) may lead to hirsutism due to a mild increase of adrenal androgen production. Acromegaly results in coarsening of preexisting hairs, as does hypothyroidism. Some congenital anomalies are associated with hirsutism. Hirsutism also accompanies porphyria cutanea tarda, in which repeated irritation of the skin leads to increased blood flow, and thereby stimulation of the hair follicles.

With Virilization

Women may develop hirsutism with virilization when they receive androgens or some progestational agents that are capable of stimulating the hair follicle and other androgen-sensitive structures. Virilizing ovarian tumors, polycystic ovary disease, congenital adrenal hyperplasia, adrenal carcinomas and adenomas, and incomplete testicular feminization syndrome may also result in hirsutism with virilization. These conditions have been discussed previously.

Clinical Evaluation

One should obtain a history of the age of onset of hair growth as well as the amount, duration, distribution, and rate. Symptoms of virilization such as deepening of the voice, change in libido, and increased odoriferous perspiration should also be sought. The family history including the racial background and country of origin is necessary to diagnose the racial and familial forms of this disorder. Menstrual and fertility history, as well as drug history, should also be obtained. Hair growth that begins around the time of puberty and is slowly progressive is most compatible with idiopathic hirsutism, racial and familial hirsutism, and polycystic ovary disease. The rapid onset of progressive hirsutism and virilization at any age suggests an ovarian or adrenal neoplasm. Normal menstrual function is compatible with the racial and familial varieties, as well as with idiopathic hirsutism, whereas menstrual disturbances are more commonly seen with organic ovarian disorders.

Physical examination should include a measurement of height in order to eliminate congenital adrenal hyperplasia as a cause of hirsutism and virilization, a measurement of blood pressure to rule out adrenal 11-hydroxylase deficiency, and assessment of the hair distribution, presence or absence of acne, degree of muscle development, laryngeal development, and female secondary sex characteristics. Abdominal and pelvic masses should be sought, and a measurement of clitoral size obtained. The degree of hirsutism can then be classified as: mild, which includes fine, pigmented hair over the face, extremities, chest, and abdomen; moderate, with coarse pigmented hair over the face (not the complete beard), chest, abdomen, and perineum; severe, with coarse pigmented hair over the face (total beard), ears, nose, and proximal interphalangeal joints; and virilization with temporal hair recession, deepening of the voice, clitoromegaly, and male muscle development.

Laboratory Evaluation

In the normal female, four 17β-hydroxysteroids present in the blood provide virtually the total androgenic activity. These four are testosterone, dihydro-testosterone, androstenediol, and androstanediol (3-α, 3-β). Of these, testosterone accounts for approximately 50% of the total androgen activity in the blood. Despite variation in testosterone concentrations during the menstrual cycle, approximately half of the testosterone emanates from the ovary and the other half from the adrenal gland. The adrenal gland produces the 17β-hydroxysteroids from androgen precursors, the 17-ketosteroids, which include dehydroepiandrosterone and androstendione. In all conditions in which the adrenal gland produces excessive testosterone, levels of the androgen precursors (17-ketosteroids) are elevated. On the other hand, the ovaries are capable of secreting large amounts of testosterone efficiently, and severely elevated levels of testosterone may be found with little or no elevation of 17-ketosteroids in ovarian disorders. The activity of the circulating androgen depends on its concentration, potency, and degree of binding to protein. The major protein that binds androgens is testosterone-estradiol binding globulin (TeBG). Because the free androgen is the biologically active material, a situation in which the TeBG level is decreased results in a greater concentration of free androgen, whereas an elevation of TeBG results in a lowered concentration of free androgen.

The laboratory evaluation of hirsutism should include a measurement of serum testosterone (preferably free testosterone) as well as a measurement of adrenal androgen secretion. The latter may be performed by measuring 17-ketosteroid concentration in a 24-hour urine or by measuring the plasma DHEA-S level. Because 90 to 96% of DHEA-S arises from the adrenal gland, its level serves as a useful parameter of adrenal androgen secretion. Generally, these 2 measurements are the only requisites in the evaluation of hirsutism without virilization. Mildly elevated testosterone or 17-ketosteroid levels are usually of little significance, whereas moderately or severely elevated levels require further studies of ovarian or adrenal function.

These further tests include a dexamethasone suppression test (2 mg dexamethasone taken orally each day for 6 days), with testosterone and DHEA-S levels measured before and during the last day of suppression. Inability to suppress is suggestive of an adrenal neoplasm. Severely elevated levels that do suppress with dexamethasone are more compatible with congenital adrenal hyperplasia. Administration of ethinyl estradiol (40 μg/day for 25 days) with medroxyprogesterone acetate (10 mg/day orally during the last 5 days) may be sufficient to suppress serum LH levels; this suppression in turn decreases ovarian androgen secretion. However, because the estrogen may stimulate the liver to produce more globulins, including TeBG, the total serum testosterone level at the end of this suppression may be elevated. A more direct way of determining the androgen production site is by selective ovarian and adrenal venous catheterization with blood sampling for the androgens. Ancillary studies include determination of serum LH and FSH levels when considering the polycystic ovary syndrome, intravenous pyelography and arteriography or venography for adrenal neoplasms, and laparoscopy for suspected ovarian neoplasms.

Approximately 10% of patients with significant hirsutism have normal levels of testosterone, perhaps from an increase in the free fraction of testosterone due to a decrease in TeBG, increased turnover of testosterone, increased levels of other active androgens such as dihydrotestosterone, increased conversion of weaker androgens such as DHEA to testosterone, or idiopathic end-organ sensitivity to the androgens.

Therapy

Surgical removal of virilizing ovarian or adrenal neoplasms usually causes a prompt regression of hirsutism. Other therapeutic procedures include cosmetic approaches and medical therapy. Excessive hair may be removed by a variety of means including shaving, wax stripping, or chemical depilation. None of these procedures stimulate hair growth, but since they do not destroy the hair follicle, the growth of hair continues. Mild hirsutism may be treated cosmetically by bleaching the hairs, while more severe hirsutism may be treated permanently by electrolysis. During electrolysis the electrologist attempts to destroy the hair follicle, with either chemicals or electrical current. If the hair follicle is destroyed, no further hair grows from that follicle. However, because of the curvature of the hair shaft, it is difficult to successfully eliminate each follicle treated. If an ovarian or adrenal neoplasm is present, complete surgical removal is curative.

Medical therapy includes suppression of adrenal androgen secretion by glucocorticoids, suppression of ovarian androgen secretion by a combination of estrogens and progestogens, and combined adrenal and ovarian suppression. Approximately a third of individuals with familial, idiopathic, or polycystic ovary disease as a cause of hirsutism respond to adrenal suppression, whereas approximately half respond to ovarian suppression. As noted, the prolonged administration of estrogens may increase the TeBG level and may thereby decrease the amount of free androgen available to the hair follicles. Experimental therapies include the use of peripheral antagonists to androgens, such as cyproterone acetate, spironolactone, cimetidine, and medroxyprogesterone acetate. These medical therapies for hirsutism require a minimum of 3 to 6 months of trial before the patient notices a decrease in the rate of hair growth. This long duration of therapy is needed because approximately 10% of the hairs at any one time are in a resting stage, so 3 months pass before the hair falls out and a new hair is formed. Therefore, it takes about 30 months before the androgen-sensitive hairs are turned over.

CLINICAL PROBLEMS

Patient 1. This patient was the product of a full-term uncomplicated gestation. At birth, the patient had transient generalized edema (Bonnevie-Ullrich syndrome) and webbing of the neck.

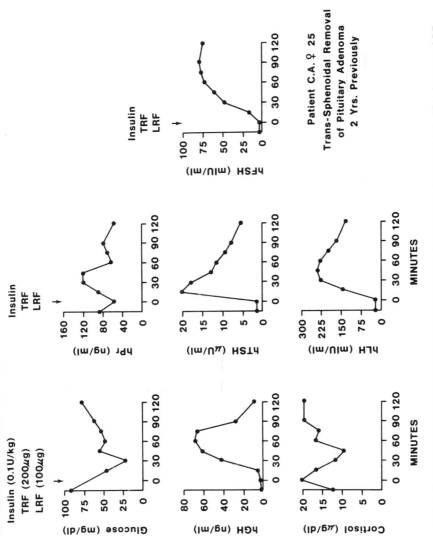

Figure 6–5. Responses of 25-year-old woman (patient 3) to combined test with LRH, TRH (same as LRF and TRF), and insulin.

At age 3, a buccal smear analysis revealed no Barr bodies, and the diagnosis of Turner's syndrome was entertained. At the age of 8 years, her parents became concerned because of her short stature, and when examined at age 11, she was noted to have short stature (52 inches), webbed neck, wide-spaced nipples, cubitus valgus, micrognathia, and a high-arched palate. A chromosome analysis revealed 45 XO and both urinary gonadotropins and serum LH and FSH were elevated in comparison to age-matched controls. At the age of 14, she was begun on low-dose ethinyl estradiol therapy, which was gradually increased to a full estrogen replacement dosage (40 μg/day). This dose was given for 25 days of each month, and during the last 5 days medroxyprogesterone acetate, 10 mg/day, was added. This therapy resulted in cyclic bleeding on a monthly basis. After institution of the estrogen therapy, the patient noted growth of her breasts, as well as a 2-inch spurt in height.

QUESTIONS

1. If this patient's mother were a carrier of classic hemophilia (an X-linked recessive disorder), could the patient have clinical hemophilia?
2. Does this patient need to have her dysgenetic gonads removed?
3. Should the estrogen therapy have been instituted earlier in this patient?

Patient 2. This 46-year-old Caucasian woman was in excellent health until October, 1975, when she first noted puffiness of her hands and feet. Shortly afterward, she developed a large amount of coarse facial hair, acne, and oily skin. During the next 2 months she gained approximately 6 pounds, developed pedal edema, and noted deepening of her voice.

PHYSICAL EXAMINATION. She was found to be hypertensive and was referred to an endocrinologist in December, 1975. At that time, her blood pressure (BP) was 170/100, her height was 5 feet 2 inches, weight 142 pounds, and her face demonstrated coarse hair in the beard area and on the chin and neck. A marked facial plethora was also noted. Her fat distribution was normal, and she did not exhibit easy bruisability or violaceous striae.

LABORATORY DATA. Laboratory evaluation included baseline serum cortisols, both morning and evening, of 30 μg/100 ml. After 1 mg dexamethasone taken at midnight, an 8:00 A.M. plasma cortisol was 24 μg/100 ml. A plasma testosterone was 83 ng/dl (normal, <60 ng/dl), and a serum LH was 11 mIU/ml (normal). A 24-hour urine for pregnanetriol was 7.8 mg/24 hours (normal, less than 4.0). A 2 and 8 mg dexamethasone suppression test was carried out, and the results are shown below:

Urine	17-ketosteroids (mg/24 hr)	17-hydroxysteroids (mg/24 hr)
Baseline 1	33	67
2	52	76
Dexamethasone 2 mg	66	80
Dexamethasone 8 mg	47	77

Because of these abnormal laboratory findings, the patient was hospitalized and underwent an intravenous pyelogram, which demonstrated a large left suprarenal mass. This growth was confirmed by ultrasound of the area and by arteriography, which demonstrated a 13-cm mass with neovascularization. In January, 1976, a left adrenalectomy was performed, and a 13 × 13 × 9-cm adrenocortical carcinoma was removed.

QUESTIONS

1. Why did this patient's 17-hydroxysteroids fail to suppress on 8 mg dexamethasone given for 2 days?
2. If the patient noted a strong family history of hirsutism, would the diagnostic considerations be different?
3. Why was this patient virilized with only a moderate elevation of her serum testosterone concentration?
4. If a patient with a similar problem were pregnant when she developed the tumor, what would be the effects on the fetus?

Patient 3. This 25-year-old Argentinian woman was well until the age of 14, at which time she developed irregular menstrual periods, headaches, and emotional instability. Visual field disturbances at the age of 22 prompted an evaluation, which revealed a pituitary tumor. A chromophobe adenoma was removed through a transsphenoidal approach at the age of 23. She received approximately 4000 rads of irradiation to the pituitary-hypothalamic area postoperatively. Her postoperative endocrine evaluation, performed in Argentina, reportedly was normal, including normal responses to LRH, TRH, and insulin-induced hypoglycemia. At the age of 25, she moved to Los Angeles and sought endocrine consultation because of her oligomenorrhea, orthostatic hypotension, and persistent galactorrhea, which had been noted since the time of surgery. She denied weight loss, excessive urination, nocturia, loss of axillary or pubic hair, change in the color of her skin, visual defects, or symptoms of hypothalamic dysfunction.

PHYSICAL EXAMINATION. The examination revealed an alert, thin, Caucasian woman in no acute distress. BP was 140/80, both supine and upright. Pertinent physical findings included normal visual fields to confrontation, a normal funduscopic examination, and a normal pelvic examination. Bilateral galactorrhea was present.

LABORATORY DATA. The patient was admitted to the hospital and underwent a combined LRH, TRH, and insulin tolerance test, the results of which are shown in Figure 6–5. Her GH, ACTH, and TSH secretory capacities were normal. Her LH and FSH response was supranormal, and she demonstrated basal hyperprolactinemia, which increased even further after TRH stimulation. Her estradiol level was in the normal range for the mid-cycle peak at 40 ng/100 ml, and she demonstrated a normal rise in 11-desoxycortisol after metyrapone (patient's response, 10.3 µg/100 ml; normal, greater than 7). Serum thyroid hormone levels were in the normal range and formal visual fields were normal. Her skull roentgenogram revealed some calcification within the sella turcica, but was otherwise normal.

QUESTIONS

1. Is there any evidence that this patient has residual pituitary tumor?
2. If this patient were desirous of pregnancy, what therapy may be required in order to induce ovulation? What effect will pregnancy have on this patient's residual normal pituitary or on any residual chromophobe adenoma?
3. Is adrenal insufficiency responsible for this patient's complaint of orthostatic dizziness?

SUGGESTED READING

Normal Menstrual Cycle

Abraham, G.E., et al.: Simultaneous radioimmunoassay of plasma FSH, LH, progesterone, 17-hydroxyprogesterone, and estradiol-17β during the menstrual cycle. J. Clin. Endocrinol. Metab., *34*:312, 1972.

Korenman, S.G., Sherman, B.M., and Korenman, J.C.: Reproductive hormone function: the perimenopausal period and beyond. Clin. Endocrinol. Metab., 7:625, 1978.

Lenton, E., and Cooke, I.D.: Other disorders of ovulation. Clin. Obstet. Gynecol., *1*:313, 1974.

Moghissi, K.S., Syner, F.M., and Evans, T.N.: Composite picture of the menstrual cycle. Am. J. Obstet. Gynecol., *114*:405, 1972.

Shaw, R.W.: Neuroendocrinology of the menstrual cycle in humans. Clin. Endocrinol. Metab., 7:531, 1978.

Sherman, B.M., and Korenman, S.G.: Hormonal characteristics of the human menstrual cycle throughout reproductive life. J. Clin. Invest., *55*:699, 1975.

Wentz, A.C.: Physiologic and clinical considerations in luteal phase defects. Clin. Obstet. Gynecol., 22:169, 1979.

Yen, S.S.C.: Neuroendocrine regulation of the menstrual cycle. Hosp. Pract., *14*:83, 1979.

Amenorrhea

Braunstein, G.D., and Odell, W.D. (eds.): Symposium on adolescent gynecology and endocrinology. West. J. Med, *131*:401, 1979; *131*:516, 1979; *132*:39, 1980.

Frisch, R.E., Wyshak, G., and Vincent, L.: Delayed menarche and amenorrhea in ballet dancers. N. Engl. J. Med., *303*:17, 1980.

Gilson, M.D., and Knab, D.R.: Primary amenorrhea: a simplified approach to diagnosis. Am. J. Obstet. Gynecol., *117*:400, 1973.

Griffin, J.E., and Wilson, J.D.: The syndromes of androgen resistance. N. Engl. J. Med., *302*:198, 1980.

McDonough, P.G.: Gonadal dysgenesis and its variants. Pediatr. Clin. North Am., *19*:631, 1972.

Shaw, R.W.: Ovary. Clin. Endocrinol. Metab., *8*:511, 1979.

Hirsutism

Casey, J.H.: Hirsutism: pathogenesis and treatment. Aust. N.Z. J. Med., *10*:240, 1980.

Ginsburg, J., and White, M.C.: Hirsutism and virilisation. Br. Med. J., *280*:369, 1980.

Kirschner, M.A., and Bardin, C.W.: Androgen production and metabolism in normal and virilized women. Metabolism., *21*:667, 1972.

Muller, S.A.: Hirsutism: a review of the genetic and experimental aspects. J. Invest. Dermatol., *60*:457, 1973.

Rosenfield, R.L.: Relationship of androgens to female hirsutism and infertility. J. Reprod. Med., *11*:87, 1973.

Shapiro, G., and Evron, S.: A novel use of spironolactone: treatment of hirsutism. J. Clin. Endocrinol. Metab., *51*:429, 1980.

CHAPTER 7

Male Reproductive Abnormalities

Ronald S. Swerdloff and Allan R. Glass

NORMAL REPRODUCTIVE HORMONAL AXIS

The reproductive hormonal axis in the adult male consists of four main components: (1) the hypothalamus, (2) the pituitary gland, (3) the testes, and (4) the gonadal sensitive end organs. The components of this system function in a closely regulated manner resulting in the concentrations of testosterone required for maintenance of secondary sexual characteristics and male sexual behavior. The reproductive axis also regulates the orderly maturation of sperm necessary for normal fertility.

The hypothalamus is the site of production of biogenic amines that regulate the synthesis and secretion of a small hypothalamic peptide hormone, luteinizing hormone releasing hormone (LRH). LRH is transported via a hypophyseal portal venous system to the pituitary gland where it stimulates secretion of luteinizing hormone (LH) and follicle-stimulating hormone (FSH). LH is the predominant stimulus for testicular steroid secretion by the Leydig cell. Recent evidence has suggested that FSH, GH, and prolactin (PRL) may modulate testosterone secretion by enhancing the Leydig cell response to LH.

Spermatogenesis is the orderly maturation of germinal cells in the spermatogenic tubules from spermatogonia to sperm. Most evidence indicates that FSH and LH are both required for the initiation of this process at puberty. The effect of LH is probably indirect in that it causes high intratesticular testosterone levels, which in turn act on the spermatogenic tubules to stimulate spermatogenesis. After puberty, spermatogenesis may be maintained by adequate intratesticular testosterone concentration.

The secreted gonadal androgens, testosterone and dihydrotestosterone, act on numerous end organs, cause the secondary sexual characteristics of "maleness," and are responsible for male sexual behavior.

Secretion of LH and FSH is regulated by the negative feedback effects of testicular hormones. Testosterone is believed to be the predominant inhibitor of LH secretion and a major controller of FSH secretion. Estradiol is secreted by the testis (30%) and is produced in peripheral tissues (70%) by conversion from precursors such as testosterone and estrone. The role of estrogens in the feedback control of gonadotropin secretion is controversial, but estrogens may be involved in this process. An additional peptide substance produced in the spermatogenic tubules has been implicated in the inhibition of FSH secretion. This hormone, named inhibin, has been tentatively characterized as having a molecular weight of approximately 20,000. Support for a physiologic role of inhibin arises from the demonstration that selective damage to the germinal epithelium results in moderate increases in serum FSH without affecting either serum testosterone or LH.

Normal male adult serum levels of LH, FSH, testosterone, and estradiol are shown in Table 7–1.

LABORATORY TESTS

Serum Testosterone

Serum testosterone is now routinely measured by radioimmunoassay. Its level should be determined in all patients with hypogonadism. The measurement of serum testosterone includes both protein-bound and free testosterone. Only the unbound (or free) testosterone is biologically active, and this free testosterone concentration is only about 1% of the total testosterone concentration. Thus, hypogonadism (underandrogenization) may be associated with a low free testosterone but a normal total plasma testosterone level. Serum testosterone has a circadian rhythm with a peak in the early morning. Normal total serum testosterone values in adult men are 300 to 1100 ng/100 ml.

Serum LH and FSH

Serum LH is now routinely measured by radioimmunoassay; normal values vary from laboratory to laboratory. Elevated levels usually indicate a primary failure of the testis to produce testosterone, while low levels may indicate hypothalamic or pituitary failure. Levels of LH fluctuate widely in the blood, varying two- or threefold over a two-hour period. Thus, several samples must be drawn and assayed to give a reasonable measure of the mean level of plasma LH.

Table 7–1. Serum LH, FSH, Testosterone, and Estradiol Levels in Normal Adult Males

Hormone	Level
LH	1–15 mIU/ml
FSH	<1–15 mIU/ml
Testosterone	300–1100 ng/100 ml
Estradiol	<40 pg/ml

Serum FSH is routinely measured by radioimmunoassay and is elevated as is LH in patients with primary hypogonadism. In addition, it can be selectively increased in patients with primary damage to the spermatogenic tubules. Since much less variation exists in the plasma levels of FSH than of LH, multiple sampling is not needed. However, in many laboratories some normal men have undetectable serum FSH, making it difficult to separate those with normal FSH from those with low FSH.

Serum Estradiol

Serum estradiol is measured by radioimmunoassay; normal values in men are 40 pg/ml or less. Measurement of serum estradiol is helpful in cases of gynecomastia or feminization.

LRH

LRH is a ten-amino-acid peptide hormone normally secreted by the hypothalamus to stimulate pituitary release of FSH and LH; synthetic LRH is now availabile on an investigational basis. Administration of 100 μg LRH intravenously causes a tripling of serum LH within an hour in normal men; the rise of serum FSH is inconstant and of smaller magnitude. Patients with hypogonadism secondary to pituitary destruction or tumor generally have no increase in serum LH after administration of LRH. Patients with hypothalamic disorders resulting in hypogonadism may have normal or impaired responses to LRH; an impaired LRH response may return to normal if LRH is given on a long-term basis in a pulsatile fashion. In primary testicular causes of hypogonadism, the loss of the normal inhibitory effect of testosterone results in an exaggerated rise in serum LH after LRH administration. In practice, testing with a single injection of LRH has not been a reliable method for separating hypothalamic from pituitary causes of hypogonadism.

Clomiphene

Clomiphene citrate is a compound that stimulates the release of LH and FSH, probably by blocking the inhibitory effect of testosterone and estrogen on the hypothalamus. In normal men, administration of 150 mg clomiphene per day for 10 days causes a doubling of serum LH. A failure to respond to clomiphene coupled with normal pituitary function indicates a probable hypothalamic cause of hypogonadism. Since the ability to respond to clomiphene does not develop until stage III of puberty, this test has usually not been helpful in assessing disorders of delayed puberty. It is also used as a general test of hypothalamic-pituitary function.

HCG

Administration of human chorionic gonadotropin (HCG), which has biologic activity similar to LH, directly stimulates the testes to secrete testosterone. Normal men double their serum testosterone after 2 injections of 2000 IU of HCG; patients with primary testicular causes of hypogonadism may have either no reponse or a blunted response. Patients with pituitary or hypothalamic causes of hypogonadism may have a small rise in serum testosterone after HCG, but prolonged administration of HCG may restore this response to normal.

Semen

Spermatogenesis depends on the integrity of the hypothalamic-pituitary-Leydig cell axis. Normal spermatogenesis requires the presence of testosterone; however, spermatogenesis may be defective independently of testosterone production. Semen analysis (as a test for evaluation in infertility) is optimally performed by examination of a specimen obtained after 48 to 72 hours of abstinence. Normal men have at least 20 million spermatozoa per milliliter with 60% motility and 60% normal forms. Specific abnormalities may be associated with specific disorders; e.g., the presence of a large number of tapered forms suggests varicocele.

Buccal Smear and Karyotype

Examination of buccal smear for Barr bodies and karyotyping of peripheral blood lymphocytes enable determination of sex chromosome composition and are indicated when a congenital defect may exist. It is especially indicated when serum FSH or LH are elevated, since the most common cause of hypergonadotropic hypogonadism in adult males is Klinefelter's syndrome.

Microscopic examination of epithelial cells from the buccal mucosa reveals the presence of Barr bodies (dark chromatin clumps) in patients who have more than one X chromosome per cell. The Barr body represents the heterochromatin of the extra X chromosome; the number of Barr bodies per cell is one less than the number of X chromosomes. Normal males have Barr bodies in fewer than 5% of their buccal mucosal cells; in normal females, Barr bodies are present in more than 20% of buccal mucosal cells. A more specific method of determining sex chromosome composition is by karyotyping, i.e., examination of photomicrographs of the metaphase plates of cultured peripheral blood lymphocytes. In these preparations, the Y chromosome can be located by its characteristic fluorescence when exposed to quinacrine. Recently, it has become possible to determine the presence of a Y chromosome without karyotyping by looking for the presence of a specific "Y antigen" on the surface of cells.

HYPOGONADISM

Clinical Manifestations

Dependence on Age at Onset

Hypogonadism or impaired testicular function may be reflected clinically as underandrogenization, infertility, or a combination of the two. The clinical features of decreased testosterone secretion depend on the degree of deficiency and the age of onset of the disorder. Deficiencies occurring during early fetal development result in pseudohermaphroditism; those first manifest during late gestation may result in micropenis.

The clinical onset of testosterone deficiency prior to puberty will result in eunuchoid proportions and female hair distribution. Eunuchoid proportions include an arm span two inches greater than height and an upper-lower body ratio of less than one. (These proportions may be normal for Negro men of east African derivation.) Patients with hypogonadism acquired after puberty have normal body proportions and male temporal hair recession, but show other clinical signs of hypogonadism (Fig. 7–1).

Facies

The distribution of facial beard in normal males depends on the person's racial background. Deviations from the racially determined norm indicate the presence of hypogonadism. Normal hair distribution varies from that on the cheek, moustache, chin, and neck requiring shaving at least once a day to that on the upper lip and chin requiring shaving every two to three days. The former is normal for most Caucasian subraces while the latter may be normal for men of Black, Oriental, or American Indian extraction. Detailed questioning of other male family members is helpful in assessing the clinical status of a suspected hypogonadal patient. Hypogonadism is also associated with increased fine wrinkling of the skin about the mouth and eyes.

Body Hair Distribution

Body hair distribution also varies with racial background. Many normal Black, Oriental, and Indian men have body hair limited to the axillary, pubic, and sternal areas while many Caucasian men have additional pectoral, back, and flank hair. The male pubic hair distribution is diamond-shaped with hair extending up toward the umbilicus. When the pubic hair has an inverted triangle appearance, it is described as a female escutcheon. Severe long-standing hypogonadism results in absence of chest hair and sparseness of pubic hair. Less severe defects produce more subtle changes, which should be evaluated with the patient's racial and family hair patterns as a guide.

Testicular Size

Ninety percent of the normal testis volume consists of spermatogenic tubules. The testes should be measured in all patients; testes greater than 4.0 cm in length or greater than 15 ml in volume (measured with a Prader orchidometer) are normal in size. Most patients with hypogonadism have smaller than normal testes. If the onset of the lesion is prepubertal, the testes are often infantile in size. Hypogonadism beginning after puberty results in testicular size varying from small, soft organs to those that are near normal. Severe tubular injury not associated with underandrogenization may result in small testes and normal Leydig cell function.

Classification

Hypogonadism occurs in three main categories: (1) hypothalamic-pituitary defects (hypogonadotropic), (2) primary gonadal defects (hypergonadotropic), and (3) defective androgen action. Each of these categories consists of multiple subcategories described next. (Some rare disorders have not been included.)

1. Abnormalities in Hypothalamic-Pituitary Function
   a. Panhypopituitarism (congenital or acquired)
   b. Hypothalamic syndromes (acquired or congenital)
      Structural Defects (neoplastic or inflammatory)
      Prader-Willi syndrome (mental retardation, hypogonadism, hypotonia, and obesity)
      Laurence-Moon-Biedl syndrome (mental retardation, hypogonadism, retinitis pigmentosa, and hand anomalies)
   c. Isolated LH or FSH deficiency (may be associated with anosmia [Kallmann's syndrome])
   d. Hyperprolactinemia (chromophobe adenoma, most common cause)
   e. Malnutrition and anorexia nervosa
   f. Drug-induced suppression of LH (androgens, estrogens, tranquilizers, antidepressants, antihypertensives, barbiturates, and opiates)
2. Primary Gonadal Abnormalities
   a. Acquired (irradiation, orchitis, castration)
   b. Chromosomal
      Klinefelter's and variants
      True hermaphroditism
   c. Defective androgen synthesis
      20α-hydroxylase (cholesterol 20,22-desmolase) deficiency
      17,20-desmolase deficiency
      3β-hydroxysteroid dehydrogenase deficiency
      17α-hydroxylase deficiency
      17 keto reductase (17β-hydroxysteroid dehydrogenase) deficiency
      5α-reductase deficiency
   d. Testicular agenesis
   e. Selective seminiferous tubular disease
   f. Miscellaneous
      Noonan's syndrome (short stature, pulmonary valve stenosis, hypertelorism, and ptosis)
      Streak gonads
      Myotonia dystrophica
      Cystic fibrosis
3. Defects in Androgen Action (Pseudohermaphroditism)
   a. Complete androgen insensitivity (also called testicular feminization)
   b. Incomplete androgen sensitivity
      Testosterone receptor defect
      Testosterone postreceptor defect
      5α-reductase deficiency

From a clinical standpoint it is important to: (1) define the anatomic site of the defect; (2) determine whether the defect has additional serious consequences to the patient such as would occur in patients with hypothalamic or pituitary tumors, panhypopituitarism, hypothalamic syndromes, and many congenital adrenal and testicular enzymatic defects; (3) determine whether a genetic disorder requires genetic counseling to the family; and (4) characterize the site of the defect in order to give better therapy. (Patients with hypogonadotropic hypogonadism could be treated with testosterone to produce virilization, but fertility requires treatment with gonadotropins.)

Localization of Site of Defect

Evaluation of patients with clinical evidence of underandrogenization should begin with measurements of basal or static serum testosterone, LH, and FSH levels. In almost all such cases, serum testosterone concentrations are lower than normal, thus confirming the diagnosis of hypogonadism. In such patients, the serum LH and FSH concentrations separate the patients into two main categories: hypergonadotropic (high LH and FSH) or hypogonadotropic (low or inappropriately normal LH and FSH).

Hypogonadotropic hypogonadism may be further dissected into the hypothalamic and pituitary abnormalities. Ability to smell should be tested in all hypogonadotropic patients because its absence suggests a congenital hypothalamic cause of hypogonadism (Kallmann's syndrome). Skull roentgenograms including special views of the sella turcica must be obtained in such patients. These films will detect: (1) enlargement of the sella turcica, suggesting an intrapituitary or suprasellar mass; (2) calcification in or above the sella, suggesting a craniopharyngioma; and (3) evidence of increased intracranial pressure.

Additional laboratory tests should be done in hypogonadotropic patients. Serum prolactin measurements are required because a marked elevation suggests a prolactinoma. Lesser elevations of prolactin may occur in many disorders (see Chap. 2). Hyperprolactinemia may suppress LH and FSH secretion in the absence of anatomic damage to the LRH- and gonadotropin-secreting cells. Lowering prolactin levels with a dopamine agonist (bromocriptine) will reverse the hypogonadotropic state. All hypogonadotropic patients should have a complete assessment of hypothalamic-pituitary function. Additional tests of the reproductive function may be indicated to characterize the lesion. The response to clomiphene is abnormally low in patients with either hypothalamic or pituitary disease. LRH administration increases LH and FSH levels in most patients with hypothalamic disease and fails to do so in most patients with a pituitary cause of hypogonadism. Unfortunately, the ability of this test to determine the site of the defect is not 100%. Some patients with pituitary disease respond normally, and others with a hypothalamic problem respond only after prolonged treatment with LRH.

Hypergonadotropic Hypogonadism

Patients with low serum testosterone and elevated serum LH and FSH have a primary testicular disorder. In some patients with borderline testosterone levels, an HCG test may demonstrate the presence of impaired Leydig cell reserve.

The clinical history frequently indicates whether there has been infection or trauma. Chromosome analysis identifies patients with disorders such as Klinefelter's syndrome and its variants (see next section). Most defects of testosterone biosynthesis result in pseudohermaphroditism. (Diagnoses of such disorders are discussed in an earlier section.) Other rare disorders can be identified by their clinical characteristics, e.g., Noonan's syndrome and myotonia dystrophica.

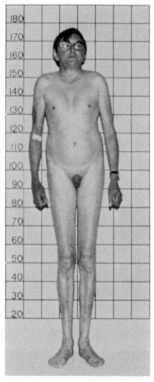

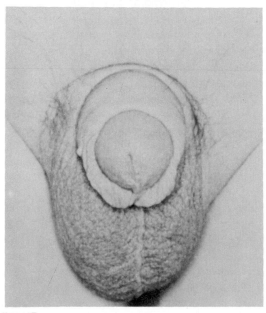

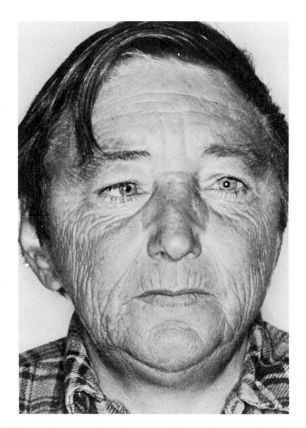

Figure 7–1. A 43-year-old man with hypogonadotropic hypogonadism due to a chromophobe adenoma. Prepubertal onset is apparent from the eunuchoidal proportions. The sparse pubic hair, absence of beard (never shaved), infantile genitalia, and increased facial wrinkling indicate severe androgen deficiency.

Testicular function is often abnormal in an aged male population. This abnormality is usually associated with elevated serum LH and FSH levels, which indicate a primary defect at the level of the testis. Some controversy exists as to whether the testicular failure seen in the aged is a normal consequence of growing older or a result of concomitant disease processes.

End-Organ Resistance

Some patients may have signs of underandrogenization and yet have normal or elevated serum testosterone levels. These patients often come to the clinic with male pseudohermaphroditism manifest by a broad range of physical appearances. In the most severe form (testicular feminization), the phenotypic appearance is female. In less severe forms the patients may have hypospadias and gynecomastia. The several defects described include inability to convert testosterone to dihydrotestosterone (DHT) (5α-reductase deficiency) and unresponsiveness to testosterone and DHT in androgen-sensitive tissues (testosterone receptor defect). In the latter case, estradiol levels are usually above the normal male range, serum testosterone and LH levels are normal or high, and FSH is usually normal or low.

Klinefelter's Syndrome

Klinefelter's syndrome, the most common cause of male hypogonadism, is a congenital disorder characterized by the presence of XXY sex chromosome composition in the testis. The abnormal testicular function resulting from this genetic defect is responsible for the manifestations of Klinefelter's syndrome seen in the reproductive tissues. In addition, the abnormal sex chromosome composition may also be found in other body tissues (e.g., buccal mucosa and skin fibroblasts) or may be associated with mosaicism with variable cell sex chromosome composition. These mosaics may show features of Klinefelter's syndrome to a variable degree, but they all possess at least one or more cell lines containing two X chromosomes and one Y chromosome. The incidence of Klinefelter's syndrome is approximately 0.2% of live male births. The cause of the disorder is thought to be nondisjunction, and like some other chromosomal disorders, it seems to be associated with advanced maternal or paternal age.

The cardinal physical finding in patients with Klinefelter's syndrome is small, firm testes, which on biopsy show germ cell loss, hyalinization of spermatogenic tubules, and Leydig cell clumping and hyperplasia. These abnormalities usually result in azoospermia and infertility, but the temporal pace of germ cell loss and tubular hyalinization allows a broad range in testicular size and consistency on physical examination. Androgen deficiency, as manifested by such factors as decreased facial and pubic hair growth, reduced muscle mass, small penis size, and impaired sexual potency, is usually present in Klinefelter's syndrome, but some patients may appear normally virilized. Gynecomastia, as evidenced microscopically by hyperplasia of the interductal breast tissue, is another condition in many patients. These individuals tend to have tall stature and long legs, in association with the typical eunuchoidal proportion of upper segment:lower segment ratio less than one. In contrast with other disorders resulting in eunuchoidal proportions, however, Klinefelter's patients may have an arm span less than their height.

Klinefelter's syndrome is also associated with a number of nonreproductive abnormalities, including diabetes, chronic bronchitis, breast cancer, thyroid abnormalities, and mental retardation in as many as 15 to 25% of patients. The association with mental retardation is confirmed by noting that the prevalence of Klinefelter's syndrome in institutions for the mentally retarded is 1%, which is higher than that in the general population.

Laboratory findings in Klinefelter's syndrome reflect both the genetic and hormonal abnormalities. The XXY chromosomal composition may be detected by examining a buccal smear for the presence of Barr bodies. More definitive diagnosis requires complete karyotyping of peripheral blood lymphocytes, and the presence of mosaicism may in some cases be detected only by determining the karyotype of several cell lines. Semen analysis in these patients usually shows azoospermia. Plasma testosterone levels are usually low normal or reduced, and the loss of inhibitory feedback is reflected by high normal or frankly elevated serum levels of LH and FSH. Some patients may have selective damage to the germinal elements and come to the clinic with elevated serum levels of FSH and normal testosterone and LH concentrations. Most patients, however, show impaired testicular steroid reserve when challenged with injections of HCG.

INFERTILITY

The evaluation of an infertile couple requires an assessment of both partners. In the initial evaluation a semen analysis should be obtained on the male partner. Patients with decreased sperm counts (less than 20,000,000/ml) should have serum LH, FSH, and testosterone values determined; patients with panhypogonadism have low serum levels of testosterone. Many oligospermic or azoospermic patients do not show evidence of Leydig cell dysfunction. Hormonal parameters are normal, or an isolated increase in FSH is seen. A few patients may have had previous testicular injury, infection, chemotherapy, or irradiation, which would explain the isolated germinal element damage. Some patients have unsuspected sex or autosomal chromosome abnormalities. Significant numbers of patients have obstruction to the ductal system. Obstruction to the semen excretory ductal system is strongly suggested by normal serum FSH levels in a patient with azoospermia. Varicoceles (worm-like dilatation of the spermatic venous system) may be associated with infertility; an increased number of tapered forms on morphologic examination of the sperm suggests such a possibility. The role of autoimmunity, sperm and cervical mucus, and female antibody incompatibility with sperm is under investigation. In the majority of oligospermic and azoospermic patients the pathogenic cause of impaired spermatogenesis cannot be determined.

GYNECOMASTIA

Gynecomastia is defined as an increase in the nonfatty tissue of the male breast. This increase may be in either the parenchymal or stromal elements and may be bilateral or unilateral. Breast enlargement in the male is seen in many clinical situations, some of which are:

1. Puberty (seen in 50 to 70% of normal boys).
2. Cirrhosis (especially after recovery from hepatic decompensation).
3. Chronic renal failure with chronic hemodialysis.
4. Drugs (estrogens, digitalis, spironolactone, marijuana, reserpine, and other drugs known to act on the central nervous system).
5. Hyperthyroidism or, rarely, hypothyroidism.
6. Rapid weight gain (especially after previous weight loss).
7. Primary testicular failure (including Klinefelter's syndrome).
8. Hypogonadotropic hypogonadism (less common than in primary testicular failure).
9. Cancer
   a. with overproduction of estrogens.
   b. with production of an HCG-like peptide hormone.

The mechanisms producing gynecomastia are diverse. The relationship between an increase in the estrogen/androgen ratio and breast enlargement is well known, and the mechanism of gynecomastia in men taking estrogens for prostatic carcinoma or those with estrogen-producing adrenal carcinoma is obvious. In hyperthyroidism and cirrhosis, the total plasma levels of estrogens and androgens may be normal, but abnormalities of the globulin that binds them in plasma may lead to an increase in the physiologically active free estrogen/free androgen ratio and consequent gynecomastia. On the other hand, spironolactone seems to block the attachment of androgens to their receptors on target tissues (including the breast) and leads to an increase in the estrogen/androgen ratio at the cellular level. Similarly, in patients with testicular feminization, these androgen receptors on the target tissues may be entirely absent. The mechanism producing gynecomastia in normal boys during puberty remains controversial; some investigators find elevated plasma estrogen levels and others do not.

When evaluating a patient with gynecomastia, one must keep in mind that most cases are either pubertal or idiopathic. Careful history and physical examination identifies most of the known causes of gynecomastia listed previously. Special attention should be paid to history of sexual functioning and examination for signs of virilization, since most patients with normal libido, potency, and virilization do not have a life-threatening underlying disorder. Normal levels of plasma LH, FSH, testosterone, and estradiol are often found and are typical of the idiopathic cases. Serum LH should be measured in all cases of gynecomastia because high levels may indicate primary hypogonadism (e.g., Klinefelter's syndrome) or HCG production by choriocarcinoma of the testis or other tumor. (HCG cross-reacts in the usual LH radioimmunoassay.) In the latter case, the presence of β-HCG in the serum, as determined by specific radioimmunoassay, would confirm the diagnosis of tumor since β-HCG is not normally present in males. A high level of plasma estradiol may suggest a feminizing adrenal carcinoma. Idiopathic or pubertal gynecomastia usually regresses spontaneously.

CLINICAL PROBLEMS

Patient 1. A 17-year-old male high-school student is brought in by his mother, who is concerned about his delayed puberty and poor social adjustment at school, though his academic work has been satisfactory. When questioned, the patient concedes that he has been worried that he was not turning into a man. He reports that he began to develop a small amount of pubic hair at age 15, but he has rarely had an erection, though he may have had 1 or 2 nocturnal emissions. He has shaved 2 or 3 times per month since the age of 15 with no recent increase in frequency. His mother relates that his neonatal and childhood development were normal.

PHYSICAL EXAMINATION. His height is 73 inches (upper segment 35 inches, lower segment 38 inches) with an arm span of 71 inches. He has minimal facial hair and no temporal recession of his hairline. Mild gynecomastia is present. Axillary hair is present; pubic hair is sparse. The penis is small, and the testes are small and firm. Remainder of the physical exam is normal.

LABORATORY DATA. He brings the results of blood tests obtained by his referring physician; these show a serum testosterone of 250 ng/100 ml, serum LH of 18 mIU/ml, serum FSH of 24 mIU/ml, and serum estradiol of 40 pg/ml.

QUESTIONS

1. What do you think is the most likely diagnosis at this point? How common is this disorder?
2. What simple test could be done to confirm this diagnosis?
3. A buccal smear shows that 15% of his cells contain Barr bodies (normal females, greater than 20%; normal males, less than 5%). Does this change your diagnosis, and how would you follow this up?
4. What are the chances his 8-year-old brother has the same disorder? If he did, what would you expect the results of his laboratory tests to be?
5. Is a skull roentgenogram necessary?
6. Will the patient ever be fertile?
7. Why does he have gynecomastia?
8. A repeat serum LH is 14 mIU/ml. How do you explain this change from his previous value?
9. What other endocrine systems might be defective?
10. As part of an experimental protocol, you decide to administer LRH intravenously. How would his response compare to the response of a normal male?
11. As part of the same protocol, you administer HCG. How would his response compare to that of a normal male?

Patient 2. A 15-year-old boy is referred to you because of short stature and delayed puberty. He attends a special school because of congenital nerve deafness. His parents have noted that he has not developed any male secondary sexual characteristics and he is shorter than all his classmates. The patient states he has had no erections, no ejaculations, and no desire for sex. His father is 70 inches tall; his mother is 64 inches tall.

PHYSICAL EXAMINATION. The examination reveals the boy's height is 58 inches (upper segment 28 inches, lower segment 30 inches) and his arm span is 60 inches. There is slight hair on the upper lip, but no other facial hair and no temporal recession of the hairline. Axillary hair is sparse; pubic hair is absent. The testes are infantile and the penis is small. A repaired cleft palate is present. Examination of his growth curve shows that he was following the fifth percentile until approximately age 10, when his growth rate began to fall off, though he continued to grow slowly.

LABORATORY DATA. Serum testosterone is 150 ng/100 ml and serum FSH and LH are both undetectable.

QUESTIONS

1. What are the most likely diagnostic possibilities? What physical finding might establish a specific cause?
2. Is a skull roentgenogram important in the initial evaluation?
3. What would you expect the bone age to be?
4. What accounts for the relative slowdown in growth rate at age 10? How will his eventual stature compare with normal?
5. Would his younger brother be similarly affected?
6. Would his plasma LH increase normally after a single injection of LRH? After pulsatile, long-term administration of LRH?
7. Would his plasma testosterone increase normally after 2 injections of HCG? After daily injection for 2 months?

SUGGESTED READING

Reproductive Hormone Physiology
Baker, H.W.G., et al.: Testicular control of follicle-stimulating hormone secretion. Recent Prog. Horm. Res., *32*:429, 1976.
Longcope, C., Kato, T., and Horton, R.: The conversion of blood androgens to estrogens in normal adult men and women. J. Clin. Invest., *48*:2191, 1969.
Santen, R.J., and Bardin, D.W.: Episodic luteinizing hormone secretion in man. Pulse analysis, clinical interpretation, physiologic mechanisms. J. Clin. Invest., *52*:2617, 1973.
Swerdloff, R.S.: Physiology of male reproduction—the hypothalamic-pituitary axis. *In* Campbell's Urology. 4th Ed. Edited by J.H. Harrison, et al. Philadelphia, W.B. Saunders, 1979.

Infertility
Sherins, R.J., and Howards, S.S.: Male infertility. *In* Campbell's Urology. 4th Ed. Edited by J.H. Harrison, et al. Philadelphia, W.B. Saunders, 1979.
Swerdloff, R.S., and Boyers, S.P.: Evaluation of the male partner of an infertile couple. JAMA., *247*:2418, 1982.

Hypogonadism
de Kretser, D.M., and Swerdloff, R.S.: Eunuchoidism. Int. Med., *1*:308, 1981.
Franks, S., Jacobs, H.S., Martin, N., and Nabarro, J.D.: Hyperprolactinemia and impotence. Clin. Endocrinol., *4*:277, 1978.
Imperato-McGinley, J., and Peterson, R.E.: Male pseudohermaphroditism: the complexities of male phenotypic development. Am. J. Med., *61*:251, 1976.
Lubs, H.A.: Testicular size in Klinefelter's syndrome in men over fifty. N. Engl. J. Med., *267*:325, 1962.
Marshall, J.C.: Investigative procedures. Clin. Endocrinol. Metab., *4*:545, 1975.
Odell, W.D., and Swerdloff, R.S.: Abnormalities of gonadal function in men. Clin. Endocrinol., *8*:149, 1978.
Santen, R.J., and Paulsen, D.A.: Hypogonadotropin eunuchoidism. I. Clinical study of mode of inheritance. J. Clin. Endocrinol. Metab., *36*:47, 1973.

Aging and Reproductive Function
Harman, S.M., and Tsitouras, P.D.: Reproductive hormones in aging men. J. Clin. Endocrinol. Metab., *51*:35, 1980.
Sparrow, D., Bosse, R., and Rowe, J.W.: The influence of age, alcohol consumption, and body build on gonadal function in men. J. Clin. Endocrinol. Metab., *51*:508, 1980.
Swerdloff, R.S., and Heber, D.: Effects of aging on male reproductive function. *In* The Endocrinology of Aging. Edited by S. Korenman. New York, Elsevier North-Holland, 1982.

Gynecomastia
Carlson, H.E.: Gynecomastia. N. Engl. J. Med., *303*:795, 1980.
Knorr, D., and Bidlingmaier, F.: Gynecomastia in male adolescents. Clin. Endocrinol. Metab., *4*:157, 1975.
Nuttal, F.Q.: Gynecomastia as a physical finding in normal men. J. Clin. Endocrinol. Metab., *48*:338, 1979.

CHAPTER 8

Diabetes Mellitus and Hypoglycemia

Mayer B. Davidson

This chapter describes the pathophysiology, diagnosis, and treatment of adult hypoglycemia and diabetes mellitus. The metabolic pathways that characterize the fasting and fed states are reviewed, so that hypoglycemia and hyperglycemia (diabetes mellitus) can be discussed in terms of specific departures from these normal homeostatic mechanisms.

It is important to have a solid understanding of the disorders of carbohydrate metabolism. No matter which area of medicine students choose to enter, they will encounter some aspect of the many problems presented by the diabetic. On the other hand, some practitioners contend that hypoglycemia is responsible for many modern ills, such as alcoholism, sexual inadequacy, allergies, drug addiction, depression, learning disorders, and behavior problems. Clearly, hypoglycemia is not the problem in these situations; however, it is important for any physician who cares for patients to know how to make a bona fide diagnosis of hypoglycemia and to determine which of many conditions may be responsible for it.

NORMAL METABOLISM

Fasting State

The metabolic machinery of mammals is geared to handle a wide variety of metabolic situations. For instance, a Peruvian miner working at high altitude may ingest 5000 calories a day and maintain a stable normal weight. A neurotic individual living at sea level with no unusual caloric expenditure eating 5000 calories a day may gain 115 lb in a year. An extremely obese individual undergoing a protein-sparing diet may lose 115 pounds in one year. The Eskimo eating approximately 2000 calories a day, 80% of which is in the form of fat, has a normal body composition. All these individuals are able to function normally, a testimony to our amazing versatility in adjusting to various metabolic conditions.

Metabolic homeostasis during fasting is shown in Figure 8–1. Under fasting conditions (12 to 24 hours after eating), only a few tissues depend entirely on glucose for energy. The most important of these obligate glucose consumers is the brain, which uses approximately 115 g glucose per day. The red blood cells, the next most avid glucose consumer, use approximately 25 g glucose per day. Platelets, leukocytes, peripheral nerves, and the renal medulla account for approximately 12 g glucose consumed per day. The rest of the tissues in the body use predominantly free fatty acids (FFA) for energy.

The liver is the sole source of glucose production during the usual fasting situation. The liver produces glucose through 2 pathways. The first involves the breakdown of glycogen (glycogenolysis). Glycogen contributes only a small amount of glucose, and in approximately 8 to 12 hours this reserve is depleted. The major source of glucose production by the liver occurs through the metabolic pathway of gluconeogenesis (the production of new glucose from noncarbohydrate precursors). There are 3 gluconeogenic precursors, 2 of which make minor contributions to glucose production. One is lactate, which is produced from glucose utilization by the red blood cells and brain and is channeled back to the liver. Glucose conversion to lactate by the peripheral tissues with subsequent synthesis of glucose from the generated lactate is termed the Cori cycle. The other minor gluconeogenic precursor is glycerol, which is supplied by the breakdown of adipose tissue triglyceride (lipolysis). The major gluconeogenic precursors are amino acids derived from muscle. Of all the glucogenic amino acids, alanine is of particular importance.

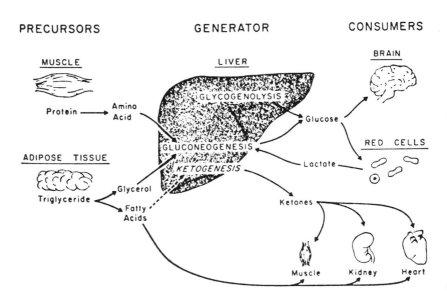

Figure 8–1. Fasting homeostasis. (From Arky, R.A.: Pathophysiology and therapy of the fasting hypoglycemias. Edited by Harry F. Dowling.: DM, February, 1968. Year Book Medical Publishers, Inc., Chicago.)

A transamination pathway in muscle allows conversion of pyruvate to alanine and subsequent delivery of alanine to the liver. The rate-limiting step for gluconeogenesis seems to be the amount of substrate presented to the liver.

Most stored energy is contained in adipose tissue triglycerides. The breakdown of triglyceride yields FFA and glycerol. As stated earlier, glycerol is a gluconeogenic precursor, whereas FFA are the main source of energy for most tissues in the fasting state. The FFA delivered to the liver have three metabolic fates. First, they can be re-esterified back into triglycerides. Second, they can be used as an energy source for the liver through β-oxidation to acetyl-coenzyme A (CoA) with subsequent metabolism through the Krebs cycle. Third, the acetyl-CoA can be channeled into ketone bodies, acetoacetate, and β-hydroxybutyrate.

Although the molar ratio of insulin to glucagon in the portal vein influences ketogenesis, the most important control of hepatic ketone body formation is the amount of FFA delivered to the liver. After synthesis, the ketone bodies are released into the general circulation, where they can be used to some extent by the peripheral tissues. The amount that can be taken up by peripheral tissues is limited, however, and after 12 to 24 hours without food, the ketone bodies spill over into the urine (ketonuria). This condition is known as starvation ketosis and must be carefully distinguished from diabetic ketosis, described later. Ketosis can also be seen in subjects ingesting low carbohydrate diets. When dietary carbohydrate is limited (fewer than approximately 50 to 100 g/day), lipolysis increases, enhancing FFA delivery to the liver and thus increasing ketone body formation.

The body has powerful homeostatic mechanisms to maintain glucose concentrations during total starvation so that the obligate glucose consumers can continue to function normally. When calories are totally withheld, an initial drop of glucose concentration by 15 to 20 mg/100 ml usually stabilizes after approximately 3 days. Some individuals of normal weight undergoing total caloric deprivation (especially women) may have glucose levels as low as 35 to 40 mg/100 ml but remain asymptomatic. During the next several weeks, hepatic glucose production is equal to glucose utilization by the brain and red blood cells; therefore, glucose concentrations remain stable. Insulin levels uniformly decrease and glucagon concentrations increase. FFA concentrations are approximately doubled while ketone body concentrations rise some two-hundredfold. Glucogenic amino acid levels (especially alanine levels) decrease to approximately one-third of their prefast value with a concomitant increase in hepatic extraction of these precursors. Plasma lactate and pyruvate concentrations show no change.

After 3 to 4 weeks of starvation, the body makes certain alterations in an attempt to conserve the protein stores. If continued breakdown of muscle protein were to occur in order to supply the glucogenic amino acids, a severe depletion of protein would ensue. To counteract this continued drain, the brain adapts so that ketone bodies can be used for energy. Thus, less glucose is required for the most important (and avid) obligate consumer, with consequent sparing of protein. At this point, the kidney (the other tissue capable of gluconeogenesis) begins to contribute glucose to the general circulation. Prior to this time, glucose synthesized by renal gluconeogenesis was used locally by the renal tissue itself, and the kidney did not supply glucose for other tissues.

Fed State

Dietary carbohydrates are ingested in the form of simple carbohydrates (disaccharides, e.g., sucrose, lactose, and maltose) and complex carbohydrates (starches). Both types are broken down in the intestine and absorbed primarily as monosaccharides, chiefly glucose. Glucose stimulates insulin secretion into the portal vein. Therefore, the newly released insulin goes first to the liver where approximately 50% of the insulin is degraded on each passage. The rest is degraded in the periphery, mostly by the kidney. The half-life of insulin in the peripheral circulation is 5 to 10 minutes. Insulin binds to specific insulin receptors in muscle and adipose tissue where the hormone may exert its effect for several hours after the initial binding.

Dietary carbohydrate can also be stored as triglyceride. Glucose is metabolized through glycolysis to glycerol, which serves as the backbone for the triglyceride molecule. Further metabolism of glucose through the glycolytic pathway produces acetyl-CoA, which can be synthesized into fatty acids (lipogenesis). This process provides the other component of the triglyceride molecule. These triglycerides are released from the liver and are stored in adipose tissue by a complicated series of reactions that are not germane to the present discussion. Adipose tissue triglyceride may also be synthesized directly from glucose by the same pathways as outlined for the liver, although some controversy exists whether fatty acid carbons can be derived from the glucose molecule in human adipose tissue. The remainder of the glucose that escapes into the periphery is stored as muscle glycogen or is used by non-insulin-dependent tissues, mainly brain and red blood cells.

HYPOGLYCEMIA

Definition

Hypoglycemia is a biochemical abnormality that has many causes. First, one has to document the low glucose concentration. Then, one systematically determines which condition is responsible for it.

The glucose concentration measured in whole blood is approximately 15% lower than that measured in plasma or serum because approximately 30% of the red cell is composed of solid material that is not capable of dissolving glucose. Thus, when whole blood is used, glucose is distributed in only 85% of the volume tested (assuming a hematocrit of 50%). Since this result is expressed per milliliter, the value for whole blood is actually 15% (not 15 mg/100 ml) less than that for plasma or serum. In adults, plasma or serum glucose concentrations of less than 50 mg/100 ml (and of whole blood less than 40 mg/100 ml) are abnormally low following oral glucose. In the fasting state, plasma glucose concentrations of less than 60 mg/100 ml (50 mg/100 ml for whole blood) signify hypoglycemia.

Hormonal Responses

Glucoreceptors in the hypothalamus initiate certain hormonal responses to hypoglycemia or to a rapidly falling glucose concentration that has not yet reached hypoglycemic levels. The four responses are summarized in Table 8–1. One of the signals emanating from hypothalamic centers, increased sympathetic nervous system activity, may cause glycogenolysis directly via sympathetic nerve endings located in the liver. Additionally, epinephrine secretion by the adrenal medulla is rapidly stimulated. Although it is generally held that epinephrine causes hepatic glycogenolysis, this is probably not true as the studies upon which this hypothesis is based were carried out using pharmacologic (not physiologic) amounts of epinephrine. Recent evidence suggests that epinephrine may stimulate glucagon secretion, which affects hepatic glycogenolysis. Epinephrine directly increases glucose concentrations by decreasing tissue utilization of glucose. This process may occur through a stimulation of muscle glycogenolysis, which causes a buildup of intracellular glucose-6-phosphate. This action in turn would inhibit phosphorylation of free intracellular glucose with a subsequent feedback inhibition on glucose transport into muscle. Epinephrine also counteracts hypoglycemia by increasing gluconeogenesis and by inhibiting endogenous insulin secretion (through an α-adrenergic effect).

Glucagon secretion is also rapidly stimulated. This effect may result from sympathetic nervous system activation through fibers originating in the hypothalamus and terminating in the pancreas; in addition, it may be secondary to circulating epinephrine, or it may occur through a direct metabolic effect of glucose deprivation in the α-cell. Glucagon increases glucose concentra-

Table 8–1.   Hormone Responses to Hypoglycemia

Hormone	Secretion	Action	Mechanism(s)
Epinephrine	Rapid	Rapid	Stimulates glucagon secretion
			Inhibits insulin secretion
			Inhibits glucose utilization by muscle
			Increases hepatic gluconeogenesis
Glucagon	Rapid	Rapid	Stimulates hepatic glycogenolysis
			Increases hepatic gluconeogenesis
Cortisol	Delayed	Probably immediate	Increases hepatic gluconeogenesis
			Inhibits glucose utilization by muscle(?)
Growth hormone	Delayed	Delayed	Inhibits glucose utilization by muscle
			Increases hepatic gluconeogenesis(?)

tions by stimulating hepatic glycogenolysis and gluconeogenesis. This hormone has no effect on peripheral tissue utilization of glucose.

Secretion of growth hormone (GH) and cortisol in response to hypoglycemia is delayed. During an insulin tolerance test, secretion of these two hormones occurs one half to one hour after the nadir of the glucose level. Hypoglycemia stimulates the hypothalamic releasing hormones, corticotropin-and GH-releasing factors. The latter factor acts directly on the pituitary to stimulate GH release. Corticotropin-releasing factor stimulates pituitary ACTH secretion, which in turn increases glucocorticoid output from the adrenal cortex.

The most important effect of cortisol is to increase gluconeogenesis, probably by stimulating glucogenic amino acid delivery to the liver. Cortisol also decreases peripheral tissue utilization of glucose. The most important effect of GH is to impair glucose utilization by peripheral tissues. It may also increase gluconeogenesis. Note that the effect of GH is delayed one to two hours after its secretion, but the effect lasts up to six hours. Thus, the body has a nicely orchestrated response to hypoglycemia: 2 hormones being secreted rapidly, both having a rapid effect that is quickly dissipated, and two hormones showing a delayed secretion, one of which has a further delay in its effect. Antihypoglycemic factors are working almost immediately after the perception of hypoglycemia by the hypothalamus until four to six hours later.

Signs and Symptoms

The signs and symptoms of hypoglycemia are due to both increased autonomic nervous system activity and depressed central nervous system activity. Since the hypothalamic glucoreceptors sense a decrement in glucose concentrations, signs and symptoms due to increased autonomic nervous system activity may occasionally be present with normoglycemia or even mild hyperglycemia, for example, in a diabetic with hyperglycemia who is given fast-acting insulin. On the other hand, if glucose concentrations decrease gradually, the autonomic nervous system may not be stimulated, and only the signs and symptoms of depressed central nervous system function may be present.

The signs and symptoms of increased autonomic nervous system activity include weakness, tingling of the fingers and around the mouth, sweating, tachycardia, feelings of anxiety, tremor, nervousness, and occasionally nausea and vomiting. Depressed central nervous system activity usually occurs only with an absolutely low level of glucose. The mild signs and symptoms associated with this situation include headache, visual disturbances, feeling of faintness, and mental confusion. More profound signs and symptoms are loss of consciousness, primitive movements such as sucking, grasping, or grimacing, tonic-clonic spasms, and hyperresponsiveness to pain. As the depth of hypoglycemic coma proceeds, positive Babinski signs, extensor spasm, decorticate posture, deep coma, shallow respiration, bradycardia, miosis followed by fixed dilated pupils, absent corneal reflexes, and finally death occur. Although mental deterioration, schizophrenia, hemiparesis or hemiplegia, aphasia, choreiform movements, epilepsy, narcolepsy, and Parkinsonism have been reported as possible permanent sequelae of hypoglycemia, it should be stressed that these conditions occur infrequently and only after repeated hypoglycemic episodes.

Classification

A functional classification of the common causes of adult hypoglycemia is given in Table 8–2. This classification separates the causes into fasting and fed hypoglycemias, a useful approach in the work-up of individual cases. It is extremely important to ascertain whether the hypoglycemia occurs in the fasting state (i.e., after an overnight fast or when a meal is missed) or only after eating. The fasting hypoglycemias occur much less frequently and are potentially much more serious than the fed hypoglycemias.

Fasting

The most common form of fasting hypoglycemia is due to drug ingestion. Most frequently this hypoglycemia is secondary to insulin administration in diabetics. Sulfonylurea drugs also cause hypoglycemia. Salicylates (in large amounts) are probably the next most common drug associated with hypoglycemia. They stimulate insulin secretion. Other drugs that are occasionally associated with hypoglycemia are monoamine oxidase inhibitors (which stimulate insulin secretion, at least in vitro), propranolol (which probably facilitates glucose utilization in the periphery), and oxytetracycline (unknown mechanism). Drug-induced hypoglycemia is often seen in the clinical setting of restricted carbohydrate intake (including missed meals), liver or renal dysfunction, and ethanol ingestion. The diagnosis is usually made by a careful history, and the treatment is to discontinue or decrease the drugs and/or to normalize food intake.

Ethanol interferes with hepatic gluconeogenesis even in the absence of liver disease. If alcohol is infused into normal subjects after an overnight fast, it has little effect on plasma glucose levels. However, after a 3-day fast in these same normal subjects, ethanol infusions caused a 30% decrease in fasting glucose levels. This decrease occurs because, after 3 days of caloric restric-

Table 8–2.   Differential Diagnosis of Hypoglycemia in the Adult

Fasting	Fed (Reactive)
Drug ingestion	Hyperalimentation
Ethanol ingestion	Impaired glucose tolerance*
Hepatic failure	Idiopathic reactive hypoglycemia ("functional")
Adrenal insufficiency ———————————————→	
Non β-cell tumors	
β-cell tumors ——————————————→	
(insulinomas)	

*Formerly called latent or chemical diabetes mellitus.

tion, maintenance of plasma glucose levels is critically dependent on hepatic gluconeogenesis. Any interference with this process leads to hypoglycemia. Many cases of drug-induced hypoglycemia are associated with ethanol intake, even in children. The diagnosis is made by a careful history, and the treatment is to reduce ethanol ingestion and to normalize food intake.

An important cause of fasting hypoglycemia is adrenal insufficiency. The mechanism by which this hormonal deficiency causes hypoglycemia is decreased hepatic gluconeogenesis. A high index of suspicion is often necessary for consideration of the diagnosis, which is made by appropriate testing of the pituitary-adrenal axis. Replacement with glucocorticoids is an effective treatment. Because patients with pituitary insufficiency who are treated with glucocorticoids do not have difficulties with hypoglycemia, it is unlikely (at least in the adult) that GH deficiency causes hypoglycemia.

Although hepatic failure is common, it is an unusual cause of fasting hypoglycemia because the liver has a remarkable ability to produce glucose. If the liver parenchyma has been destroyed to such a degree that hepatic glucose production is impaired, the prognosis for the patient is extremely poor. The diagnosis is usually not difficult as associated clinical signs and symptoms of hepatic failure are apparent. Grossly abnormal liver function tests confirm the diagnosis. Treatment consists of maintaining the patient on intravenous glucose with the hope that the liver will eventually regenerate.

Tumors that do not contain pancreatic β-cells are an important cause of fasting hypoglycemia. The most common are rare large mesenchymal tumors, which account for approximately 50 to 65% of the cases reported. These tumors weigh at least a kilogram and are located in the thorax, retroperitoneal space, or pelvic area. These mesenchymal tumors, many of which are benign, include mesotheliomas, fibrosarcomas, neurofibromas, neurofibrosarcomas, spindle cell sarcomas, leiomyosarcomas, and rhabdomyosarcomas. The next most common tumor causing hypoglycemia is hepatocellular carcinoma (hepatoma), which accounts for approximately 20 to 25% of the hypoglycemia associated with tumors. Adrenal carcinomas, gastrointestinal tumors, and lymphomas account for 5 to 10% each. Most other tumors have occasionally been associated with hypoglycemia. The most common of these are kidney and lung tumors, anaplastic carcinoma, and carcinoid tumors.

There is no agreement concerning the mechanisms whereby any of these non-β-cell tumors cause hypoglycemia. Although it is commonly held that glucose use by the large mesenchymal tumors eventually exceeds the ability of the liver to produce glucose and thereby leads to hypoglycemia, good evidence for this sequence of events is lacking. A possible explanation for many cases of tumor hypoglycemia is the synthesis and release of certain polypeptide growth factors that also induce hypoglycemia. A number of these compounds have both growth-promoting and insulin-like activities, some of which have been called somatomedins. Increased amounts of certain of these compounds have been found in the plasma of some patients with tumor hypoglycemia.

The diagnosis can be difficult. Large retroperitoneal tumors may cause deviation of the ureters that can be visualized by intravenous pyelography. Newer ultrasound and computerized scanning techniques may also prove helpful in diagnosing these tumors. Hepatic tumors may be diagnosed by hepatic scans and liver function tests. Adrenal carcinomas are sometimes associated with elevated urinary 17-ketosteroids (levels over 50 mg/day). Treatment of non-β-cell tumor-induced hypoglycemia may be difficult. Surgical removal is often helpful for the large mesenchymal tumors because enough tumor can be removed to ameliorate hypoglycemia for significant periods of time even though complete excision is usually not possible. Glucocorticoids or diazoxide, discussed later, can also be helpful in individual cases.

Although insulinomas (β-cell tumors) are rare, they are an important cause of fasting hypoglycemia. They are potentially curable and may have devastating effects on the patient if the diagnosis is missed. Of these patients, 80 to 90% have single tumors while 10 to 20% have multiple ones. Approximately 90% of these tumors are benign and 10% are malignant, although histologically this distinction can be difficult. Hyperplasia of the β-cell, as part of the multiple endocrine adenomatosis type I syndrome, is also seen rarely. The mechanism of the hypoglycemia is uncontrolled secretion of insulin.

The key to the diagnosis is the demonstration of an inappropriately high insulin level in the presence of an abnormally low glucose concentration. Therefore, the best test is a fast for up to 3 days, with glucose and insulin measurements taken every 2 to 4 hours while the patient is awake and 4 to 6 hours during sleep. This practice is in keeping with the basic endocrinologic tenet of diagnosing hyperfunctioning glands by suppression tests and hypofunctioning glands by stimulation tests. Fasting is an effective way to suppress the activity of the β-cell. A glucose (mg/100 ml)-insulin (μU/ml) ratio of less than 2.5 is suspicious. Because plasma glucose levels are 50 to 70 mg/100 ml and insulin concentrations are 5 to 10 μU/ml after 3 days of fasting in normal subjects, a false-positive glucose-insulin ratio of less than 2.5 would be unlikely. Hypoglycemia occurs within 24 hours in approximately two-thirds of patients with insulinomas. Within 48 hours over 95% of them manifest hypoglycemia. Fewer than 5% of patients with β-cell tumors need 3 days of total caloric deprivation to manifest hypoglycemia.

Proinsulin (see Fig. 8–7) normally constitutes less than 20% of the total plasma immunoreactive insulin concentration in the fasting state. In many patients with insulinoma, the proinsulin content of the fasting plasma may be 25 to 50% of the total insulin level. Patients with malignant insulinoma may have the highest amounts of proinsulin, 50 to 70% of the total insulin concentration. In the rare patient with an insulinoma in whom the glucose-insulin ratio during fasting does not meet the criteria previously discussed, the diagnosis can be made by demonstrating an elevated proinsulin level.

Although evaluating the glucose and insulin responses to intravenous tolbutamide, glucagon, and calcium as well as to oral leucine has been advocated to help diagnose an insulinoma, false-positive and false-negative results are common. Because normal, diabetic, and flat oral glucose tolerance test results are all seen in patients with β-cell tumors, this test is distinctly unrewarding in this situation and should be avoided.

If an insulinoma is suspected by virtue of the preceding tests, pancreatic arteriography should be carried out. It is positive in approximately 50% of the patients and may be helpful for the surgeon because many of these tumors are less than 2 centimeters in diameter. The inaccuracies of localizing insulinomas by arteriography have led to more sophisticated techniques. In some specialized centers, vessels draining parts of the pancreas are catheterized by a transhepatic approach, and samples are collected for measurement of insulin concentration. Much higher levels are present in the veins draining the tumor.

The treatment for insulinoma (assuming β-cell hyperplasia is not suspected because of associated tumors of the parathyroid and pituitary glands) is surgical extirpation. If the tumor cannot be localized at operation, a two-thirds distal pancreatectomy is usually recommended as these tumors are often so small that they can be found only by careful dissection in the pathology laboratory.

If surgical removal fails to cure the patient or metastatic disease is present, several drugs can be helpful. The one most commonly used is diazoxide (Proglycem), a benzothiadiazine that directly inhibits insulin secretion by the β-cell and blocks glucose utilization by stimulating catecholamine secretion from the adrenal medulla. For this purpose the drug is given orally, 100 mg 3 to 4 times a day. (An intravenous preparation of diazoxide, Hyperstat, is used to treat hypertensive crises.) The oral preparation has several side effects. In spite of its close molecular structure to the thiazide diuretics, diazoxide causes sodium retention, and a diuretic often has to be given with it. It also causes hyperuricemia, unexplained tachycardia, and excessive hair growth. If the tumor is malignant, an antitumor agent, streptozotocin, can be administered intravenously. It localizes in the β-cells of both the pancreas and metastatic tissue and destroys them. Even in the absence of treatment, metastatic insulinoma often progresses slowly.

Several rare causes of fasting hypoglycemia are not listed in Table 8–2. Hypothyroidism, a common endocrine disorder, has been associated with a few reported cases of hypoglycemia. Another cause is chronic renal failure, a common metabolic disorder, in which fasting hypoglycemia has been recognized occasionally. Isolated case reports document hypoglycemia in sepsis, in congestive heart failure associated with hepatic congestion, and in patients who inexplicably form autoantibodies against either their tissue insulin receptors or their endogenous insulin molecule.

Fed

The fed or reactive hypoglycemias are much more common than the fasting hypoglycemias. Of the five recognized causes, two can be dispensed with quickly. Although reactive hypoglycemia may occur in adrenal insufficiency

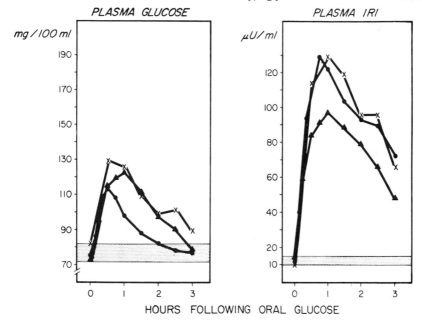

Figure 8–2. Plasma glucose and insulin responses to oral glucose in nonobese normal subjects. ●–●, n = 21; ▲–▲ ,n = 9; x – x, n = 17. (Results of three separate studies reviewed by Freinkel, N., and Metzger, B.F.: Reprinted, by permission, from N. Engl. J. Med., *280*:820, 1969.)

and with insulinomas, almost invariably the fasting component is also present. Therefore, the differential diagnosis of strictly fed hypoglycemia resides among three causes that are easily distinguished from each other.

The normal responses to an oral glucose challenge are peak glucose and insulin concentrations at one half to one hour, with a subsequent return toward fasting levels (Fig. 8–2). In the fed hypoglycemia seen after gastrectomy or a drainage procedure on the stomach (labeled in Fig. 8–3 as alimentary hyperglycemia), the mechanism appears to be the rapid absorption of glucose from the small intestine. This rapid absorption of glucose leads to an excessive insulin response and subsequent hypoglycemia occurring usually within two hours. The initial glucose levels are often high, sometimes exceeding 300 mg/100 ml. A diagnosis is easily made by taking a careful history.

The second cause of fed hypoglycemia is impaired glucose tolerance (formerly called latent or chemical diabetes mellitus and labeled in Figure 8–3 as diabetes.) The mechanism seems to be a delayed rise of insulin that peaks late (see Fig. 8–3). This delayed peak drives down the glucose concentration between 3 and 5 hours after carbohydrate ingestion. That the early glucose concentrations are higher than normal suggests the diagnosis of impaired glucose tolerance.

The third cause of reactive hypoglycemia is the most controversial. Formerly called functional hypoglycemia, it has recently been the subject of

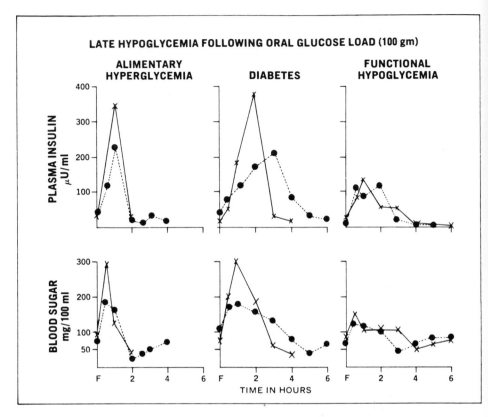

Figure 8–3. Glucose and insulin responses in reactive hypoglycemia. Each curve represents an individual patient. (From Conn, J.W., and Pek, S.: Current concepts: on spontaneous hypoglycemia. Scope monograph published by The Upjohn Co., Kalamazoo, Mich., 1970. Reproduced with permission.)

much publicity in the lay press. A better term is idiopathic reactive hypoglycemia. The pattern is one of normal glucose concentrations early in the glucose tolerance test with later hypoglycemia occurring 3 to 5 hours after oral administration of glucose (see Fig. 8–3). The mechanism is uncertain. Excessive insulin secretion can be shown in some patients and increased intestinal absorption of glucose in a few others. However, in most patients, the mechanism remains unknown. Idiopathic reactive hypoglycemia is uncommon. Overdiagnosis is due to the fact that low glucose levels 3 to 5 hours after oral glucose are a normal occurrence in the healthy population. Up to one-third of normal subjects, especially if they are young and overweight, have plasma glucose levels below 60 mg/100 ml after an oral glucose load. The reason for the overdiagnosis is that the signs and symptoms of anxiety and hypoglycemia are similar since they are both due, in large part, to excessive epinephrine secretion. Both patient and doctor, in seeking an organic cause for the various symptoms of psychoneurosis, have equated the commonly occurring low plasma glucose concentrations with the many psychogenic symptoms, which, unfortunately, are also common in our population. A flat oral glucose tolerance test, which is defined as less than a 20 mg/100 ml rise in glucose concentration at any time (including the $^1/_2$-hour sample) after oral carbohydrate, occurs in approximately 20% of the normal population and therefore does not indicate hypoglycemia.

To make a valid diagnosis of idiopathic reactive hypoglycemia, four criteria have to be met:

1. Hypoglycemia has to be documented (a plasma glucose level below 50 mg/100 ml or a whole blood glucose level below 40 mg/100 ml).
2. Symptoms of which the patient complains must occur at this time.
3. These symptoms have to be relieved quickly (within 10 to 20 minutes, not 1 to 2 hours) by eating.
4. This pattern (symptoms of hypoglycemia after meals, relieved quickly by eating) must be regular, rather than an isolated occurrence. If these criteria are followed, idiopathic reactive hypoglycemia occurs infrequently.

The treatment for all forms of reactive hypoglycemia is primarily dietary. A high protein, low carbohydrate diet (35% of calories derived from carbohydrate) is the treatment of choice. Simple carbohydrates must be avoided. Multiple feedings (5 to 6 times a day) are sometimes necessary, especially after a gastrectomy. Weight loss in patients with impaired glucose tolerance, who are often obese, is important. If these dietary measures fail, several drugs have been successful. Anticholinergic agents can be helpful, but their unpleasant side effects limit their use. Recently, propranolol has been found to be effective, for unknown reasons. Diazoxide and phenytoin (Dilantin), both of which directly inhibit insulin secretion, have occasionally been used.

DIABETES MELLITUS

Definition

Diabetes mellitus is a syndrome with both metabolic and vascular components that are probably interrelated. The *metabolic syndrome* is characterized by an inappropriate elevation of blood glucose concentrations associated with alterations in lipid and protein metabolism. The *vascular syndrome* consists of a nonspecific macroangiopathy (atherosclerosis) and a more specific microangiopathy, particularly affecting the eye and the kidney. The peripheral nervous system is also affected in a great many patients, although it is not certain whether this problem occurs on a vascular or metabolic basis. Evidence exists that both play a role.

Pathophysiology of Signs and Symptoms

To appreciate the pathophysiology of the signs and symptoms of the metabolic syndrome of diabetes mellitus, it is helpful to describe a gradual wors

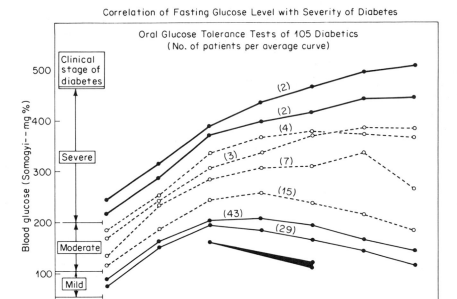

Correlation of Fasting Glucose Level with Severity of Diabetes

Figure 8–4. Oral glucose tolerance tests in 105 diabetics with varying degrees of carbohydrate abnormality. (The numbers in parentheses on each curve represent the number of patients per average curve.) (From Seltzer, H.S.: Diagnosis of diabetes. *In* Diabetes Mellitus: Theory and Practice. Edited by M. Ellenberg and H. Rifkin, 1970. Used with permission of McGraw-Hill Book Co.)

ening of glucose tolerance: from normalcy through mild to moderate glucose intolerance, progressing to fasting hyperglycemia, ketosis, and finally ketoacidosis. Most patients do not show this sort of progression. Many patients have impaired glucose tolerance and are asymptomatic. Some manifest fasting hyperglycemia and may be symptomatic. Most of these patients never become ketotic. A smaller number have ketosis, which may progress to frank ketoacidosis if not treated with insulin.

Oral glucose tolerance tests on diabetic patients with many degrees of carbohydrate abnormality are shown in Figure 8–4. The heavily shaded line between one and two hours is the upper limit of normal for blood glucose concentrations following a glucose challenge. The bottom two curves depicted in solid lines are examples of impaired glucose tolerance. These patients have no symptoms attributable to diabetes mellitus itself, but often manifest the signs and symptoms of accelerated atherosclerosis.

Moderate Glucose Intolerance

The patients whose glucose tolerance curves are depicted by dashed lines in Figure 8–4 have moderate glucose intolerance. These patients may complain of *fatigue*. If their postprandial glucose concentration exceeds the renal tubular threshold (T_m) for glucose (approximately 180 mg/100 ml in the presence of a normal glomerular filtration rate), they show glucosuria at that time. Remember, however, that the curves in Figure 8–4 depict the response to a large amount of simple carbohydrate, which is a much greater challenge to the pancreas than the usual meal containing much smaller amounts of complex carbohydrate. The sequence of events to be described concerns patients ingesting their usual diets. Patients who have enough effective insulin to keep their fasting glucose concentrations normal (lower two dashed curves in Fig. 8–4) usually do not have positive tests for glucose in the urine and are relatively asymptomatic.

Fasting Hyperglycemia

On the other hand, if patients have fasting hyperglycemia (upper two dashed curves in Fig. 8–4), their glucose concentrations during the day often exceed their T_m. Consequently, glucosuria may be a chronic condition and may lead to presence of glucose in the renal tubules that causes an osmotic diuresis. This mechanism accounts for a prevalent symptom in uncontrolled diabetes, *polyuria*. The resultant fluid loss through the kidneys leads to a mild state of

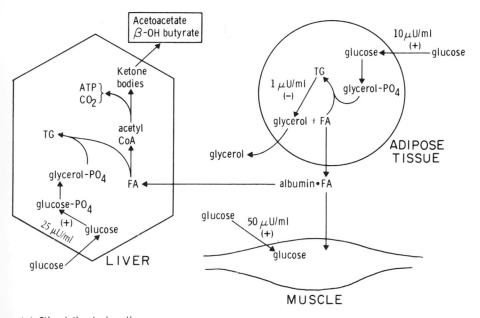

(+) Stimulation by insulin
(−) Inhibition by insulin
TG Triglyceride
FA Fatty acid

Figure 8–5. Pathophysiology of ketosis. (+), Stimulation by insulin; (−), inhibition by insulin; TG, triglyceride; FA, fatty acid. See text for discussion.

dehydration that the patient tries to correct by increasing water intake. This measure causes the second prevalent symptom of uncontrolled diabetes, *polydipsia*. Because of the decreased amount of effective insulin, the body is not able to use sufficient calories; this inability leads to the third prevalent symptom of uncontrolled diabetes, *polyphagia* (increased appetite) in the face of persistent weight loss. At this point, patients may show increased susceptibility to certain *infections*. Especially prominent are infections due to *Staphylococcus aureus,* which are marked by recurrent furuncles or carbuncles, and fungus infections, usually moniliasis, which appear as candidiasis of the vagina, nails, or occasionally the mouth (oral thrush). These patients may also have *blurring of vision* due to alterations in the shape of the lens that probably occur because of osmotic changes secondary to the hyperglycemia.

Ketosis

As the metabolic syndrome worsens because of less and less effective insulin, ketosis appears. Its mechanism is depicted in Figure 8–5. Insulin stimulates glucose uptake and utilization by muscle, liver, and adipose tissue. In muscle and adipose tissue, insulin stimulates glucose transport into the cells. The situation in the liver is more complex. Insulin increases the phosphorylation of glucose rather than its transport. In addition, through mechanisms that are not entirely clear, insulin also inhibits hepatic glucose production. In vitro studies have shown that concentrations of insulin that increase glucose utilization by tissues range from 10 to 50 μU/ml.

Insulin also plays a critical role in controlling lipolysis of adipose tissue triglyceride. This reaction is sensitive to insulin. In vitro studies show that only 1 μU/ml insulin is necessary to inhibit lipolysis. As discussed previously, the controlling factor for the production of ketone bodies is the amount of FFA delivered to the liver. Therefore, only when no effective insulin is left does uncontrolled lipolysis occur, flooding the liver with FFA and leading to an overproduction of ketone bodies. Put another way, as the amount of effective insulin becomes less and less, postprandial hyperglycemia supervenes because of the failure of glucose utilization by the tissues. Fasting hyperglycemia occurs when the amount of effective insulin remaining is unable to control hepatic glucose production. As long as any effective insulin is left, however, lipolysis is controlled and ketone body production remains normal. When an overproduction of ketone bodies does occur, effective insulin is essentially absent.

As more and more ketone bodies are produced, the peripheral tissues that use them soon become overwhelmed. They begin to accumulate and the patient then becomes ketotic. The only change in the signs and symptoms at this point is that polyphagia is no longer present because ketone bodies cause anorexia and mild nausea. Ketone bodies are acidic and therefore have to be buffered. As the body bases become depleted, the patient becomes acidotic. The acidosis due to an accumulation of ketone bodies is termed ketoacidosis, which is almost invariably due to diabetes mellitus.

Ketoacidosis

The pathophysiology of diabetic ketoacidosis is shown in Figure 8–6. This condition is the result of insulin deficiency affecting all three aspects of metabolism—carbohydrate, protein, and fat. Insulin deficiency decreases glucose uptake, which causes hyperglycemia and thus intensifies the osmotic diuresis that occurs with uncontrolled diabetes. Increased water loss ensues, producing dehydration. The osmotic diuresis also causes electrolyte depletion as sodium and potassium are swept along the renal tubules and cannot be reabsorbed. Insulin deficiency causes increased protein catabolism that leads to nitrogen loss (reflected clinically by weight loss) and increased circulating levels of amino acids. These serve as excellent gluconeogenic precursors, which tend to exacerbate the hyperglycemia. Insulin deficiency also causes uncontrolled lipolysis resulting in increased concentrations of both glycerol and FFA. Glycerol also serves as a gluconeogenic precursor leading to more hyperglycemia. Increased delivery of FFA to the liver results in increased ketone body production (ketogenesis) which soon leads to significant levels of ketone bodies in the circulation (ketonemia). These increased concentrations of ketone bodies spill over into the urine; this process exacerbates the electrolyte depletion as cations must be excreted with them. Most important, continued overproduction of ketone bodies leads to acidosis as the body bases become more and more depleted.

The symptoms of diabetic ketoacidosis are an intensification of the symptoms of uncontrolled diabetes (polyuria, polydipsia, weakness, and finally *anorexia* due to the ketosis) plus *nausea, vomiting,* and *abdominal pain.*

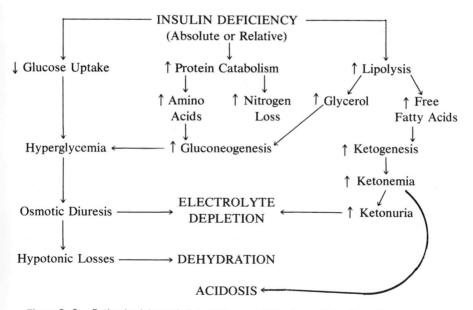

Figure 8–6. Pathophysiology of diabetic ketoacidosis. See text for discussion.

Diabetic ketoacidosis can cause severe gastrointestinal signs that may mimic a surgical emergency. In addition, patients may complain of *headache,* myalgia, and shortness of breath. In reality, they are simply overbreathing rather than experiencing significant dyspnea. The acidosis drives the respiratory center so that the resulting respiratory alkalosis helps compensate for the metabolic acidosis.

The signs of ketoacidosis are hypothermia (a fever usually indicates the presence of a significant infection), hyperpnea, or Kussmaul's respiration (the depth of respiration is important, not the rate, which is termed tachypnea), acetone odor on the breath, dehydration (intravascular volume depletion), hyporeflexia (associated with a low serum potassium), "surgical abdomen," hyptonia proceeding to stupor, coma, incoordination of ocular movements, fixed dilated pupils, and finally, death. The signs of dehydration are flat neck veins when lying horizontally (lack of filling of the neck veins from below to less than halfway up to the angle of the jaw) and orthostatic changes in blood pressure. Soft eyeballs, dry mouth, and "tenting" of the skin are late signs of dehydration in the adult.

The magnitude of urinary loss in a diabetic totally without insulin for 24 hours is considerable. Two kinds of experiments have been performed to assess this loss. In one, the amounts of fluid and electrolytes to replenish patients in diabetic ketoacidosis were measured. In the other kind, insulin therapy was discontinued temporarily in ketosis-prone diabetics and the actual losses were measured. The approximate amounts within 24 hours were: water—6.5 L, sodium—500 mEq, potassium—400 mEq, chloride—400 mEq, magnesium—50 mEq, and phosphorus—70mM.

Laboratory findings in patients with ketoacidosis are: increased glucose concentrations (usually between 300 and 800 mg/100 ml), ketonemia, decreased bicarbonate concentrations and pH, increased blood urea nitrogen (BUN) and creatinine (which may be prerenal, reflecting intravascular volume depletion), leukocytosis (even in the absence of infection), increased amylase (in the absence of documented pancreatitis), and increased plasma osmolality (up to 340 mOsm/kg). Potassium and sodium concentrations are variable. They may be low, normal, or high even though total body sodium and potassium stores are severely depleted.

The detailed treatment for this condition is beyond the scope of this chapter, but includes insulin, fluids (saline solution), and potassium. The need to administer a base (bicarbonate) remains controversial. The prognosis for patients in diabetic ketoacidosis is good. The mortality rate is approximately 5 to 10%, and a poor outcome is usually due to a complication rather than to the ketoacidosis itself. The prognosis is not correlated with the amount of acidosis, level of glucose, or any other biochemical parameter. It seems to correlate best with the age of the patient and the level of consciousness at the time of examination.

Patients who are in diabetic ketoacidosis need insulin therapy permanently. However, some patients who are initially in ketoacidosis may go through a "honeymoon" period. On recovery from the initial episode, their insulin requirements gradually decrease, and some are able to discontinue insulin entirely. During this period, the pancreatic β-cell partially recovers its ability to secrete insulin. This recovery is only temporary, and virtually all patients require insulin again, usually within 3 to 6 months.

Hyperosmolar Nonketotic Coma

Some patients are in hyperosmolar nonketotic coma rather than in diabetic ketoacidosis. The pathophysiology for this condition is also shown in Figure 8–6. If enough insulin is present to regulate lipolysis, the chain of events shown on the right side of the figure (i.e., increased lipolysis leading to ketogenesis and ketonuria with subsequent development of acidosis) does not occur. Insulin lack would affect carbohydrate and protein metabolism and would lead only to electrolyte depletion and dehydration. In the absence of the gastrointestinal symptoms caused by ketosis and ketoacidosis, patients may not seek medical attention. Then this sequence of events (hyperglycemia leading to dehydration and electrolyte depletion) occurs over a much longer period of time and leads to severe dehydration, which eventually impairs renal plasma flow. Less glucose is presented to the kidney, and renal losses of glucose do not keep pace with hepatic overproduction. Glucose concentrations may become high, sometimes exceeding 2000 mg/100 ml.

The signs and symptoms of hyperosmolar, nonketotic coma are marked polyuria, polydipsia, and lethargy. Most of these patients have an altered state of consciousness. In addition, many of them have *focal* neurologic findings; in fact many are diagnosed as having had a cerebrovascular accident. All have severe dehydration, and some may have abdominal tenderness.

The laboratory results are similar to diabetic ketoacidosis except that the glucose levels are usually higher, as explained previously. As expected, serum osmolalities are also more elevated (up to 450 mOsm/kg). The contribution of circulating glucose to serum osmolality can be calculated by dividing the glucose concentration by 18 (the molecular weight of glucose is 180). Bicarbonate concentrations and pH are often normal; however, there may be a mild decrease in pH and bicarbonate levels because classic hyperosmolar nonketotic coma and diabetic ketoacidosis simply represent 2 ends of a spectrum. Some patients may have mild ketoacidosis, but severe hyperglycemia. Evidence suggests that increased osmolality inhibits fat cell lipolysis independent of insulin. Therefore, the high plasma osmolalities attained probably contribute to the lower FFA levels and the lack of ketosis and acidosis in the syndrome of hyperosmolar nonketotic coma.

The prognosis in hyperosmolar nonketotic coma is usually not as good as in diabetic ketoacidosis because many of these patients are older and have other complicating diseases. Thrombosis with resultant emboli is an important complication. Of those patients who survive, a large percentage can be treated eventually with either oral hypoglycemic agents or diet alone. The treatment reflects that these patients are able to secrete some endogenous insulin and that, with proper attention to diet, their glucose levels can be controlled without exogenous insulin.

Classification

This classification of diabetes mellitus and other categories of glucose intolerance was developed by the National Diabetes Data Group of the National Institutes of Health. It is based on abnormalities of carbohydrate metabolism and does not consider the presence or absence of vascular disease. Patients with minimal glucose intolerance may have the large- and, much less commonly, small-vessel angiopathy associated with diabetes mellitus.

Diabetes Mellitus

Diabetes mellitus can be divided into three general types: an insulin-dependent type (IDDM) and non-insulin-dependent types (NIDDM). Former terminology for IDDM included juvenile-onset diabetes, ketosis-prone diabetes, and unstable diabetes. The new (rather nondescriptive) name is *type 1 diabetes mellitus*. The important metabolic characteristic of this type of diabetes is the presence of ketosis in the absence of treatment. Although the onset of type 1 diabetes is more frequent in childhood, adolescence, and young adulthood, it can also occur in the older patient.

Former terminology for NIDDM included adult-onset diabetes, maturity-onset diabetes, ketosis-resistant diabetes, and stable diabetes. When the disorder occurred in childhood and adolescence, it was termed maturity-onset diabetes of youth.The new name is *type 2 diabetes mellitus*. The important metabolic characteristic of this type of diabetes is the absence of ketosis. Although type 2 diabetes mellitus is much more common in individuals over the age of 40 years, it does occur in younger subjects. Most (80 to 90%) ketosis-resistant diabetics are obese. An occasional type 2 diabetic may temporarily become ketotic under great stress (trauma, infection, myocardial infarction), but this phenomenon is distinctly unusual.

The third kind of diabetes is now termed *other types*. It was formerly called secondary diabetes and included: (a) diseases of the pancreas that destroyed the β-cells (e.g., hemochromatosis, pancreatitis, cystic fibrosis); (b) hormonal syndromes (e.g., acromegaly, Cushing's syndrome, pheochromocytoma) that interfere with insulin secretion and/or inhibit insulin action; (c) drugs that may interfere with insulin secretion (e.g., phenytoin) or may inhibit insulin action (e.g., glucocorticoids, estrogens); (d) rare conditions involving abnormalities of the insulin receptor; and (e) a variety of rare genetic syndromes in which diabetes mellitus inexplicably occurs more frequently than in healthy persons.

Impaired Glucose Tolerance

The results of oral glucose tolerance tests in patients falling in this category are higher than normal, but fail to meet the criteria for diabetes mellitus. Former terminology included chemical, latent, subclinical, borderline, and asymptomatic diabetes. When the subjects are retested with an oral glucose challenge, even after many years, approximately 30% will have reverted to normal, 50% will continue to show impaired glucose tolerance, and the remaining 20% will be diabetic. Progression to overt diabetes in this latter population occurs at a low rate, 1 to 5% per year. Recent evidence suggests that patients with impaired glucose tolerance are unlikely to develop microangiopathic complications—retinopathy and nephropathy—of diabetes. However, these patients are prone to the macroangiopathic complications—coronary artery, peripheral vascular, and cerebrovascular disease.

Gestational Diabetes

The term *gestational diabetes* is reserved for women with the onset or the initial recognition of diabetes during pregnancy. Thus, diabetics who subsequently become pregnant are not included in this class. The precipitation of diabetes in susceptible women is thought to be due to the production of insulin-antagonistic hormones by the placenta. This disorder is associated with increased perinatal risks to the offspring and an increased risk to the mother for progression to diabetes mellitus within the next five to ten years. When the pregnancy ends, these patients will require reclassification into previous abnormality of glucose tolerance, impaired glucose tolerance, or diabetes mellitus, depending on the results of their postpartum evaluation.

Previous Abnormality of Glucose Tolerance

This class is restricted to persons whose glucose tolerance test at one time fulfilled the criteria for impaired glucose tolerance or diabetes mellitus, either spontaneously or in response to an identifiable stress, but who are currently normal. This group was formerly termed latent diabetes or prediabetes. Gestational diabetics are an obvious source for this class, as are formerly obese patients who have lost weight. Subjects undergoing acute stress due to trauma or illness may experience transient hyperglycemia and would fit into this category. With the exception of gestational diabetics, there has been little systematic study of the propensity of these subjects to subsequently develop diabetes mellitus. It is likely that the risk is increased, however, and these individuals should be monitored closely when they are in stressful situations.

Potential Abnormality of Glucose Tolerance

This class is reserved for individuals who have never exhibited abnormal glucose tolerance, but who have a substantially increased risk for the development of diabetes mellitus. The former term for this class was prediabetes or potential diabetes. Subjects who are at increased risk for type 1 diabetes include (in decreasing order of risk): persons with islet-cell antibodies; the monozygotic twin of a type 1 diabetic; the sibling of a type 1 diabetic, especially one with identical HLA haplotypes; and the offspring of a type 1 diabetic.

Individuals who are at increased risk for type 2 diabetes include (in decreasing order of risk): monozygotic twin of a type 2 diabetic; first-degree relative (sibling, parent, or offspring) of a type 2 diabetic; mother of a baby weighing more than 9 pounds at birth; obese subjects; and members of racial or ethnic groups with a high prevalence of type 2 diabetes (e.g., a number of Indian tribes). The actual degree of risk for any of these circumstances is not well established at the present time, however.

Diagnosis

It is important for physicians to be familiar with the site of sampling, the methods of measuring glucose used by the laboratory, and the nutritional and clinical (presence or absence of stress) status of the patient. They must also know whether plasma (or serum) or whole blood is used for the measurement of glucose before a valid interpretation of a glucose tolerance test can be made. The glucose oxidase method, which depends on an enzymatic degradation of glucose, is specific. Other methods give higher values (5 to 10 mg/ 100 ml) because certain circulating constituents (uric acid, creatinine, glutathione if the red blood cells are hemolyzed, fructose, and galactose) influence the results. However, this slight increase is not clinically important. (The older Folin-Wu method measures nonspecific reducing substances; consequently, the values are 20 to 30 mg/100 ml higher. This method should no longer be used.) Capillary blood obtained by finger or ear lobe puncture often gives higher values than those measured in venous samples because capillary samples consist, in large part, of arterial blood, and the peripheral tissues have not had a chance to extract the glucose. The difference between capillary and venous glucose levels is usually small in the fasting state, but may range up to 60 mg/100 ml (average 25 mg/100 ml) for several hours after a glucose challenge.

Diabetes Mellitus in Nonpregnant Adults

These recommendations were made by the National Diabetes Data Group for the diagnosis of diabetes mellitus in nonpregnant adults. Any of the following are considered diagnostic of diabetes:

1. Presence of the classic signs and/or symptoms of diabetes, such as polyuria, polydipsia, ketonuria, and rapid weight loss, together with gross and unequivocal elevation of plasma glucose concentrations.
2. Elevated fasting glucose concentration on more than one occasion:
   venous plasma $\geq$ 140 mg/100 ml
   venous whole blood $\geq$ 120 mg/100 ml
   capillary whole blood $\geq$ 120 mg/100 ml
   If the fasting glucose concentration meets this criterion, an oral glucose tolerance test is unnecessary because the results in virtually all patients will exceed the criteria in 3.

3. Fasting glucose concentration less than that diagnostic for diabetes, but sustained elevated glucose concentrations after an oral challenge on more than one occasion. *Both* the 2-hour value and another value obtained between the administration of the dextrose load and 2 hours later must meet the following criterion:

> venous plasma $\geqslant$ 200 mg/100 ml
> venous whole blood $\geqslant$ 180 mg/100 ml
> capillary whole blood $\geqslant$ 200 mg/100 ml

In nonpregnant subjects, the oral glucose tolerance test is carried out for only 2 hours with samples taken before ingestion of dextrose and at 30-minute intervals thereafter. The subjects should be fasted (water is allowed) for 10 to 16 hours before the administration of either 75 g glucose or 75 g carbohydrate equivalent (a more palatable solution of a mixture of polysaccharides quickly hydrolyzed to glucose in the intestine and liver). In children, the glucose challenge should be 1.75 g/kg ideal body weight up to a maximum of 75 g. The oral glucose tolerance test should be carried out in the morning; the subject should remain seated and should not smoke throughout the test. The test should only be performed in individuals who are normally active and who consume a diet containing > 150 g carbohydrate daily for at least 3 days prior to the test. Physical inactivity and low carbohydrate intake impair glucose tolerance. This response to a low carbohydrate diet has been called "starvation diabetes" and is probably secondary to impaired hepatic glucose uptake. Therefore, glucose concentrations in the peripheral blood are higher than if the normal amount of glucose had been deposited in the liver.

Impaired Glucose Tolerance in Nonpregnant Adults

Glucose concentrations must meet three criteria:

1. Fasting value:
   > venous plasma < 140 mg/100 ml
   > venous whole blood < 120 mg/100 ml
   > capillary whole blood < 120 mg/100 ml
2. Half-hour, 1-hour, or $1\frac{1}{2}$-hour value after 75 g oral glucose or its equivalent:
   > venous plasma $\geqslant$ 200 mg/100 ml
   > venous whole blood $\geqslant$ 180 mg/100 ml
   > capillary whole blood $\geqslant$ 200 mg/100 ml
3. Two-hour value after 75 g oral glucose or its equivalent:
   > venous plasma between 140 and 200 mg/100 ml
   > venous whole blood between 120 and 180 mg/100 ml
   > capillary whole blood between 140 and 200 mg/100 ml

Normal Glucose Levels in Nonpregnant Adults

Glucose concentrations must meet three criteria:

1. Fasting value:
     venous plasma $<$ 115 mg/100 ml
     venous whole blood $<$ 100 mg/100 ml
     capillary whole blood $<$ 100 mg/100 ml
2. Half-hour, 1-hour, or $1\frac{1}{2}$-hour value after 75 g oral glucose or its equivalent:
     venous plasma $<$ 200 mg/dl
     venous whole blood $<$ 180 mg/dl
     capillary whole blood $<$ 200 mg/dl
3. Two-hour glucose value after 75 g oral glucose or its equivalent:
     venous plasma $<$ 140 mg/100 ml
     venous whole blood $<$ 120 mg/100 ml
     capillary whole blood $<$ 140 mg/100 ml

Glucose values above these concentrations but below the criteria for diabetes or impaired glucose tolerance should be considered nondiagnostic, and these subjects should be followed more closely.

Gestational Diabetes Mellitus

The criteria for establishing the diagnosis of diabetes mellitus in pregnancy were not changed by the National Diabetes Data Group. A 100-g glucose (or its equivalent) load was retained, as well as sampling times before administration of the carbohydrate challenge and 1, 2, and 3 hours thereafter. The criteria that must be met to make a diagnosis of gestational diabetes mellitus are summarized in Table 8–3. Note that the fasting glucose concentration in pregnancy is lower than in the nonpregnant state. Therefore, fasting glucose values exceeding 140 mg/100 ml in plasma and 120 mg/100 ml in whole blood are certainly sufficient to diagnose diabetes in pregnancy as well as in nonpregnant individuals.

Children

The criteria for the diagnosis of diabetes mellitus in children are the same as in adults. For the diagnosis of impaired glucose tolerance in children, only the fasting and 2-hour glucose concentrations are considered, the values being

Table 8–3.   Criteria* for the Diagnosis of Gestational Diabetes Mellitus

	Venous plasma (mg/100 ml)	Venous whole blood (mg/100 ml)	Capillary whole blood (mg/100 ml)
Fasting	105	90	90
1-hr	190	170	190
2-hr	165	145	165
3-hr	145	125	145

*Two or more of the values must be met or exceeded.

the same as in adults. Normal glucose levels in children are also slightly different from those in adults, as follows:

1. Fasting value:
   venous plasma < 130 mg/100 ml
   venous whole blood < 115 mg/100 ml
   capillary whole blood < 115 mg/100 ml
2. Two-hour glucose value after 75 g oral glucose or its equivalent:
   venous plasma < 140 mg/100 ml
   venous whole blood < 120 mg/100 ml
   capillary whole blood < 140 mg/100 ml
   The National Diabetes Data Group did not include a value between 0 and 2 hours in the criteria for normalcy in children.

Two other situations deserve special mention. Persons who have undergone gastric operations have elevated glucose levels following an oral challenge (see Fig. 8–3). Therefore, an oral glucose tolerance test cannot be used to diagnose diabetes mellitus in these patients, and the fasting glucose concentration is the only criterion. Glucose tolerance deteriorates as individuals age. There is an approximate 10 mg/100 ml increase per decade an hour after a glucose challenge in adults. Many former critieria included a 10 mg/100 ml increase per decade in the upper limits of normal after the age of 50 years. The National Diabetes Data Group did not make such a recommendation, probably because their criteria are less sensitive (i.e., the glucose values are much higher) than previous ones. Fortunately, the fasting plasma glucose concentration rises only 1 to 2 mg/100 ml per decade. Therefore, as a diagnostic criterion for diabetes mellitus, it is virtually independent of age.

Pathogenesis

Type 1 diabetes is due to a profound impairment or an absence of insulin secretion secondary to β-cell destruction. Recent evidence implicates a combination of viral, immune, and genetic factors in the pathogenesis of at least some cases of this type of diabetes. It has long been suspected on clinical and experimental grounds that viral illnesses may be associated with type 1 diabetes. First, there are a number of isolated case reports of different viral syndromes preceding the onset of ketosis-prone diabetes by several weeks. Second, direct epidemiologic data relate the prevalence of new cases of type 1 diabetes in the winter months to seasonal changes of viral illnesses. Third, a similar direct relation exists between antibody titers to Coxsackie B virus (after viral infections, titers rise acutely and then fall) and the onset of new cases of type 1 diabetes. Fourth, certain strains of mice develop diabetes after infection with several different viruses. Direct proof that a virus may be implicated in the β-cell destruction of certain cases of ketosis-prone diabetes was furnished when a Coxsackie B virus was found in the pancreas of a ten-year-old boy who unfortunately died in the diabetic ketoacidosis that heralded the onset of his diabetes. Further, the virus isolated from his pancreas produced diabetes when injected into mice.

Obviously, most children recover fully from a viral illness and do not develop diabetes. Those who do, like the specific strain of mice that develop viral diabetes, may have a susceptibility related to their genetic constitution. Certain genes determine which surface antigens are produced by an individual's cells. These surface antigens are involved in the rejection process (when tissue from one host is transplanted into another). Their identification requires in vitro testing with white blood cells, and hence they are called human leukocyte antigens (HLA). Since many different surface antigens are possible in a population, a large number of separate genes (located on the short arm of the sixth chromosome in humans) are responsible for them. There are at least six different closely linked loci (currently called A, B, Bf, C, D, and DR) on this chromosome in the genetic region responsible for producing surface antigens. However, only a few HLA types are common in type 1 diabetics. This means that certain genes, the ones whose expression produces these HLA types, are also common in these patients and provide a marker for the genetic background that increases susceptibility to type 1 diabetes.

In Caucasian populations, type 1 diabetes is associated with an increased prevalence of HLA types B8, B15, B18, Dw3, Dw4, DRw3, and DRw4. In non-Caucasian populations, other HLA types are more commonly found in type 1 diabetics. It is unlikely that the HLA antigens themselves confer the susceptibility. Rather, they probably act as inert "markers" for the existence of disease susceptibility or immune response genes (see discussion following) that are in linkage disequilibrium with the HLA system. (Linkage disequilibrium is the tendency in a population for some alleles at closely linked loci to occur together in the same haplotype more often than expected by chance.) Further, because the association with type 1 diabetes is strongest for the D and DR alleles, it is also probable that significant increases in the HLA B alleles occur because of their proximity to the HLA D and DR regions with which they are in linkage disequilibrium. That is, the region on the short arm of the sixth human chromosome that is associated with susceptibility to type 1 diabetes seems to be closest to the HLA D and DR loci.

The HLA system in humans corresponds to the major histocompatibility system in animals. This chromosomal region consists of loci that not only control the synthesis of transplantation (surface) antigens, but also have fundamental roles in the immune process. Indeed, good evidence suggests that an immune process is active at the onset of type 1 diabetes. Lymphocytic infiltrates are seen in the islets of Langerhans of patients on whom an autopsy is performed soon after the diagnosis. Antibodies against islet cells are present in the sera of over 80% of type 1 patients if they are tested near the onset of their disease; a gradual reduction in antibody titers occurs over the ensuing year in most patients. However, islet-cell antibody titers are more likely to be sustained in diabetics with HLA types B8 and Dw3. These HLA types are also increased in patients with other autoimmune endocrine diseases (e.g., Hashimoto's thyroiditis and Addison's disease).

The following hypothesis is currently being considered. Certain individuals are susceptible to type 1 diabetes. When they contract a particular viral infection, their β-cells are damaged. Because β-cells do not have the capacity to regenerate, diabetes soon results. The insult to the β-cells could be due to the virus itself secondary to a compromised immune response. Alternatively, in the process of neutralizing the virus, the altered immune response could damage the β-cells. It is uncertain at present whether the islet-cell antibodies simply reflect damage to the β-cells or cause their destruction. This hypothesis, if true, probably does not explain all cases of type 1 diabetes; however, its importance lies in the eventual possibility of immunizing susceptible individuals, identified by HLA typing, against the viruses that could precipitate type 1 diabetes in them.

The pathogenesis of type 2 diabetes mellitus remains controversial. Some investigators believe that abnormalities of insulin secretion are the primary cause. Others hold that impairment of insulin action is responsible. Since the radioimmunoassay for insulin was introduced over 20 years ago, insulin secretion in diabetes has been studied extensively. Techniques to assess insulin action in patients have recently been developed, however, and this area is currently receiving considerable attention. Because type 2 diabetes mellitus represents a heterogenous disorder, both points of view may have merit.

Insulin Secretion

Insulin is a polypeptide hormone with a molecular weight of approximately 6000 (dark structure in Figure 8–7). It consists of an A and a B chain connected by 2 disulfide bridges. In addition, a disulfide bridge within the A chain connects amino acids 6 and 11. The synthesis and secretion of insulin by the β-cell of the pancreas are shown in Figure 8–8. Insulin is first synthesized in the rough endoplasmic reticulum as a single-chain polypeptide. In the Golgi apparatus of the cell, the single-chain polypeptide is aligned in such a way that the resultant A and B chains of insulin come into opposition to each other and the disulfide bridges between the 2 chains are formed. This molecule, known as proinsulin (entire structure in Figure 8–7), has a molecular weight of approximately 9000 and consists of the final insulin molecule connected by an amino acid chain termed the connecting (C-) peptide. Proinsulin is hydrolyzed by trypsin and carboxypeptidase in the Golgi apparatus. The resulting 2 molecules, insulin and the C-peptide (light structure in Figure 8–7), are packaged into secretory granules that are released into the cytoplasm of the cell. When insulin secretion is called for, the secretory granules are transferred to the plasma membrane of the cell through microtubules (not depicted in Fig. 8–8). Through the process of emiocytosis, insulin and the C-peptide with a small amount of intact proinsulin are extruded from the cell.

Proinsulin cross-reacts with insulin antibodies and is measured in the insulin immunoassay. It has only 10 to 20% of the biologic effectiveness of insulin. No evidence exists for increased secretion of proinsulin in diabetes mellitus. The C-peptide has no known biologic activity, but does serve as a marker

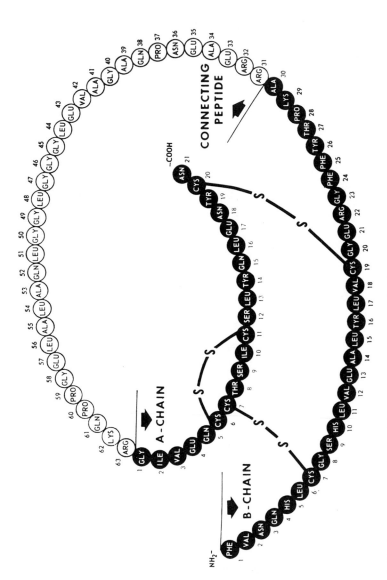

Figure 8–7. Structure of porcine proinsulin. Cleavage occurs at the straight lines, yielding equimolar amounts of the C-connecting peptide and insulin. (From Chance, R.E.: Diabetes, *21* (Suppl. 2): 461, 1972. Reproduced with permission.)

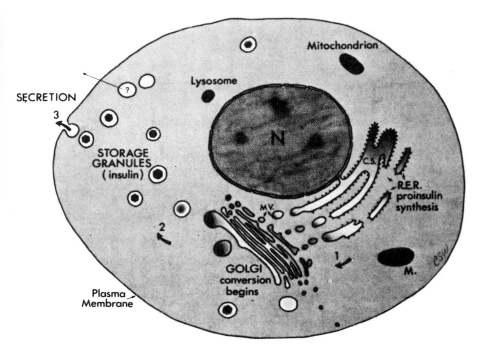

Figure 8–8. Schematic view of β-cell secretion of insulin. (M.V., microvesicle; R.E.R., rough endoplasmic reticulum; C.S., cisternal spaces of R.E.R.; 1, transport of proinsulin to Golgi apparatus; 2, transport of storage granules to plasma membrane; 3, transport of insulin into the extracellular space by emiocytosis. See text for discussion.) (From Kemmler, W., et al.: Diabetes, *21* (Suppl. 2): 572, 1972. Reproduced with permission.)

for insulin secretion because equimolar amounts are secreted by the β-cell. Insulin-treated diabetics all develop insulin-binding antibodies that interfere with the immunoassay of insulin. Therefore, measurement of C-peptide is useful for assessing insulin secretion in these patients.

Insulin stored in the granules of the pancreatic β-cells begins to be released within seconds of the receipt of the appropriate stimulus. This insulin constitutes the "quickly releasable" pool, which is emptied within minutes. Some stimuli (glucagon, intravenous tolbutamide, cyclic AMP, and isoproterenol) affect this pool only. The intravenous administration of glucose and certain amino acids also stimulates this pool; if these stimuli are continually applied, a second surge of insulin release occurs. This surge is thought to originate from a second pool, called the "slowly releasable" pool. This characteristic biphasic pattern of insulin release is depicted on the left side of Figure 8–9. In these experiments, glucose was given by a constant infusion to an isolated rat pancreas preparation. The right side of Figure 8–9 demonstrates an impairment of insulin secretion from the "slowly releasable" pool when puromycin, an inhibitor of protein synthesis, is added to the perfusate. Note that the "quickly releasable" pool is unaffected, as might be anticipated, because

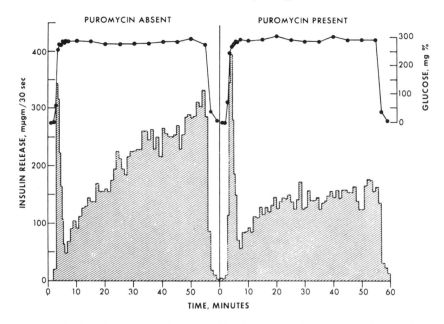

Figure 8–9. Insulin response (shaded area) to glucose perfusion (top curve) in the isolated rat pancreas. See text for discussion. (From Curry, D.L., et al.: Endocrinology, *83*:572, 1968. Reproduced with permission.)

insulin is already packaged in the granules waiting to be secreted. Therefore, continued exposure of the β-cell to glucose and amino acids results in synthesis of new insulin. This biphasic pattern of insulin release can also be demonstrated in humans after intravenous glucose and amino acids.

Insulin secretion in type 2 diabetes is variable. As shown in Figure 8–2, insulin concentrations normally reach their peak levels by 1 hr and return toward baseline values by 2 hr after an oral challenge. Because there is a delayed peak (maximal levels attained between 90 and 180 min) in many diabetic patients, both the timing and the magnitude of the response of insulin to oral stimuli are usually evaluated. The results of many studies are summarized in Table 8–4. Some of them include patients who would now be considered to have impaired glucose tolerance rather than their previous classification of latent diabetes mellitus. Although obesity, which is common in ketosis-resistant diabetes, is associated with increased insulin concentrations, this variable was taken into consideration in many of these studies. It is obvious that there are a variety of insulin responses, and controversy persists regarding a primary abnormality of insulin secretion in these patients. That type 2 diabetes probably represents a heterogenous group of disorders may explain the divergent results in Table 8–4.

Two other lines of evidence suggest that an abnormality of insulin secretion may be present in at least some of these patients. The sympathetic nervous system affects the response of the pancreatic β-cell; the α-adrenergic com-

Table 8–4.   Insulin Responses During Oral Glucose Tolerance Tests
in Patients with Type 2 Diabetes Mellitus*

Early†	Late‡
Delayed	Subnormal
Delayed	Normal
Delayed	Supernormal
Normal	Normal
Normal	Supernormal
Supernormal	Supernormal

*Some of these patients had chemical diabetes according to older classifications and would now be considered to have impaired glucose tolerance.
†Response between 0 and 60 min.
‡Response after 60 min.

ponent blocks insulin secretion while the β-adrenergic component stimulates it. A small amount of intravenous glucose injected over several minutes causes a rapid insulin response and return to baseline levels within a short period. This phenomenon probably represents secretion of insulin from the "quickly releasable" pool. No insulin response to this intravenous stimulus is present in type 2 diabetes. However, these patients do respond normally to intravenous isoproterenol (a β-adrenergic agonist), which also causes a short burst of insulin secretion. Many of them also respond normally to other nonglucose intravenous stimuli of insulin secretion, for example, tolbutamide and arginine. This response suggests that the pancreatic β-cell fails to recognize the glucose molecule, at least when administered in this manner.

The second line of evidence involves the effect of prostaglandins on insulin secretion. In humans, certain prostaglandins inhibit insulin release. When type 2 diabetics are given inhibitors of prostaglandin synthesis, their blunted insulin response to glucose returns toward normal. Thus, impaired insulin secretion may be important in the pathogenesis of some subsets of type 2 diabetes mellitus.

Insulin Antagonism

Two elegant techniques to measure insulin action in human subjects have recently been developed. In the steady state plasma glucose (SSPG) method, a solution containing glucose, insulin, epinephrine, and propranolol (a β-adrenergic antagonist) is infused intravenously. The α-adrenergic effect of epinephrine and propranolol inhibits endogenous insulin secretion. Similar steady state plasma insulin (SSPI) concentrations are attained in all subjects because the rate of exogenous insulin infusion is the same. The level at which the glucose concentrations reach a plateau is a measure of the effectiveness of the exogenous insulin. Thus, lower levels signal sensitivity to insulin, whereas higher glucose values denote an impaired response to insulin. In the second method, the euglycemic clamp technique, insulin is infused at a specified rate, and glucose concentrations are measured frequently. This information is used to adjust the rate of a glucose infusion to maintain plasma glucose concentrations at their basal levels. Because the glucose concentrations do not change, the amount of glucose infused must equal the amount of glucose disposed of by the tissues. The more glucose deposited into the tissues, the more sensitive the subject is to the infused insulin; the less glucose, the more insensitive to insulin.

Both the SSPG method (Fig. 8–10) and the euglycemic clamp technique (Fig. 8–11) demonstrate the presence of insulin antagonism in type 2 diabetics. This insensitivity to insulin seems to be above and beyond that due to the obesity that is often present. The binding of insulin to its receptor on the plasma membranes of cells, the first step in insulin action, is decreased in tissues from some of these patients. However, the assessment of insulin binding and its effects on the subsequent intracellular metabolism of glucose is extremely complex.

Investigators are finding abnormalities in insulin action and carbohydrate metabolism beyond the receptor (postreceptor defects) to explain the insulin

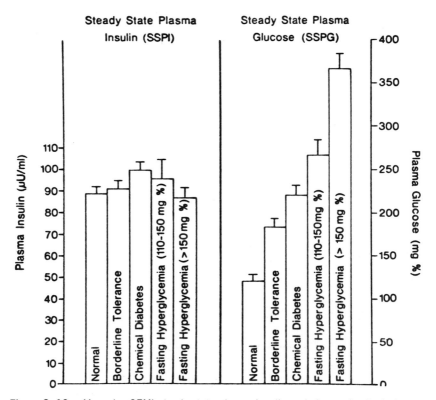

Figure 8–10. Mean (± SEM) steady-state plasma insulin and glucose levels during the infusion of epinephrine (6 μg/min), propranolol (0.08 mg/kg/min), insulin (80 μU/min), and glucose (6 mg/kg/min) in 5 groups of patients. (From Reaven, G.M. et al.: Am. J. Med., 60:80, 1976.)

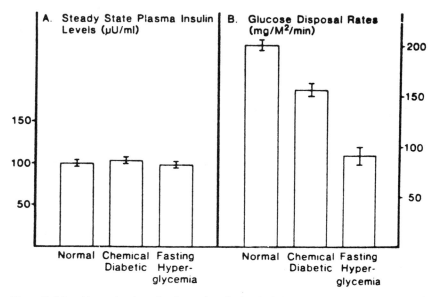

Figure 8–11. Mean steady-state plasma insulin levels *(A)* and glucose disposal rates *(B)* in normal subjects, patients with impaired glucose tolerance (chemical diabetics), and type 2 diabetics. Values obtained from euglycemic clamp studies. (From Olefsky, J.M.: Diabetes, *30*:148, 1981. Repoduced with permission from the American Diabetes Association, Inc.)

antagonism of many patients with type 2 diabetes. Thus, the results of studies evaluating both insulin secretion and insulin action suggest that type 2 diabetes mellitus is a heterogenous disorder.

Glucagon

The α-cells in the islets of Langerhans secrete glucagon, a hormone whose major function is to promote hepatic glucose production by both glycogenolysis and gluconeogenesis. Glucagon secretion is normally suppressed by glucose. In many diabetics, especially type 1 patients, basal glucagon levels are higher, and suppression of glucagon by glucose is impaired; that is, the concentration of glucagon does not decrease normally after glucose. Although it has been postulated that one of the primary abnormalities in diabetes may be an inability of the α-cell to respond normally to glucose, recent evidence suggests that the abnormality in glucagon secretion is secondary to the uncontrolled carbohydrate metabolism in diabetes. When animal and human diabetes is tightly controlled with insulin, glucagon levels and suppressibility return to normal. This finding suggests that the abnormality of glucagon homeostasis is simply secondary to the altered metabolism and does not constitute a primary lesion of diabetes mellitus.

Genetics

The inheritance of diabetes mellitus is probably the most controversial of all the many uncertainties surrounding this enigmatic syndrome. Indeed, it has been termed the "geneticist's nightmare." Familial aggregation (the tendency for diabetes to run in families) was first recorded in 1628. Modern studies have shown that overall the prevalence of diabetes is approximately fourfold higher in the parents of diabetics and ninefold higher in siblings of diabetics, as compared to nondiabetics. However, the inheritance of type 1 and type 2 diabetes is clearly different, as exemplified by the following discussion.

Monozygotic twins are genetically identical, whereas the genetic constitution of dizygotic twins is like that of any two siblings. A number of twinships have been identified in which one member has diabetes. If the other twin also has the disease, they are concordant for diabetes; if diabetes is not present, they are discordant for the trait. Monozygotic twins have a much higher concordance for diabetes than dizygotic twins. However, concordance is much different in identical twinships for type 1 and type 2 diabetics. In type 1 twinships, concordance is no more than 50%. Many of the nondiabetic twins have remained normal for 20 to 30 years; this finding strongly suggests that most of these twins will never develop diabetes. It seems probable that in type 1 diabetes, there is a genetic predisposition related to the HLA locus, as discussed previously. However, in order for diabetes to occur, an outside cause is required. In contrast, concordance in type 2 identical twinships approaches 100%, with the second twin developing diabetes shortly after the first one. As these twins are usually living apart for many years before the onset of type 2 diabetes, genetic, rather than environmental, factors must play an important role.

Thus, although the evidence is overwhelming that diabetes mellitus is "inherited," the heterogeneous nature of this disorder prevents a clearer understanding of its mode of transmission. Progress will only be made when homogeneous subsets of this syndrome can be identified and studied. This type of study was possible with young type 2 diabetics (originally called MODY—maturity-onset diabetes of the young) in whom ketosis-resistant diabetes could be traced back through 3 generations. This finding indicates an autosomal dominant inheritance in this small group of type 2 patients. In addition to heterogeneity complicating the genetic analysis of the remaining 90% of type 2 diabetics, certain environmental "stresses" (e.g., obesity, pregnancy, infection) seem to be important in the phenotypic expression of the genetic trait. This environmental influence could prevent the identification of all patients who may carry the gene(s). Until these problems can be resolved, diabetes mellitus will remain the "geneticist's nightmare."

Treatment

General Principles

Since the discovery of insulin in 1922, physicians have had an effective means of treating the metabolic aspect of the diabetic syndrome. The introduction of oral hypoglycemic agents in the 1950s and 1960s made the treatment of diabetes more convenient to the majority of patients, but did not effectively increase our means of controlling the disease. ("Control" in diabetics only refers to the lowering of glucose concentrations.) It has become more and more apparent that the vascular component of the diabetic syndrome is only imperfectly treated by present means.

When deciding upon treatment for patients with diabetes mellitus, it is helpful to divide them into two groups, those with ketosis-prone and those with ketosis-resistant diabetes. (Although ketosis-prone and ketosis-resistant diabetes are now called type 1 and type 2, respectively, the former terms will be used in this section to reinforce their metabolic difference as it pertains to treatment.) As discussed previously, ketosis-prone diabetics, those patients who routinely spill ketone bodies in their urine if left untreated, have virtually no effective endogenous insulin. Therefore, they must be treated with exogenous insulin. If insulin is withheld from these patients, they gradually slip into ketoacidosis, usually within 48 hours. Ketosis-resistant patients, those diabetics who do not have ketone bodies in their urine if left untreated, do not necessarily need insulin, although persistent hyperglycemia may require its use. The majority of these patients can be effectively treated with diet alone or with the addition of oral hypoglycemic agents. Ketosis-prone and ketosis-resistant diabetics also differ in a number of other aspects in addition to their need for insulin. These differences are summarized in Table 8–5.

The abnormality in carbohydrate metabolism is severe in ketosis-prone patients. If both food and insulin are withheld, they quickly become severely hyperglycemic and slip into ketoacidosis. Their response to stress, such as infection, is ketosis and eventually ketoacidosis. They are usually not obese, and probably for this reason are usually more sensitive to insulin than the ketosis-resistant diabetic. Because these patients have an absolute requirement for insulin, they have a negligible response to diet alone and no response to sulfonylurea agents.

The ketosis-resistant diabetic has many different characteristics. Although these patients have routinely been labeled as adult-onset or maturity-onset diabetics, these terms are misleading. A small number of adults develop ketosis-prone diabetes. Certain conditions such as pregnancy, obesity, infections, or other stress may precipitate ketosis-resistant diabetes. Probably only susceptible individuals acquire diabetes mellitus when exposed to these precipitating factors. Because significant amounts of insulin are present in these patients, it is not surprising that pancreases of ketosis-resistant diabetics contain a relatively normal amount of insulin. The carbohydrate abnormality is usually less severe. As opposed to the ketosis-prone diabetic, prolonged fasting without therapy improves their glucose metabolism. These patients respond to stress by becoming hyperglycemic, but only rarely do they become ketotic. Obesity is commonly associated with ketosis-resistant diabetes, being present in approximately 80% of patients. This factor probably explains their greater requirement for insulin than that of the ketosis-prone diabetic. These

Table 8–5. Functional Classification of Diabetes Mellitus

Characteristic	Classification	
	Ketosis-Prone *(type 1)*	Ketosis-Resistant *(type 2)*
Synonyms*	Juvenile-onset diabetes, growth-onset diabetes	Adult-onset diabetes, maturity-onset diabetes
Age of onset	Usually during growth	Usually during maturity, increasing with age
Precipitating factors	Altered immune response to certain viruses (?)	Pregnancy, obesity, "stress" (e.g., infection)
Extractable pancreatic insulin	Low	Normal
Fasting insulin level	Absent or low	Low to normal (when adjusted for weight and glucose level)
Insulin responses to glucose	Little or none	Delayed and probably low when adjusted for weight and glucose levels in some patients (see Table 8–4)
Insulin antagonism	Absent	Present (independent of obesity)
Fasting glucose level	Markedly elevated	Often near normal
Carbohydrate intolerance	Severe	Moderate to severe
Response to prolonged fast	Hyperglycemia, ketoacidosis	Normal adjustment established
Response to stress	Hyperglycemia, ketoacidosis	Hyperglycemia without ketosis
Associated obesity	Absent	Commonly present (~80%)
Sensitivity to insulin	Sensitive	Relatively resistant because of associated obesity
Response to diet alone	Negligible	Present to some degree
Response to sulfonylurea agents	Absent	Present to some degree

*Although these terms have been used classically to refer to the two types of diabetes mellitus, they are inaccurate because some children and adolescents are ketosis-resistant and some adults are ketosis-prone.

(Modified from Goodner, C.J.: New Concepts in Diabetes Mellitus, Including Management. Edited by H.F. Dowling. Disease-a-Month, September, 1965. Copyright 1965 by Year Book Medical Publishers, Inc., Chicago.)

patients always respond somewhat to diet, and many of them also respond to the oral hypoglycemic agents.

The prevalence of ketosis-prone and ketosis-resistant diabetes among the diabetic population is shown in Figure 8–12. Ketosis-prone diabetics are only a minority. In addition, only a small percentage of ketosis-resistant diabetics become symptomatic if not treated with insulin. Although these are often the

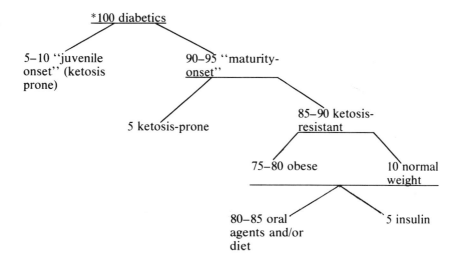

Figure 8–12.   Distribution of ketosis-prone versus ketosis-resistant diabetes in hypothetic population of 100 patients.
*Recently recognized that ketosis-resistant diabetes occurs in older children and adolescents (MODY). These patients and their families may account for up to 10% of all type 2 diabetics. Prevalence of this is unknown at present.

normal-weight patients, they are not always. Therefore, the majority of the diabetic population should be treated with diet alone. If they fail on this therapy, they may be candidates for oral hypoglycemic agents. Only a minority requires insulin.

Diet

This key element in the therapy of the diabetic has a different role in those taking insulin as compared to those who are not. In the insulin-requiring diabetic, the primary importance of the diet is to furnish a similar number of calories at the same time each day in order to "buffer" the insulin that is absorbed from the injection site at a predetermined rate depending on the kind and amount used. It is also important to avoid large amounts of simple carbohydrates (mono- and disaccharides) that are rapidly absorbed and cause severe postprandial hyperglycemia. Since the pancreas is unable to respond to this stimulus, the patient loses these calories through glucosuria (sometimes causing polyuria). "Complex" carbohydrates (starch) are perfectly acceptable in the diabetic diet and are vitally important to it.

In the ketosis-resistant diabetic, the primary role of the diet is to reduce the number of calories in those patients (approximately 80%) who are obese. It is also important in all ketosis-resistant diabetics to avoid large amounts of simple carbohydrates for the reason just given. This factor is not as critical because the pancreas of the ketosis-resistant diabetic does respond somewhat. The overall goal of diet therapy is to provide the patient with balanced nutrition, for proper growth and development in the child and adolescent and for weight reduction in the obese diabetic.

Caloric Breakdown. The method of calculating the diet for the adolescent and adult is the same whether the patient is a ketosis-prone or ketosis-resistant diabetic. The principles of ordering diets are a neglected aspect of medical education. For this reason one method of ordering a diet for adults is described here. These principles apply to nondiabetics as well as to diabetics.

The first step is to determine the ideal body weight of the individual. For a female, 100 pounds is allowed for height of 5 feet and 5 pounds for each additional inch. In a male, 106 pounds is allowed for height of 5 feet, with 6 pounds for each additional inch. If the individual has a large frame, add 10%; for a small frame, subtract 10% from the calculated ideal body weight. The total number of calories that the individual should ingest is considered next. To maintain ideal body weight, 30 calories per kilogram (cal/kg) is allowed. In obese patients 20 cal/kg is prescribed for weight loss. For those individuals who need to gain weight, those who are in late adolescence and still have not finished growing and those with increased physical activity, 40 cal/kg is prescribed. Therefore, change the pounds of ideal weight into kilograms (1 kg equals 2.2 lb) and calculate the total calories.

Alternatively, pounds can be used directly; the corresponding number of calories is 10 cal/lb for weight loss, 15 cal/lb to maintain weight, and 20 cal/lb to gain weight, for adolescents, or for those with marked physical activity. Round off (with either method) to the nearest 50 cal. Although the total number of calories differs between calculations based on pounds and those for kilograms, this difference is of little practical importance because adherence to the diet is not that precise. It should be stressed that these are caloric requirements per unit of *ideal body weight.* Finally, the number of calories should be lowered by 10% for each decade after the age of 50 years because of the decreases in physical activity, lean body mass, and resting metabolic rates that are associated with aging (e.g., 10% for patients between 51 and 60 years, 20% for those between 61 and 70 years).

The next step is to calculate the breakdown of calories between carbohydrate, fat, and protein. One gram of carbohydrate or protein provides approximately 4 cal, whereas 1 g fat gives approximately 9 cal. In the "typical" American diet today, over 50% of the calories are derived from carbohydrate. In order to increase compliance with the prescribed diet, I routinely order a diet containing 50% carbohydrate, 17% protein, and 33% fat with limitation of saturated fat to one-third the total amount of dietary fat and cholesterol intake to approximately 300 mg/day. Much evidence suggests that this decreased intake of saturated fat and cholesterol may be helpful in preventing atherosclerosis, which is more common in diabetics. Of the 50% of calories derived from carbohydrate, 35 to 40% should be in the complex form and only 10 to 15% in the simple form. Simple or refined carbohydrate (mono-

and disaccharides, which usually constitute half the carbohydrate intake in the "typical" American diet) are absorbed quickly from the gastrointestinal tract. Because the pancreatic β-cell cannot quickly respond with effective insulin to this stimulus, plasma glucose continues to rise and leads to marked hyperglycemia. Complex carbohydrates are hydrolyzed and absorbed more slowly from the gastrointestinal tract, and this process limits postprandial hyperglycemia.

This diet falls within the guidelines suggested by the American Diabetes Association (ADA), which are that 50 to 60% of the total calories should be derived from carbohydrates, 12 to 20% from protein, and approximately 30% from fat. Simple carbohydrates, saturated fat, and cholesterol are to be limited. Many physicians simply order an ADA diet of the appropriate number of calories.

Because most diabetics are obese and therefore require a hypocaloric diet, it is important for both the physician and the patient to have realistic expectations concerning the response to such diets. The "average" sedentary person uses approximately 500 cal/day more than is provided by the hypocaloric diets calculated as described. Because 1 lb fat equals 453 g, this amount of fat will furnish approximately 4000 cal (9 × 453). Therefore, patients will lose approximately 1 lb/wk. This may not seem like much, but 50 lb/yr is a safe way to lose weight. Weight loss during the first week, however, is usually much greater because most patients are also decreasing their carbohydrate intake. Lowered dietary carbohydrate, regardless of total caloric intake, results in a diuresis. Conversely, increased carbohydrate intake leads to retention of sodium and water and causes a weight gain disproportionate to the extra caloric intake. Patients should be warned of these changes in sodium and water balance so that they neither have unrealistic expectations of weight loss after the first several weeks on a hypocaloric diet nor become discouraged by the amount of weight gain should they temporarily stray from their diets.

Under ideal circumstances, a physician should offer the patient a detailed discussion about the ingredients of the diet. In practice this discussion is not feasible because the expertise required concerning the various foods and their contents and the time needed to communicate this kind of information are not available to the physician. Therefore, effective use of dieticians is extremely important in caring for diabetic patients. The dieticians take the calculated diet and translate it into the kind and amounts of food that the diabetic should eat. Usually the dietician divides the foods into six general groups called "exchange lists" (Table 8–6). Foods in the same list contain similar amounts of carbohydrate, protein, and fat. The individual diet prescribed would contain the designated amounts of the three foodstuffs. The patient can then vary the diet without changing its overall composition simply by switching or exchanging foods within the same list. Exchange lists have been devised to account for the food preferences of different ethnic groups. In this way, the patient with diabetes is able to eat a proper diet under a variety of circumstances and with differing personal preferences.

Table 8–6.   Exchange Lists for Diabetic Diets

List	Exchange lists	Food type	Amount	Carbohydrates (g)	Protein (g)	Fat (g)	Total calories
1	Milk	Whole milk	1 cup	12	8	10	170
2A	Vegetables		Freely	0	0	0	0
2B	Vegetables		1/2 cup	7	2	0	35
3	Fruit	Orange	1 small	10	0	0	40
4	Bread	Bread	1 slice	15	2	0	70
5	Meat	Meat	1 ounce	0	7	5	75
6	Fat	Butter	1 teaspoon	0	0	5	45

(Modified from "Meal Planning with Exchange Lists." American Dietetic Association, 620 N. Michigan Ave., Chicago, IL 60611, or the American Diabetes Association, 1 W. 48th St., New York, NY 10020.)

Table 8–7.   Approximate Time-Activity Relation of Various Insulin Preparations

Kind of Insulin	Preparation	Onset of Action (hr)	Maximal Action (hr)	Total Duration of Action (hr)
Short-acting	Regular*	0.5–1	2–4†	4–6
	Semilente	1–2	3–6	8–12
Intermediate-acting	NPH‡	3–4	10–16	20–24
	Lente	3–4	10–16	20–24
Long-acting	PZI§	6–8	14–20	>32
	Ultralente	6–8	14–20	>32

*Also called crystalline zinc insulin (CZI).
†In some patients, the action of regular insulin may peak later than indicated here (between 4 and 8 hr) and may last considerably longer. Therefore, addition of regular insulin to intermediate-acting insulin may cause afternoon hypoglycemia in these patients.
‡Neutral protamine Hagedorn.
§Protamine zinc insulin.

Insulin Preparations

Insulin preparations are currently packaged as U-100 or U-40, which simply means 100 units (U)/ml or 40 U/ml. Currently, 90% of the insulin used in the United States is U-100 insulin. If a patient injects 0.2 ml U-100 insulin, he receives 20 U of insulin. Patients are not required to make this kind of calculation as the units are marked on the syringes. Thus, patients taking a specific kind of insulin must use the appropriate syringe; i.e., U-40 insulin must be drawn into a U-40 syringe.

The properties of different kinds of insulin are summarized in Table 8–7. The time intervals in the table are only approximations because individuals have significant biologic variations in their response to insulin. In the Lente series of insulins, the size of the crystals determines the rate of absorption from the injection site. Lente is seven parts of Ultralente and three parts of Semilente. With neutral protamine Hagedorn (NPH) insulin, the protamine in the preparation delays absorption. The amount of protamine is carefully titrated to equal the amount of insulin so that, if regular insulin were added to the same syringe, it would exert a rapid-acting insulin effect in the patient. (Hagedorn is the name of the man who developed this insulin preparation.) With protamine zinc insulin (PZI), an excess amount of protamine is present in the preparation that delays the absorption from the subcutaneous site even more than in the case of NPH insulin.

As long as the physician and (probably more important) the patient are knowledgeable concerning the properties of the insulin preparation(s) used, it makes little difference which insulin or combination of insulins is chosen. Many different kinds of regimens might be acceptable. I prefer the following method for treating diabetic patients with insulin. First, I usually do not use the long-acting insulin preparations, mainly because their action peaks at times of little or no food intake. Either NPH or Lente may be used for an intermediate-acting insulin since their time courses of action are virtually identical. Although theoretically the foreign protein, protamine, is a possible antigen, allergies to this constituent of the NPH preparation have been reported in only one patient. I usually use regular insulin as a short-acting insulin in the same syringe containing NPH or Lente insulin. Semilente can be used, but its greater delay in onset and its longer duration of action make it less appropriate for use as a fast-acting insulin.

Determination of Dose. The general approach is first to establish the amount of intermediate-acting insulin that is necessary to control the patient's diabetes. When the dose of intermediate-acting insulin has been established, rapid-acting insulin is added. I routinely start most patients on two injections of insulin per day for two reasons. With a split dose of insulin, not only is tighter control easier to attain, but the patient has more flexibility than if one morning injection is given. The intermediate-acting insulin (NPH or Lente) taken before breakfast has a peak activity in the late afternoon or early evening and consequently the before-supper test best reflects its effectiveness. The fasting test best reflects the activity of the NPH insulin given before supper. In general, two-thirds to three-quarters of the total intermediate-acting insulin dose is given in the morning and the remainder in the evening.

The initial dose of intermediate-acting insulin is empiric. With lean diabetics (type 1 or type 2), I usually start with 8 to 10 U NPH insulin in the morning and 4 to 5 U NPH insulin before supper. These amounts are increased gradually by 4 to 5 U depending on the results of the appropriate tests. Thus, they may be adjusted independently of each other. With obese patients ($>125\%$ of ideal body weight), I usually start with 20 U NPH insulin in the morning and 10 U of the same preparation in the evening. Adjustments are made in 8- to 10-U increments. Greater amounts are necessary because of the insulin antagonism associated with obesity.

Only when the amount of intermediate-acting insulin is established should short-acting insulin be added. As a general guide, the dose of intermediate-acting insulin is established when the fasting and before-supper plasma glucose concentrations are less than 200 mg/100 ml. At this point, the need for regular insulin is assessed. Because there is a 3- to 4-hour lag period before intermediate-acting insulin starts to work effectively, most patients require some short-acting (regular) insulin to prevent postprandial hyperglycemia after breakfast. Since regular insulin usually has a peak activity 2 to 4 hours later, the results of the before-lunch test indicate the need for it. Many patients also require a small amount of regular insulin before supper. This meal usually contains the largest number of calories, at least in the United States. Although the NPH insulin given before breakfast has a peak activity at this time, it is often insufficient to prevent postprandial (supper) hyperglycemia. The lag period of the NPH insulin injected before supper prevents it from being effective at this time. Therefore, the results of the test performed before the bedtime snack may indicate the need for some regular insulin before supper. I usually start with 4 to 5 U regular insulin in lean patients and 8 to 10 U in obese individuals (before one or both meals as required). These amounts are increased gradually (by 4 to 5 U in both types of patients), as indicated by the results of the tests carried out before lunch and before the bedtime snack.

I often start older patients on a single morning injection. Because cerebral vascular disease is more likely, hypoglycemia may be more harmful to these patients. If it is caused by the evening injection, it will occur in the middle of the night and may be unrecognized. That hypoglycemia secondary to the morning injection usually occurs during the day or evening facilitates its recognition and treatment. Both the before-supper and the following day's before-breakfast test reflect the activity of morning NPH insulin. Usually the before-supper test responds before the fasting test. Increasing the NPH insulin dose in an effort to improve the fasting test often causes hypoglycemia during the afternoon. A midafternoon snack may prevent this response. If this regimen is unsuccessful, one must either accept fasting hyperglycemia or switch the patient to two injections a day. Once the amount of morning intermediate-acting insulin is established, regular insulin is usually added to the morning injection as determined by the results of the before-lunch test.

Exercise is an important part of the treatment of diabetes because it increases muscle utilization of glucose. Recent evidence suggests that exercise releases insulin from peripheral tissues (even in nondiabetics) where apparently it is bound but ineffective. Exercise also increases the rate of absorption of insulin from the injection site. Therefore, the diabetic must be aware of the effect of exercise on glucose levels. To avoid hypoglycemia, the patient should be instructed to eat a small snack before engaging in unusual exercise. Because activity is limited in the hospital, the final adjustments of insulin dose should be made when patients are at home. In addition, differences in the amount and timing of the diet often occur when the patient returns home. Both diet and exercise are critical determinants of the insulin dosage.

Side Effects. Certain untoward effects of insulin should be kept in mind.

SOMOGYI EFFECT. Although insulin can cause hypoglycemia, too much insulin can also be associated with high blood sugar levels. This paradox is known as the Somogyi effect or posthypoglycemic hyperglycemia. The mechanism for this effect is straightforward. The hormonal responses to hypoglycemia all counteract the effect of insulin. Therefore, following an episode of hypoglycemia, the patient's diabetes is often temporarily out of control because the effect of the administered insulin is antagonized. If too much insulin is administered on a long-term basis, the diabetes remains out of control. Classically, the pattern involves unsatisfactory fasting tests due to unrecognized hypoglycemia while the patient is asleep. When the amount of intermediate-acting insulin is raised to control the unsatisfactory before-breakfast test, the situation worsens, as one might expect.

The Somogyi effect is uncommon. Most patients whose diabetes is out of control need more insulin, not less. A high index of suspicion is necessary to diagnose posthypoglycemic hyperglycemia. Several clinical clues should arouse suspicion. The most common one is rapidly changing urine tests within 4 to 6 hours. Ketonuria is often noted in this situation. Patients whose urine tests are all strongly positive for glucose almost assuredly do not have the Somogyi effect. Morning headache is a subtle clue that hypoglycemia is occurring during the night. Hypothermia is also another manifestation of hypoglycemia, but temperatures on arising are usually not taken. If the Somogyi effect is suspected, it next must be documented. The patient must wake up at night and test a double-voided urine sample. If the patient is in the hospital, a blood glucose measurement should be made at the appropriate time.

Treatment for posthypoglycemic hyperglycemia is to lower the amount of insulin—gradually. For reasons that are not entirely clear, if insulin is quickly lowered by 15 or 20 U, the diabetes often remains out of control even though the amount of insulin given is eventually found to be appropriate. For instance, if the patient is taking 80 U insulin a day and the Somogyi effect is documented, the proper response is to give 5 U less each day until the appropriate amount is reached. If the amount of insulin is lowered from 80 to 55 U, the diabetes stays out of control, and the insulin has to be raised again and lowered gradually.

LOCAL DERMAL REACTIONS. When patients were initially treated, they often had local reactions several hours later at the sites of insulin injections. These are 2- to 3-cm erythematous pruritic papules that gradually disappear over the next several days. This reaction seems to be a delayed sensitivity response to impurities in the insulin preparations and gradually wanes over the next several months. These reactions should become much less common with the recent increase in purity (approximately 99% pure) of the new insulin preparations.

ALLERGY. True allergy to the insulin molecule is fortunately uncommon (approximately 0.1% of insulin-requiring patients). Within 30 to 60 minutes a local reaction occurs at the site of injection and soon spreads into a generalized urticarial pattern. Insulin allergy and penicillin allergy have many features in common: occasional angioneurotic edema and/or anaphylactic shock; positive intradermal, conjunctival, and Prausnitz-Küstner tests; generation of IgE antibodies; and treatment by desensitization.

INSULIN RESISTANCE. This phenomenon should not be confused with insulin allergy. Insulin resistance is defined as an insulin requirement of over 200 U/day for several days. This definition from the early 1940s is based on the erroneous assumption that the usual amount of insulin secreted was approximately 200 U/day. It is now known that the normal pancreas secretes only 20 to 40 U/day insulin. However, the preceding definition has stood the test of time. Conditions associated with insulin resistance are: infection, gross obesity, Cushing's syndrome, acromegaly, hemochromatosis, lipoatrophic diabetes, acanthosis nigricans, and Werner's syndrome.

Infection and gross obesity are well-documented causes of insulin antagonism and are responsible for most cases of insulin resistance. The mechanisms by which they interfere with the action of insulin are unknown. Cushing's syndrome (excess glucocorticoid) and acromegaly (excess GH) are occasionally associated with high insulin requirements. Insulin resistance has been reported in a few cases of hemochromatosis. Lipoatrophic diabetes is an unusual form of diabetes in which patients show absence of subcutaneous fat, hyperlipidemia, hepatomegaly, and insulin resistance with no tendency to develop ketosis. In several cases of insulin resistance associated with acanthosis nigricans, thousands of units of insulin have been administered with little effect. An antibody to the insulin receptor that blocks the action of insulin is present in some of these cases. Werner's syndrome is a rare inherited disorder characterized by short stature, slender extremities but stocky trunk, premature grayness and baldness, scleroderma with ulceration over the fingers, heels, and toes, cataracts, diabetes, and premature death due to atherosclerosis; the diabetes is usually mild, but resistance is frequently present.

In the absence of any of these conditions, immune-mediated insulin resistance is present. This resistance is the most frequent kind after that caused by obesity and infection and is often associated with intermittent insulin therapy (as is insulin allergy). When insulin is injected over a period of several months, insulin-binding (IgG) antibodies are generated in the recipient—in animals, in nondiabetic humans, and in all diabetics taking insulin. Recently insulin preparations of greater than 99% purity have been shown to possess few antigenic properties. Thus, it is the impurities in the insulin preparation that probably trigger antibody formation. Occasionally, these antibody titers in patients rise to high levels for unknown reasons. This rise is the cause of the high insulin requirement in immune-mediated insulin resistance, which fortunately occurs rarely (in approximately 0.1% of patients taking insulin).

Several approaches may be taken to the patient with immune-mediated insulin resistance. The one I use is simply to keep up with the insulin requirements in an attempt to keep the patient relatively asymptomatic and out of ketoacidosis. Special preparations of U-500 insulin are available for this purpose because, with this high requirement, inordinate volumes would have to be injected if the usual concentrations of insulin were used. Although the U-500 preparations contain regular insulin, a prolonged course of action occurs because of the patient's high antibody titers. Two injections a day usually give an effective response over a 24-hour period. The high antibody titers decrease, again for unknown reasons, usually within several months up to a year. Hypoglycemia can then become a problem as the large amounts of insulin bound to the antibody are released.

A second approach is to switch insulin preparations. The primary structure of mammalian insulins differ principally in the amino acids located at positions 8, 9, and 10 in the A chain and at position 30 in the B chain (Table 8–8). Beef insulin, the most common source for commercial insulin preparations, has a primary structure different from that of human insulin by 3 amino acids. Pork insulin, the second most common insulin preparation, differs from human insulin by only the amino acid in the 30 position in the B chain. As expected, beef insulin is the more antigenic of the two. Therefore, occasionally switching from beef insulin to pork insulin may be helpful in treating insulin resistance. In my experience, however, antibodies directed against beef insulin almost always bind pork insulin. Two other insulin preparations are fish insulin and sulfated beef insulin. In the latter preparation, beef insulin is treated with sulfuric acid, which deposits sulfate radicals on the tyrosine amino acids in the A chain. Since the resultant molecule does not react with antibodies to beef insulin, this locus of the insulin molecule must be an important part of the antigenic site. Unfortunately, neither preparation is available in the United States.

Table 8–8. Species Differences in Amino Acid Sequence of Mammalian Insulins

	Positions			
	A Chain			B Chain
	8	9	10	30
Beef	Alanine	Serine	Valine	Alanine
Pork	Threonine	Serine	Isoleucine	Alanine
Human	Threonine	Serine	Isoleucine	Threonine
Other Species				
Dog	Threonine	Serine	Isoleucine	Alanine
Sperm whale	Threonine	Serine	Isoleucine	Alanine
Rabbit	Threonine	Serine	Isoleucine	Serine
Horse	Threonine	Glycine	Isoleucine	Alanine
Sheep	Alanine	Glycine	Valine	Alanine
Sei whale	Alanine	Serine	Threonine	Alanine

A third approach to the problem of immune-mediated insulin resistance is to use glucocorticoid therapy. Forty to fifty milligrams of prednisone are administered daily. Insulin requirements usually increase during the first week as the insulin antagonistic effect of prednisone becomes manifest. Then insulin requirements decrease, and the dose of prednisone is tapered rapidly. The mechanism is not completely clear, but it is suspected that the glucocorticoid decreases IgG production.

OTHER SIDE EFFECTS. Both the loss and excessive deposition of subcutaneous fat can occur at the site of insulin injection. An atrophic response, probably secondary to impurities in the insulin preparation, is more common than a hypertrophic response. The latter, presumably due to the local lipogenic effect of insulin, may cause erratic absorption.

Oral Hypoglycemic Agents

Sulfonylurea compounds lower glucose concentrations, except in animals that have undergone pancreatectomy and in ketosis-prone diabetics. When these drugs are first given, insulin concentrations increase in both the portal and peripheral circulations. Therefore, functioning pancreatic β-cells are necessary for sulfonylurea agents to be effective. Although increased insulin levels can be measured during the first several weeks of therapy, insulin concentrations usually return to pretreatment levels in approximately a month,

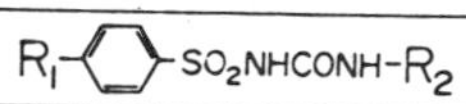

$$R_1 - \langle \rangle - SO_2NHCONH - R_2$$

FIRST GENERATION COMPOUNDS

NAME	R_1	R_2	DOSAGE RANGE (mg)	TABLET SIZE (mg)
TOLBUTAMIDE (Orinase)	CH_3-	$-(CH_2)_3CH_3$	500 – 3000	500
CHLORPROPAMIDE (Diabinese)	$Cl-$	$(CH_2)_2CH_3$	100 – 500	100, 250
TOLAZAMIDE (Tolinase)	CH_3-	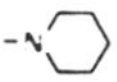 $-N\langle \rangle$	100 – 750	100, 250, 500
ACETOHEXAMIDE (Dymelor)	CH_3CO-	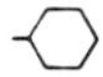 $-\langle \rangle$	500 – 1,500	250, 500

SECOND GENERATION COMPOUNDS

NAME	R_1	R_2	DOSAGE RANGE (mg)	TABLET SIZE (mg)
GLIBENCLAMIDE	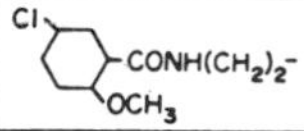 Cl— $\langle \rangle$—CONH(CH$_2$)$_2$— OCH$_3$	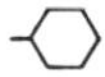 $-\langle \rangle$	2.5 – 20	5
GLIPIZIDE	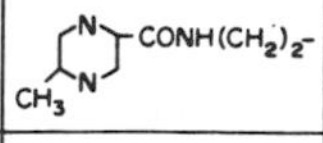 CH$_3$—pyrazine—CONH(CH$_2$)$_2$—	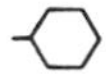 $-\langle \rangle$	2.5 – 45	5
GLIBORNURIDE	CH_3-	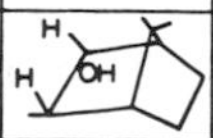 H, H, OH bicyclic	12.5 – 100	12.5

Figure 8–13. Characteristics of current sulfonylurea drugs. (Modified from Lebovitz, H.E., and Feinglos, M.N.: Diabetes Care, *1*:189, 1978. Reproduced with permission from the American Diabetes Association, Inc.)

even though blood glucose values remain lower. Recent evidence suggests that sulfonylurea agents sensitize the β-cells so that they can respond to lower concentrations of glucose. For example, before treatment, glucose levels of 350 mg/100 ml might be required to elicit a maximum insulin response. Under the continued influence of these drugs, a similar response might be seen with glucose concentrations of 200 mg/100 ml. However, sulfonylurea compounds also exert extrapancreatic effects. The most important one is to enhance the effect of the secreted insulin, possibly by increasing insulin binding to its receptor, the critical first step in insulin action.

The structure and some properties of these oral hypoglycemic agents are shown in Figure 8–13. The sulfonylurea structure ($-SO_2-NH-CO-NH-$) is the active component of the molecule. The other components of the molecular structures are responsible for the differing metabolic fates of the individual drugs. The four sulfonylurea compounds currently available in the United States, called first-generation agents, are listed in the upper part of Figure 8–13. Several second-generation drugs, shown in the lower part of Figure 8–13, are commonly used in Europe. Two of them, glibenclamide and glipizide, will soon be introduced in the United States.

Tolbutamide is carboxylated in the liver. Since the product is inactive, it has a short duration of action (6 to 12 hours), so patients need several doses a day. Chlorpropamide is bound to serum proteins and is excreted in the urine mostly unchanged. Therefore, it has a long duration of action (up to 60 hours) and should be given only once per day. It should be avoided in patients with renal insufficiency. Acetohexamide is hydroxylated in the liver, but the product is a more potent hypoglycemic agent than the parent compound. Therefore, although the half-life of the drug itself is short, the total hypoglycemic effect is much longer (12 to 24 hours) and one dose a day is often sufficient. Tolazamide is metabolized to 6 major by-products, 3 of which have hypoglycemic activity. This agent too can usually be given only once a day because its duration of action is similar to that of acetohexamide. When maximum doses of these 2 last drugs are given, however, they should be taken twice a day.

All these drugs are usually well tolerated, with only a 3 to 5% prevalence of side effects, most of which are minor. Although these drugs are the second most common cause of hypoglycemia in diabetics (after insulin), this hypoglycemia represents a therapeutic effect, not a side effect. Hypoglycemia is most common in elderly patients who are eating poorly and are taking a longer-acting sulfonylurea agent. The most common side effects are skin rash, anorexia, epigastric discomfort, and occasionally nausea, vomiting, and diarrhea. Photosensitivity has also been reported. A rare but serious side effect is the hematologic reaction of leukopenia, thrombocytopenia, pancytopenia, or occasionally agranulocytosis. A reversible cholestatic jaundice has been reported, most commonly with chlorpropamide but also with acetohexamide. In elderly patients taking chlorpropamide (and usually diuretics), an inappropriate ADH syndrome may occur. These patients have hyponatremia, lethargy, and confusion, sometimes progressing to frank coma. Discontinuance of the drug and water restriction usually reverse the process. Rarely, intolerance to alcohol (through a disulfiram-like reaction) can be associated with these drugs, especially with chlorpropamide.

No discussion of sulfonylurea agents would be complete without mentioning the University Group Diabetes Program (UGDP) study. In the early 1960s, a prospective study was initiated to evaluate the long-term effects of tolbutamide and insulin on the complications of diabetes. Approximately 800 ketosis-resistant patients were randomized into 4 treatment groups: placebo, tolbutamide (1.5 g/day in divided doses), insulin-variable (changing doses of insulin in an attempt to regulate glucose concentrations), and insulin-standard (a small amount of insulin, 10 to 16 U/day, which did not lower glucose levels). In 1970, tolbutamide was dropped from the study because of a higher rate of cardiovascular deaths in this group as compared to patients receiving placebo.

Many objections have been raised about the validity of this conclusion, including: (a) a greater prevalence of cardiovascular risk factors in the tolbutamide group as compared to the placebo group upon entrance into the study; (b) a spuriously low mortality rate of the placebo group during the first part of the study; (c) the classification of some patients as tolbutamide deaths even though they had not received this medication up to several years prior to the terminal event; and (d) the inappropriate use of the drug because the excess cardiovascular deaths occurred only in patients whose diabetes remained uncontrolled, with fasting glucose concentrations exceeding 200 mg/100 ml. Furthermore, 3 other long-term prospective studies using tolbutamide

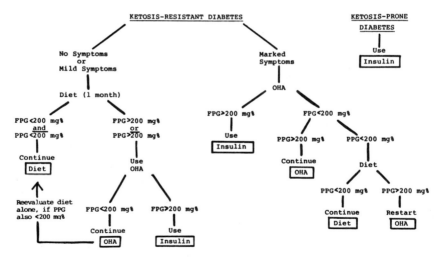

Figure 8–14. General guidelines for decisions regarding treatment of patients with diabetes mellitus. FPG: fasting plasma glucose concentration; PPG: 1- to 2-hr postprandial glucose concentration on patient's usual diet; OHA: oral hypoglycemic agent (sulfonylurea compound). (From Davidson, M.B.: Diabetes Mellitus: Diagnosis and Treatment. New York, John Wiley & Sons, 1981.)

with similar follow-up periods (5 to 8 years) failed to confirm these results. Therefore, most diabetologists do not accept the conclusion of the UGDP study that tolbutamide therapy is associated with an increased risk of cardiovascular mortality and do continue to use these oral hypoglycemic agents.

General Approach to Therapy

The general approach to treating diabetic patients is outlined in Figure 8–14. Ketosis-prone patients must be treated with insulin. If ketosis-resistant patients are symptomatic when first seen, they can be given maximal doses of a potent sulfonylurea compound (chlorpropamide or tolazamide). If the patient's fasting plasma glucose level does not decrease to below 200 mg/ 100 ml within several weeks, the patient should be switched to insulin. Most ketosis-resistant patients, however, have few or no symptoms when diagnosed. They should be treated with an appropriate diet for at least one month. If their fasting or postprandial glucose concentrations remain above 200 mg/ 100 ml, oral hypoglycemic agents are introduced. The dose is gradually increased until either the postprandial glucose level falls below 200 mg/100 ml or the maximal amount is reached. If the fasting glucose concentration is less than 200 mg/100 ml, the patient is maintained on the sulfonylurea agent. If this value exceeds 200 mg/100 ml, the patient is switched to insulin therapy.

Therapeutic Goals

Having reviewed the various modalities of diabetic treatment, it is now appropriate to discuss the goals of therapy. This seemingly simple subject is an extremely controversial one. No one would question the aim of rendering the diabetic asymptomatic, controlling the polyuria and polydipsia, reversing the weight loss, and preventing the increased susceptibility to infection. This goal can be achieved with relative ease in the ketosis-prone diabetic by the judicious use of insulin and, in the ketosis-resistant diabetic, by the use of oral hypoglycemic agents and/or diet. Indeed many ketosis-resistant diabetics are asymptomatic without treatment. Therefore, the crucial question that determines the goals of therapy is whether control of the plasma glucose level in any way affects the dreaded complications of diabetes mellitus.

I believe that the microvascular complications (retinopathy and nephropathy) as well as the neuropathy are directly related to the altered metabolism of diabetes. Therefore, I conclude that control of these metabolic abnormalities should help ameliorate these sequelae of diabetes. The evidence for this position is as follows:

1. In animals rendered diabetic by agents that destroy the β-cells of the pancreas, retinal, renal, and neuropathic changes consistent with the abnormalities observed in human diabetes can be seen.
2. Renal, retinal, and neuropathic abnormalities disappear in diabetic rats whose diabetes is either cured by pancreatic transplantation or controlled tightly with insulin.

3. Diabetic dogs, whose glucose levels were well controlled for five years through multiple injections of regular insulin throughout the day, had only mild cataracts and vascular changes in the eye, kidney, and muscle, whereas their counterparts treated with suboptimal daily injections of intermediate-acting insulin and with poorly controlled diabetes had severe changes.
4. Normal rat kidneys transplanted into inbred diabetic rats developed the vascular changes of diabetes.
5. Vascular abnormalities in kidneys of diabetic rats improved after transplantation into normal inbred rats.
6. In patients with diabetes secondary to pancreatitis or hemochromatosis, typical diabetic complications occur at a rate similar to that observed in other diabetic patients. This finding proves that the microvascular complications do not follow a separate genetic course, but are due to the abnormal metabolic status.
7. In large-scale studies in which thousands of patients were analyzed over several decades, statistical evidence of an association between good control and fewer diabetic complications is beginning to emerge.
8. Swedish diabetics treated with a free diet and one daily injection of long-acting insulin had a six- to sevenfold higher prevalence of severe retinopathy and glomerulosclerosis as compared to a Swedish group treated with a strict diet and multiple injections of short-acting insulin. (The latter group was presumably more tightly controlled.)
9. Normal human kidneys develop vascular lesions when transplanted into diabetics.
10. Two diabetic kidneys with vascular changes showed clearing of these lesions after inadvertent transplantation into nondiabetic recipients.
11. Several prospective studies have shown less progression of retinopathy, neuropathy and nephropathy when patients are maintained in strict control as compared to a more poorly controlled group.
12. Early lesions of retinopathy, neuropathy and nephropathy are reversible when strict control of diabetes is instituted, but more advanced lesions are not helped.

On the other hand, some patients have few recognizable complications despite poor control of their diabetes for many years, and a few patients with only mild carbohydrate abnormalities manifest severe diabetic complications. In the individual case it may be difficult to correlate control and the presence of complications. This problem may relate to our inability to maintain the diabetic's glucose concentrations anywhere near the normal level under the present regimens of therapy. Thus, we may be comparing complications in patients whose glucose levels usually range between 150 and 300 mg/100 ml throughout the day ("well-controlled" group) to those whose values lie between 250 and 400 mg/100 ml ("poorly-controlled" group). It may be unrealistic to expect to see any differences in diabetic complications between these two groups of patients.

Given this controversial situation, what is an appropriate goal for patients and their physicians? Because normal glucose concentrations (i.e., in nondiabetics) are not associated with diabetic microvascular complications and

Table 8–9. Degrees of Diabetic Control*

1. All preprandial urine tests negative for glucose.
2. Fasting and before supper plasma glucose concentrations <200 mg/100 ml.
3. Fasting and before supper plasma glucose concentrations <150 mg/100 ml.
4. All postprandial urine tests negative for glucose.
5. Postprandial plasma glucose concentrations <200 mg/100 ml.
6. Postprandial plasma glucose concentrations <150 mg/100 ml.

*Listed in order of increasing strictness.

these changes can be prevented or reversed in diabetic animals whose abnormal metabolism can be returned to euglycemia or close to it, a lowering of glucose levels toward normal in the diabetic should be helpful in delaying or ameliorating these complications.

Table 8–9 lists various parameters of assessing diabetic control in increasing order of strictness. Most patients are able to attain the first and second levels of control. Two exceptions are a few unstable type 1 diabetics and obese patients who cannot lose weight and who need insulin therapy. The third level of control is reached only by a minority of those requiring insulin, but by many more non-insulin-dependent patients. The fourth and fifth levels are even more difficult, and few patients attain them. These two criteria may not be different, depending on the renal threshold for glucose. Finally, the strictest level of control (approaching euglycemia) is only reached by special techniques (e.g., multiple injections of regular insulin or insulin infusion pumps). I attempt to achieve the highest degree of control possible without seriously disrupting the patient's usual life style. An occasional mild hypoglycemic reaction should be tolerated in order to obtain the maximum degree of diabetic control.

Impact of Diabetic Complications

Although a clinical and pathologic description of the complications (neuropathy, retinopathy, nephropathy, and atherosclerosis) of diabetes mellitus is beyond the scope of this chapter, these processes exact the heaviest toll from the diabetic population. Figure 8–15 illustrates the profound influence of the discovery of insulin on the diabetic population. After 1922, the percentage of diabetics dying in ketoacidotic coma abruptly decreased. Today a fatal outcome is unusual and often preventable. Over three-fourths of all deaths in diabetics are now due to one of the vascular complications, which do not usually occur until many years after the diagnosis is made.

Diabetes mellitus has a tremendous impact on the health care system. Diabetes now affects 5% of the population of the United States or approximately 10 million people. Estimates are that an equal number of patients remains undiagnosed. In 1974, 600,000 new cases were diagnosed. The incidence of diabetes is allegedly increasing at 6% per year, which translates into a doubling of the diabetic population every 15 years. Diabetes directly caused 38,000 deaths in the United States during 1974, making it the fifth

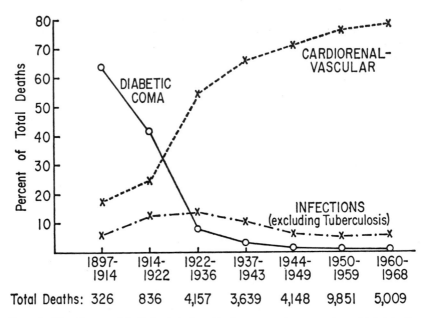

Figure 8–15. Causes of death in diabetic patients expressed as percentage of total deaths. (From Marble, A.: Diabetes, *21* (Suppl. 2):632, 1972. Reproduced with permission.)

leading cause of death. Because the complications of diabetes are also responsible for 300,000 deaths annually, it is really the third leading cause of death. Only cardiovascular disease and cancer are more lethal. Diabetes is the leading cause of new blindness in this country. Diabetics are 25 times more likely to develop blindness, 17 times more likely to develop gangrene, and twice as likely to develop heart disease as nondiabetics. Five out of 6 major amputations performed in the United States occur in diabetics. Fourteen percent of the diabetic population (usually older patients) are bedridden for an average of 6 weeks per year. No other chronic disease causes so many days in bed. The total economic impact of diabetes mellitus in the United States is currently estimated as more than 8 billion dollars per year.

At the turn of the century, Sir William Osler stated that to know syphilis was to know all of medicine. Because diabetes mellitus can affect almost all the organ systems in the body, it is not too much of an exaggeration to state that to know this disease is to know all of internal medicine. Although many of the complications cannot be entirely prevented, their onset can be delayed and their impact ameliorated by proper medical care. Helping the diabetic patient live a nearly normal life can be both challenging and satisfying for the physician.

CLINICAL PROBLEMS

Patient 1. A 34-year-old man was admitted to the emergency room in a combative, disoriented state. When his children woke him for breakfast, he was abusive and responded inappropriately.

When examined in the emergency room, this modestly obese man was oriented to name only, had no focal neurologic signs, and had a regular pulse rate of 120 beats/minute. The rest of the examination was negative. The astute emergency room physician suspected hypoglycemia, drew a plasma glucose (which returned at 23 mg/100 ml) and injected 50 ml of 50% glucose intravenously. Within 5 minutes, the patient calmed down, became completely oriented, and gave the following history. He had been to a party the night before and consumed a moderate amount of alcohol; he then drove home and went to sleep. The next thing he remembered was waking up in the emergency room. His wife recalled that he had often been difficult to arouse the morning following a party. On questioning, the patient reported that he ate frequently during the day to avoid intense hunger pains and occasional feelings of weakness. This practice had been going on for at least 3 years and had been associated with a 50-pound weight gain. His only exercise was mowing his lawn; this often caused palpitations, profuse sweating, and profound weakness, which was relieved by eating. He could not remember the last time he had missed a meal. He denied taking any drugs except aspirin for an occasional headache. His review of systems was negative except for nocturia thrice nightly. His physical exam revealed only mild hypertension (150/100) and obesity.

QUESTIONS

1. What kind of hypoglycemia does this man have?
2. His hypoglycemia is potentiated by two factors mentioned in the history. What are they, and what are their mechanisms?
3. What is the differential diagnosis of fasting hypoglycemia? Based on what you know so far, what are the possible causes for this patient's problem?
4. The following endocrinologic data were obtained:
   Twenty-four hour urine for 17-hydroxysteroids—10.8 mg/24 hours (normal 3 to 10). Symptoms of hypoglycemia appeared after 24 hours of fasting; at this time his plasma glucose concentration was 23 mg/100 ml and his insulin level, 35 μU/ml. Interpret these data.
5. In the routine work-up on this patient, a panel of blood chemistries revealed a serum calcium of 12 mg/100 ml. What is the probable diagnosis?

Patient 2. This patient was given an oral glucose tolerance test (OGTT) in which the following plasma glucose concentrations were measured: F, 85 mg/100 ml; 1 hour, 130 mg/100 ml; 2 hours, 108 mg/100 ml; 3 hours, 65 mg/100 ml; 4 hours, 43 mg/100 ml; 5 hours, 68 mg/100 ml.

QUESTIONS

1. What would the results have been if whole blood glucose had been measured?
2. List the differential diagnosis of reactive hypoglycemia.
3. Construct an OGTT representing hyperalimentation.
4. Construct an OGTT representing impaired glucose tolerance.
5. Construct an OGTT representing idiopathic reactive hypoglycemia.
6. What additional information is necessary to make a diagnosis of idiopathic reactive hypoglycemia?
7. What is the treatment of each cause of reactive hypoglycemia?
8. What is the most likely diagnosis in the person with the OGTT depicted in this problem?

Patients 3 and 4. One patient has diabetic ketoacidosis and the other has hyperosmolar nonketotic coma.

QUESTIONS

Which of the following findings are similar in the two conditions and which are different? Give reasons for your choices.
1. Polyuria
2. Polydipsia
3. Prodromal period
4. Respiratory rate
5. Neurologic examination
6. Serum ketone levels
7. Serum bicarbonate concentrations
8. Total body sodium

9. Total body potassium
10. Plasma volume
11. Arterial pH
12. Arterial P_{CO_2}
13. Initial fluid treatment
14. Prognosis
15. Treatment after discharge

Patient 5.

1. A 28-year-old, 5'11" salesman sees you during your morning office hours because of fatigue and a 10-pound weight loss during the past month. He currently weighs 165 pounds. You elicit a history of increased thirst and urination, which also awakens him 2 to 3 times a night. His appetite is "better than ever" in spite of his recent weight loss. His urine test in the office reveals 2% glucosuria and strong ketonuria. A blood sample is taken, centrifuged, and the plasma tested for ketone bodies. The results show *trace* ketone bodies in the undiluted specimen. What is your diagnosis? (More than one answer may be correct.)
   a. Starvation ketosis
   b. Type 1 diabetes mellitus
   c. Type 2 diabetes mellitus
   d. Diabetic ketoacidosis
   e. Hyperosmolar nonketotic coma

2. You arrange for the patient to be hospitalized that afternoon and leave orders for glucose and electrolytes to be measured as soon as he arrives. The laboratory phones the following results to you at 4:30 P.M. Glucose—381 mg/100 ml; Na—133 mEq/L; K—4.5 mEq/L; HCO_3—23 mEq/L. Which of the following would be appropriate to include in your admission orders? (More than one answer may be correct.)
   a. Start intravenous infusion of 1 L normal saline solution containing 20 mEq KCl to run in at 250 ml per hour.
   b. Instruct patient in a 2600-cal ADA diet
   c. Instruct patient in an 1800-cal ADA diet
   d. Give patient 5 U NPH insulin immediately
   e. Give patient 5 U NPH insulin and 5 U regular insulin immediately
   f. Have diabetes teaching nurse begin instruction tomorrow

3. You order 10 U NPH insulin before breakfast and 5 U NPH before dinner for the following day (hospital day 2) as well as plasma glucose determinations before breakfast and before supper each day. The before-supper result returns at 289 mg/100 ml. What insulin dose should you order for the morning of hospital day 3?
   a. 15 U NPH insulin
   b. 20 U NPH insulin
   c. 15 U NPH insulin and 5 U regular insulin
   d. 15 U NPH insulin plus 500 mg tolazamide (Tolinase)
   e. 10 U NPH insulin

4. By the afternoon of hospital day 5, the patient is taking 25 U NPH insulin before breakfast and 10 U NPH insulin before supper. His fasting glucose concentration is 152 mg/100 ml and his before-supper value on hospital day 4 was 185 mg/100 ml. His urine tests are as follows:

Hospital day	Before breakfast glucose/ketones	Before lunch glucose/ketones	Before supper glucose/ketones	Before bed glucose/ketones
4	neg/neg	2%/neg	neg/neg	½%/neg
5	neg/neg	2%/neg		

What would an appropriate plan be?
   a. Discharge him on 25 U NPH insulin before breakfast and 10 U NPH insulin before supper.
   b. Discharge him on 25 U NPH insulin and 5 U regular insulin before breakfast and 10 U NPH insulin before supper.
   c. Discharge him on 30 U NPH insulin before breakfast and 15 U NPH insulin before supper.

    d. Keep him hospitalized and attempt to reduce his before-breakfast and before-supper glucose concentrations to <150 mg/100 ml by cautiously increasing his dose of NPH insulin.

    e. Keep him hospitalized and add 5 U regular insulin to the morning dose of insulin to improve his before-lunch tests.

Patient 6. A 48-year-old man is referred to you because of difficulty in controlling his diabetes. He is on 80 U NPH insulin and 15 U regular insulin in the morning, and he says his urine tests are erratic. He is feeling fairly well except for intermittent nocturnal sweating and waking up with a headache. His urine tests for the 3 days before seeing you are:

Before breakfast	*Before lunch*	*Before supper*	*Before bed*
glucose/ketones	glucose/ketones	glucose/ketones	glucose/ketones
2%/mod	neg/weak	$1/4$%/neg	neg/neg
2%/strong	trace/mod	neg/neg	$1/4$%/mod
2%/strong	neg/weak	2%/neg	2%/strong

Match the following changes in therapy (number) with the probable result (letters).
1. Increase NPH insulin to 90 U in the morning.
2. Add sulfonylurea agent.
3. Decrease total insulin dose to 50 U NPH and 5 U regular in the morning.
4. Decrease total insulin to 70 U NPH and 5 U regular in the morning.
    a. No change in symptoms or urine tests
    b. Patient passes out just before supper
    c. Nocturnal sweating and morning headache disappear, urine tests consistently negative to $1/2$% for glucose, and ketones disappear
    d. Nocturnal sweating and morning headache disappear, urine tests consistently 1 to 2% for glucose, and ketonuria diminishes considerably, but is still intermittently present

SUGGESTED READING

Metabolism
Cahill, G.F., Jr.: Physiology of insulin in man. Diabetes, *20*:785, 1971.
Cahill, G.F., Jr.: Starvation in man. N. Engl. J. Med., *282*:668, 1970.
Levine, R., and Haft, D.E.: Carbohydrate homeostasis. N. Engl. J. Med., *283*:175, 237, 1970.
Oliva, P.B.: Lactic acidosis. Am. J. Med., *48*:209, 1970.

Insulin Secretion
Cerasi, E.: Insulin secretion: mechanism of the stimulation by glucose. Q. Rev. Biophys., *8*:1, 1975.
Fajans, S.S., et al.: Heterogeneity of insulin responses in latent diabetes. Trans. Assoc. Am. Physicians, *87*:83, 1975.
Genuth, S.M.: Insulin secretion in obesity and diabetes: an illustrative case. Ann. Intern. Med., *87*:714, 1977.
Kipnis, D.M.: Insulin secretion in diabetes mellitus. Ann. Intern. Med., *69*:891, 1968.
Kitabchi, A.E.: Proinsulin and C-peptide: a review. Metabolism, *26*:547, 1977.
Luft, R., et al.: On the pathogenesis of maturity-onset diabetes. Diabetes Care, *4*:58, 1981.
Robertson, R.P., and Chen, M.: A role of prostaglandin E in defective insulin secretion and carbohydrate intolerance in diabetes mellitus. J. Clin. Invest., *60*:747, 1977.
Robertson, R.P., and Porte, D., Jr.: The glucose receptor. A defective mechanism in diabetes mellitus distinct from the beta-adrenergic receptor. J. Clin. Invest., *52*:870, 1973.
Rubenstein, A.H., et al.: Clinical significance of circulating C-peptide in diabetes mellitus and hypoglycemic disorders. Arch. Intern. Med., *137*:625, 1977.
Savage, P.J.: Hyperinsulinemia and hypoinsulinemia. Insulin responses to oral carbohydrate over a wide spectrum of glucose tolerance. Diabetes, *24*:362, 1975.

Hypoglycemia
Arky, R.H.: Pathophysiology and therapy of fasting hypoglycemias. D.M., February, 1968.
Davidson, M.B.: Hypoglycemia. *In* Diabetes Mellitus: Diagnosis and Treatment. New York, John Wiley & Sons, 1981.
Fariss, B.L.: Prevalence of post-glucose-load glycosuria and hypoglycemia in a group of healthy young men. Diabetes, *23*:189, 1974.

Ford, C.V., et al.: A psychiatric study of patients referred with a diagnosis of hypoglycemia. Am. J. Psychiatry, *133*:290, 1976.
Freinkel, N., and Metzger, B.E.: Oral glucose tolerance curve and hypoglycemia in the fed state. N. Engl. J. Med., *280*:820, 1969.
Hofeldt, F.D.: Reactive hypoglycemia. Metabolism, *24*:1193, 1975.
Jung, Y., et al.: Reactive hypoglycemia in women. Results of a health survey. Diabetes, *20*:428, 1971.
Nolan, S., et al.: Low profile (flat) glucose tolerance. Am. J. Med. Sci., *264*:33, 1972.
Permutt, M.A.: Postprandial hypoglycemia. Diabetes, *25*:719, 1976.
Seltzer, H.S.: Statement on hypoglycemia. J.A.M.A., *223*:682, 1973.
Seltzer, H.S.: Drug-induced hypoglycemia. A review based on 473 cases. Diabetes, *21*:955, 1972.
Yager, J., and Young, R.T.: Non-hypoglycemia is an epidemic condition. N. Engl. J. Med., *291*:907, 1974.

Diabetes Mellitus
Arieff, A.I., and Carroll, H.J.: Nonketotic hyperosmolar coma with hyperglycemia: clinical features, pathophysiology, renal function, acid-base balance, plasma-cerebrospinal fluid equilibria and the effects of therapy in 37 cases. Medicine, *51*:73, 1972.
Bloom, M.E., Mintz, D.H., and Field, J.B.: Insulin-induced posthypoglycemic hyperglycemia as a cause of "brittle" diabetes. Clinical clues and therapeutic implications. Am. J. Med., *47*:891, 1969.
Cahill, G.F., Jr., and McDevitt, H.O.: Insulin-dependent diabetes mellitus: the initial lesion. N. Engl. J. Med., *304*:1454, 1981.
Clements, R.S., Jr., and Vourganti, B.: Fatal diabetic ketoacidosis: major causes and approaches to their prevention. Diabetes Care, *1*:314, 1978.
Craighead, J.E.: Current views on the etiology of insulin-dependent diabetes mellitus. N. Engl. J. Med., *299*:1439, 1978.
Cudworth, A.G.: Type 1 diabetes mellitus. Diabetologia, *14*:281, 1978.
Davidson, M.B.: Diabetes Mellitus: Diagnosis and Treatment. New York, John Wiley & Sons, 1981.
Fajans, S.S.: Etiologic aspects of types of diabetes. Diabetes Care, *4*:69, 1981.
Fajans, S.S., et al.: The various faces of diabetes in the young. Arch. Intern. Med., *136*:194, 1976.
Kreisberg, R.A.: Diabetic ketoacidosis: new concepts and trends in pathogenesis and treatment. Ann. Intern. Med., *88*:681, 1978.
National Diabetes Data Group: Classification and diagnosis of diabetes mellitus and other categories of glucose intolerance. Diabetes, *28*:1039, 1979.
Pyke, D.A.: Diabetes: the genetic connections. Diabetologia, *17*:333, 1979.
Reaven, G.M., and Olefsky, J.M.: The role of insulin resistance in the pathogenesis of diabetes mellitus. Adv. Metab. Disord., *9*:313, 1977.
Rotter, J.I., and Rimoin, D.L.: Heterogeneity in diabetes mellitus—update, 1978. Evidence for further genetic heterogeneity within juvenile-onset insulin-dependent diabetes mellitus. Diabetes, *27*:599, 1978.

Oral Hypoglycemic Agents
Feldman, R., et al.: Oral hypoglycemic drugs prophylaxis in asymptomatic diabetes. *In* Diabetes. Edited by W.J. Malaisse and J. Pirart. Amsterdam, Excerpta Medica/American Elsevier, 1974.
Keen, H., Jarret, J.R., and Fuller, J.H.: Tolbutamide and arterial disease in borderline diabetics. *In* Diabetes. Edited by W.J. Malaisse and J. Pirart. Amsterdam, Excerpta Medica/American Elsevier, 1974.
Lebovitz, H.E., and Feinglos, M.N.: Sulfonylurea drugs: mechanism of antidiabetic action and therapeutic usefulness. Diabetes Care, *1*:189, 1978.
Paasikivi, J.: Long-term tolbutamide treatment after myocardial infarction. Acta. Med. Scand., *507* (Suppl.):1, 1970.
Tzagournis, M., and Reynertson, R.: University group diabetes program: a study of the effects of hypoglycemic agents on vascular complications in patients with adult-onset diabetes. II. Mortality results. Diabetes, *19* (Suppl. 2):789, 1970.

Complications of Diabetes Mellitus

Colwell, J.A., et al.: Pathogenesis of atherosclerosis in diabetes mellitus. Diabetes Care, *4*:121, 1981.

Davidson, M.B.: The case for control in diabetes mellitus. West. J. Med., *129*:193, 1978.

Engerman, R., et al.: Relationship of microvascular disease in diabetes to metabolic control. Diabetes, *26*:760, 1977.

Eschwege, E., et al.: Delayed progression of diabetic retinopathy by divided insulin administration: a further follow-up. Diabetologia, *16*:13, 1979.

Job, D., et al.: Effect of multiple daily injections on the course of diabetic retinopathy. Diabetes, *25*:463, 1976.

Johnsson, S.: Retinopathy and nephropathy in diabetes mellitus. Comparison of the effects of two forms of treatment. Diabetes, *9*:1, 1960.

Kilo, C., Vogler, N., and Williamson, J.R.: Muscle capillary basement membrane changes related to aging and to diabetes mellitus. Diabetes, *21*:881, 1972.

McMillan, D.E.: Deterioration of the microcirculation in diabetes. Diabetes, *24*:944, 1975.

Mauer, S.M., et al.: Development of diabetic vascular lesions in normal kidneys transplanted into patients with diabetes mellitus. N. Engl. J. Med., *295*:916, 1976.

Mauer, S.M., et al.: Studies of the rate of regression on the glomerular lesions in diabetic rats treated with pancreatic islet transplantation. Diabetes, *24*:280, 1975.

Miki, E., et al.: Relation of the course of retinopathy to control of diabetes, age, and therapeutic agents in diabetic Japanese patients. Diabetes, *18*:773, 1969.

Pirart, J.: Diabetes mellitus and its degenerative complications: a prospective study of 4,400 patients observed between 1947 and 1973. Diabetes Care, *1*:168, 252, 1978.

Raskin, P.: Diabetic regulation and its relationship to microangiopathy. Metabolism, *27*:235, 1978.

Takazakura, E., et al.: Onset and progression of diabetic glomerulosclerosis based on serial renal biopsies. Diabetes, *24*:1, 1975.

Tchobroutsky, G.: Relation of diabetic control to development of microvascular complications. Diabetologia, *15*:143, 1978.

CHAPTER 9

Disorders of Calcium and Phosphate and Metabolic Bone Diseases

D.A. Henry and J.W. Coburn

PHYSIOLOGY OF CALCIUM REGULATION

Calcium (Ca) homeostasis involves the precise control of ionized blood calcium, the maintenance of the structural integrity of the skeleton, and the regulation of intracellular Ca movement. This last component of Ca regulation is complex and involves factors beyond those regulating the blood calcium; intracellular Ca regulation is not considered here.

The principal regulators of blood Ca include (1) parathyroid hormone (PTH); (2) vitamin D, or its active hormonal form, 1,25-dihydroxy-vitamin D_3 $(1,25(OH)_2D_3)$; (3) calcitonin (CT); and (4) the serum level of inorganic phosphate (PO_4). Large stores of both Ca and PO_4 are found in bone, and it is generally believed that interchange between bone and the extracellular fluid (ECF) is the principal flux regulating the blood Ca and PO_4. Large amounts of Ca and PO_4 enter the glomerular filtrate and must be reclaimed by tubular reabsorption, however. Variation in the renal tubular reabsorption of Ca may be important in the control of blood Ca in man, particularly when skeletal turnover is low. The intestinal Ca absorption is stimulated by $1,25(OH)_2D_3$, and this hormone controls the rate of Ca absorption. Moreover, a reciprocal relationship exists between the blood levels of PO_4 and Ca, related in a large part to the solubility product of $CaHPO_4$; increasing blood PO_4 causes a fall in Ca with deposition of Ca and PO_4 into bone and soft tissues.

Parathyroid Hormone

Parathyroid hormone, which exists in the parathyroid glands as a prohormone, is secreted as an 84-amino-acid chain, with a molecular weight (M.W.)

228

of 9500 daltons. Once secreted in response to a fall in blood Ca, PTH is rapidly degraded in the kidney and liver, with generation of inactive carboxyl-terminal fragments, M.W. 5000 to 7000. These carboxyl (C) terminal fragments are more slowly degraded than intact PTH and are detected by many immunoassays for PTH. The amino (N) terminal fragment of PTH and intact PTH, itself, are degraded rapidly. They become bound to the target tissues where they activate adenylate cyclase, which converts adenosine triphosphate (ATP) to cyclic adenosine-3',5'-monophosphate (cAMP). The cAMP activates a protein kinase, which initiates the intracellular events characteristic of PTH action. It is also believed that PTH enhances the intracellular flux of Ca independent of cAMP.

The actions of PTH on bone and kidney increase the blood level of Ca and reduce the level of PO_4. In bone, PTH increases reabsorption by stimulating the activity of both osteoclasts and osteocytes; this action releases both Ca and PO_4 into the blood. In the kidney, PTH reduces the tubular reabsorption of PO_4 and augments the net tubular reabsorption of Ca. The fall in serum PO_4, which results from the phosphaturia, permits greater stimulation of bone resorption by PTH; otherwise, an increase in serum PO_4 from bone resorption would inhibit the skeletal action of PTH. PTH also reduces the tubular reabsorption of amino acids and bicarbonate; this action contributes to aminoaciduria and/or mild hyperchloremic acidosis seen with excess action of PTH. In the kidney, PTH also stimulates the conversion of 25-hydroxy-vitamin D_3 to $1,25(OH)_2D_3$; the latter acts to augment the intestinal absorption of Ca and, to a smaller extent, PO_4.

Vitamin D

It is now clear that vitamin D should really be considered a "prohormone," and the scheme of vitamin D metabolism is shown in Figure 9–1. Thus, vitamin D_3, which originates in the skin or diet, is converted in the liver to $25(OH)D_3$ (calcifediol). The latter, which undergoes enterohepatic circulation and is reabsorbed from the gut, is the major circulating form of vitamin D. Its plasma half-life is 20 to 25 days, and its turnover rate is 2 to 3 µg/day. It is converted to $1,25(OH)_2D_3$ (calcitriol) by a mitochrondrial enzyme system in the cells of the proximal convoluted tubule. Another sterol, $24,25(OH)_2D_3$, is also produced in the kidney; its biologic effects are unknown.

The actions of vitamin D, which are mediated largely or entirely through $1,25(OH)_2D_3$, occur in the intestine to increase the absorption of Ca and PO_4 and in bone, where it may increase bone resorption (Table 9–1). Despite its apparent action to cause bone resorption, $1,25(OH)_2D_3$ stimulates bone mineralization in rickets, perhaps by elevating the blood levels of Ca and PO_4 and by improving the synthesis and maturation of the collagen. It may also act on the kidneys and parathyroid glands, but the effects of these two organs are not certain. Calcitriol is believed to act through messenger RNA to induce protein synthesis, which enhances the movement of Ca across the cell.

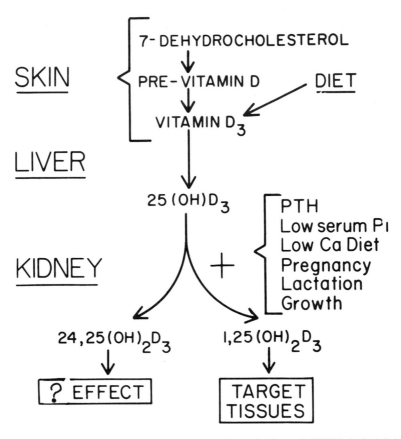

Figure 9–1. Metabolic activation of vitamin D to its active form, $1,25(OH)_2D_3$ (calcitriol). Vitamin D arises either from dietary ingestion or from conversion of 7-dehydrocholesterol in the skin through the action of ultraviolet light. Vitamin D_3 is converted in the liver to $25(OH)D_3$, (calcifediol), the circulating form of vitamin D in the blood. The active sterol, $1,25(OH)_2D_3$, is formed in the renal cortex by the enzyme, $25(OH)D_3\text{-}1\text{-}\alpha\text{-OHase}$, under the stimulus of several factors noted. The biologic effect of $24,25(OH)_2D_3$ is uncertain.

The conversion of vitamin D_3 to $25(OH)D_3$ occurs with little or no regulation, and the plasma levels of $25(OH)D_3$ increase substantially after vitamin D treatment or increased exposure to sunlight. In contrast, the conversion of $25(OH)D_3$ to $1,25(OH)_2D_3$ is under close metabolic control; it is stimulated by a low-Ca diet, a low-PO_4 diet, and by PTH. On the other hand, this conversion is reduced when dietary Ca is high and after parathyroidectomy.

Calcitonin

Calcitonin (CT) is a peptide hormone secreted by the parafollicular cells of the thyroid gland. It acts to decrease osteoclastic bone resorption, which causes blood Ca to fall as a result of continued bone accretion. Thus, this

Table 9–1.   Target Tissues and Actions of 1,25 (OH)$_2$-Vitamin D

Gut	↑ Ca absorption
	(↑ PO$_4$ absorption)
Bone	Mineralization of osteoid
	(↑ bone resorption)
	(Collagen maturation)
Kidney	(↑ Ca and PO$_4$ reabsorption)
	With high serum PO$_4$: ↓ PO$_4$
	reabsorption
Parathyroid	(↓ PTH secretion)
(Muscle)	(Improved function)

( ) Parentheses indicate that effect is quantitatively small or of questionable physiologic significance.

hypocalcemic effect is more marked when bone turnover is high. Calcitonin may act on the kidney to increase urinary excretion of Na, Ca, PO$_4$, and Mg.

The secretion of CT is stimulated by a rise of serum Ca and by gastrin and pentagastrin. The role of CT in normal physiology in man is uncertain. It may prevent an inordinate rise in serum Ca following the ingestion of a Ca-containing meal. Plasma CT levels are higher in the fetus and in infants than in adults; this difference suggests a more important role during growth. Calcitonin treatment is useful in the treatment of Paget's disease of bone and in the management of certain cases of hypercalcemia.

Feedback Regulation of Blood Calcium

When blood Ca falls, secretion of PTH increases; the latter acts on the kidney to increase Ca reabsorption and thereby to reduce urinary Ca. PTH also reduces the renal tubular resorption of PO$_4$ and causes a fall in blood PO$_4$, and it increases the synthesis of 1,25(OH)$_2$D$_3$. These effects on renal tubular transport cause a slight rise in serum Ca and a substantial fall in serum PO$_4$. In bone, PTH increases osteoclastic activity with enhanced bone resorption, releasing both Ca and PO$_4$ into the extracellular fluid. PTH has no direct effect on the gut, but acts indirectly through the increased level of 1,25(OH)$_2$D$_3$ to enhance intestinal absorption of both Ca and PO$_4$. The net results of all these effects are a fall in serum PO$_4$ and an increase in Ca. The increased blood Ca causes a decrease in PTH secretion, completing the negative feedback loop (see also Fig. 9–4).

Dietary Calcium and Net Balance for Calcium

The daily losses of Ca from the body are nearly constant in normal individuals (Fig. 9–2). Thus, the renal excretion rate of Ca is 100 to 200 mg/day, and this rate falls only slightly with restricted Ca intake. The endogenous fecal losses of Ca, i.e., Ca excreted into the bile and intestinal juices that is not reabsorbed, are constant at approximately 175 mg/day. Another 20 mg/day are lost from the skin.

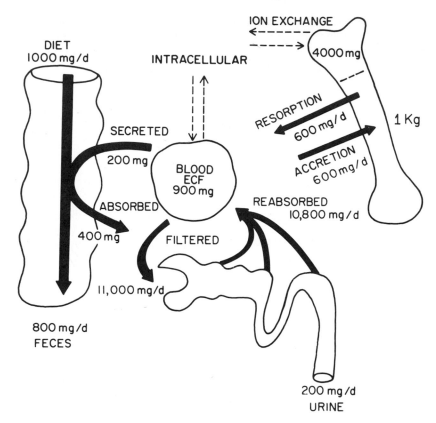

Figure 9–2. Quantitative aspects of normal calcium metabolism, showing approximate quantities of Ca moving into the blood or extracellular fluid (ECF) from various sources (heavy dark arrows). A sizable fraction of Ca in bone is freely exchangeable with extracellular and intracellular Ca; quantities of Ca are deposited into and are resorbed from bone crystals, themselves, by the active processes, accretion and resorption.

Since the only route for Ca to enter the body is through intestinal absorption, a consideration of some quantitative aspects of dietary Ca intake and absorption is pertinent. The efficiency of absorption of dietary Ca varies inversely with the amount ingested. With a low-Ca diet, such as 150 mg/day, the efficiency of absorption increases to about 60%. As dietary Ca is increased, the efficiency falls rapidly; thus, with a dietary Ca intake of 800 mg/day, which is recommended by the National Research Council, the absorption averages approximately 25%, but with a wide range among "normal" individuals. Good evidence suggests that the fraction of Ca that is absorbed is affected by $1,25(OH)_2D_3$; the plasma level of $1,25(OH)_2D_3$ correlates with the fraction of Ca absorbed in normal individuals.

Calculations based on the average losses in the urine, feces, and the skin suggest that the average adult rarely achieves a neutral or positive balance at the recommended dietary intake. Moreover, a significant fraction of the population may have an intake below the recommended daily allowance, with a slightly negative balance for Ca for most of their adult life. A low dietary Ca intake may be an important factor contributing to the osteoporosis that occurs with aging (see discussion later in this chapter).

Regulation of Bone Metabolism

Because 98 to 99% of Ca and PO_4 within the body are present in bone, it is obvious that bone has an important effect on Ca metabolism. Within both trabecular (spongy) and cortical (compact) bone, three basic types of cells are involved in the active turnover of bone: osteoclasts, osteoblasts, and osteocytes. The osteoclasts are large, multinucleated giant cells that act to resorb bone on the surface of bone trabeculae and within the haversian canals of compact bone. Following the stimulation of bone resorption by PTH and several other factors, osteoblasts accumulate; these cells synthesize new collagen and bring about the formation of new bone. In the haversian system of compact bone, the osteoblasts are then buried by the bone matrix; when this occurs they become osteocytes that interconnect by fine canaliculi. Some degree of bone resorption is stimulated by the osteocytes, a process known as osteocytic osteolysis.

Through events that are poorly understood, the activation of the osteoclasts with increased bone resorption is followed close at hand by an increase in the activity and number of osteoblasts, which then increase bone formation. Osteoclasts and osteoblasts are known to originate from different precursor cells, and the important homeostatic process by which an increase in osteoclastic activity is almost invariably followed by increased osteoblastic bone formation remains unknown.

PHOSPHATE METABOLISM

Phosphorus is an important element in the body; it is present in the extracellular fluids as inorganic phosphate, within cells as various phosphorylated compounds, many of which are critical to energy metabolism, and in bone as calcium phosphate or hydroxyapatite. Phosphate is usually abundant in the diet, with an intake of 1000 to 1500 mg/day. Forty to sixty percent of dietary PO_4 is absorbed, with little or no change in absorption in response to differing body needs. Little plasma PO_4 is bound to plasma protein, and PO_4 is freely filtered at the glomerulus, with 80 to 90% of the filtered PO_4 reabsorbed by the renal tubule. Many factors control the reabsorption of PO_4, and the kidney is the primary organ that regulates body PO_4 content. With an increase in dietary PO_4 intake, plasma PO_4 increases; this process can lower serum Ca and thereby stimulate PTH secretion. The latter enhances the renal excretion of PO_4 and restores the serum PO_4 toward normal. With ingestion of a diet low in PO_4, its tubular reabsorption increases, so that the urinary losses approach zero. Other factors that can increase PO_4 excretion include an increase in dietary Na, expansion of ECF volume, and to a smaller extent alkalosis, growth hormone, calcitonin, and perhaps glucocorticoids.

Phosphate depletion with marked hypophosphatemia can occur under several conditions including prolonged dietary deprivation, substantial protein anabolism, redeposition of calcium-phosphate salts in bone, and marked renal phosphate wasting. Short-term intracellular shifts of phosphate may occur during the infusion of large quantities of glucose and during respiratory alkalosis, although these events rarely produce "phosphate depletion."

With phosphorus depletion, a substantial deficit of intracellular phosphate may occur with impaired high-energy phosphate metabolism. Thus, there may be impaired leukocyte function, reduced platelet function, impaired muscular function, and a disorder of the central nervous system. Moreover, cardiac function can be substantially impaired. Marked hypophosphatemia and phosphate depletion can cause impaired deposition of calcium in bone, with increased bone resorption. Thus, osteomalacia can develop with prolonged phosphate depletion. Phosphate depletion can also predispose a patient to muscle dysfunction leading to rhabdomyolysis.

The most frequent cause of severe phosphate depletion in the United States, where dietary phosphate intake is usually adequate, is chronic alcoholism. Decreased dietary intake, reduced intestinal absorption, augmented urinary excretion of phosphate, and a tendency for protein anabolism during refeeding in the hospital are factors involved in the pathogenesis of hypophosphatemia in alcoholics.

The condition of phosphate excess is usually associated with decreased renal function and impaired ability to excrete phosphate. When renal function is impaired, any sudden increase in extracellular phosphate, e.g., by dietary ingestion, tissue catabolism, or the sudden lysis of tumor cells during cancer chemotherapy, can lead to hyperphosphatemia. The use of enemas containing large quantities of phosphate can also cause hyperphosphatemia in patients with decreased renal function. In those conditions, there may be a reciprocal fall in serum Ca and a substantial decrease in renal function, which is often caused by the precipitation of $CaHPO_4$ in the kidney.

MAGNESIUM METABOLISM

Magnesium is a significant extracellular cation, and it is second only to potassium as a major intracellular cation. Bone contains 60% of body Mg. Intracellular Mg is maintained constant, largely independent of plasma Mg levels. The intracellular functions of Mg include its being a cofactor for enzymes and the chelation or binding of many enzymes to subcellular structures. In bone, approximately one-third of the Mg is freely exchanged with plasma Mg; the remainder is deep within bone crystals.

The typical American diet contains approximately 300 mg Mg/day. Thirty to sixty percent of the Mg is absorbed independent of the bodily needs. The fecal losses of Mg can increase in several disorders with diarrhea or malabsorption. The kidney is the major regulator of body Mg; thus there is rapid reduction in urinary Mg when dietary Mg intake is reduced. When Mg intake is high, the maximal rate of tubular reabsorption (Tm) is reached and excess

Mg is excreted in the urine. The renal tubular reabsorption of Mg is reduced by several factors that decrease the reabsorption of Na and water, including expansion of ECF volume, osmotic diuretics, hypercalcemia, alcohol, and the "loop" diuretics, i.e., furosemide or ethacrynic acid. PTH may increase the tubular reabsorption of Mg slightly.

With Mg depletion, bone provides the major labile pool of Mg, and intracellular Mg is only minimally affected. Serum Mg is probably the best available indicator of Mg depletion, whereas intracellular Mg varies with other factors including cell potassium content and protein nutritional state. Hypomagnesemia can occur with: (1) prolonged reduction of Mg intake, (2) reduced intestinal absorption of Mg (malabsorption syndrome, diarrhea, and alcoholism), and (3) a defect in renal tubular reabsorption of Mg (primary aldosteronism, diuretic use, ethanol, or a primary tubular defect). Magnesium can also be lost as it shifts out of extracellular fluids during dialysis therapy and during the rapid restoration of bone mineral.

Magnesium excess can be produced by short-term Mg loading; it persists only while the renal ability to excrete Mg is impaired. Thus, hypermagnesemia occurs during renal insufficiency when there is a high Mg intake. PTH secretion can respond to changes in the concentration of Mg in a manner similar to the effect of Ca, but this response is usually achieved only in experimental conditions. Moreover, with prolonged and marked depletion of Mg, secretion of PTH is impaired and the action of PTH on bone may be reduced; this change leads to hypocalcemia with reduced serum immunoreactive PTH (iPTH) levels (see discussion later).

HYPERCALCEMIA

Hypercalcemia is commonly encountered in clinical practice; it varies in its severity from a life-threatening illness to an asymptomatic, long-standing condition, which is only detected accidentally by routine laboratory screening tests. The manifestations of hypercalcemia reflect both the degree of elevation of blood Ca and its duration. When serum calcium exceeds 15 mg/dl, it can constitute a serious medical emergency. A brief consideration of the general manifestations and features of hypercalcemia precede a discussion of specific pathogenic processes that cause hypercalcemia.

Several organ systems are affected by hypercalcemia, especially the kidneys and the central nervous system. The renal manifestations vary from kidney stones to reversible or even irreversible renal failure. Kidney stones usually occur as a consequence of hypercalciuria that is primarily caused by a long-standing increase in filtered load of Ca. Thus, kidney stones are most common when hypercalcemia is mild and long-standing. Other symptoms of hypercalcemia include polydipsia and polyuria; these arise because hypercalcemia causes a defect in urinary concentrating ability, presumably because of reduced renal medullary hypertonicity and a decreased permeability of the collecting ducts to water. The decreased concentrating ability and polyuria can predispose a patient to dehydration.

Calcium has a depressive effect on the nervous system. Impaired nerve conduction, hypotonia, hyporeflexia, and even paresis can occur. Reduced bowel motility can cause constipation, a frequent presenting symptom. With severe hypercalcemia, the patient's mental status may be impaired with lethargy, confusion, and even coma. Hypercalcemia can have a positive inotropic effect on the heart, and it can alter the cardiac conduction system with arrhythmias and a shortened Q-T interval. Hypercalcemia may be associated with hypertension; the possible mechanisms include alterations in the renin-angiotensin system and a direct increase in peripheral resistance. Gastrointestinal symptoms include anorexia and nausea. Moreover, there is an increased incidence of peptic ulcer disease and pancreatitis. The peptic ulcer may be related to increased gastrin release as a consequence of the increased blood Ca. Hypercalcemia may be associated with the increased deposition of calcium salts in soft tissues, with the lungs, kidneys, blood vessels, and joints being most susceptible.

Hypercalcemia, which can arise from many causes, may develop from increased bone resorption, increased intestinal absorption, or decreased urinary Ca excretion; some causes can involve more than a single mechanism. Of the causes discussed in the following sections, primary hyperparathyroidism and malignant disease are the most common.

Primary Hyperparathyroidism

Hyperparathyroidism is the cause of hypercalcemia in 10 to 30% of cases. A parathyroid adenoma, usually single, is the cause in 80 to 85% of cases, and parathyroid hyperplasia occurs in 10 to 15%, whereas parathyroid carcinoma is rarely the cause. A patient with primary hyperparathyroidism may have other associated endocrine tumors, with a syndrome referred to as "multiple endocrine adenomatosis (MEA)," type 1 or type 2.

It was originally thought that hypercalcemia arose in primary hyperparathyroidism because PTH secretion was independent of serum Ca. However, recent data indicate that PTH secretion is partially dependent on blood Ca both with a parathyroid adenoma and in primary hyperplasia. Nonetheless, the PTH secretion is greater than expected for any level of blood Ca.

Hyperparathyroidism is a disorder best managed surgically. Since this disorder can be "cured" in most instances, this diagnosis should be pursued energetically when one encounters patients with hypercalcemia. No discriminating clinical features separate the various causes of hypercalcemia, except kidney stones do occur more commonly with the mild and prolonged hypercalcemia common in patients with primary hyperparathyroidism. However, certain laboratory features can be distinctive in those patients with primary hyperparathyroidism. An understanding of these features depends upon knowledge of the actions of PTH. The findings present in characteristic cases include: (1) mild to moderate hypercalcemia in the presence of levels of iPTH that are inappropriately high; (2) the presence of indices of renal phosphate reabsorption that show a decreased tubular PO_4 reabsorption inappropriate for

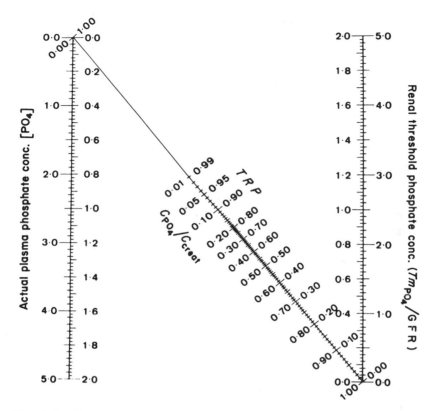

Figure 9–3. Nomogram illustrating the derivation of the renal threshold phosphate threshold (Tm$_{PO_4}$/GFR) from the serum phosphorous level and either the tubular reabsorption of phosphate (TRP) or C$_{PO_4}$/C$_{creat}$ (the ratio of phosphate clearance to creatinine clearance). The TRP is calculated from $1 - (C_{PO_4}/C_{creat})$. There are two scales: an outer scale (0.0 to 5.0) in mass units (mg/dl) and an inner scale in SI units (mMol/L). The normal range of Tm$_{PO_4}$/GFR is 2.5 to 4.2 mg/dl. A lower value suggests a decrease in capacity for tubular reabsorption of PO$_4$ and, therefore, a renal "leak" of PO$_4$. Conversely, a value above 4.2 mg/dl suggests an increased capacity for PO$_4$ reabsorption, i.e., hypoparathyroid states. (From Walton, R.J., and Bijvoet, O.L.M.: Nomogram for derivation of renal threshold phosphate concentration. Lancet, 2:309, 1975.)

the serum PO$_4$ level; (3) the finding of only mild-to-moderate hypercalciuria in the face of a substantial increase in filtered Ca—this finding implies enhanced tubular reabsorption of Ca; (4) mild hyperchloremic acidosis, produced by the action of PTH to decrease the tubular reabsorption of bicarbonate; and (5) an increased urinary excretion of cyclic AMP. This last occurs since most cyclic AMP excreted in the urine is dependent on the effect of PTH to activate the adenylate cyclase in the kidney.

The actions of PTH on the renal phosphate reabsorption have been studied in detail; the tubular reabsorption of phosphate is dependent on PTH as well as on serum phosphorus level and the general status of body phosphate stores.

To correct for the effect of serum PO_4, the determination of theoretic phosphate threshold (Tm_{PO_4}/GFR), which evaluates the percentage of tubular PO_4 reabsorption relative to the plasma PO_4 levels, provides the best clinical index of renal phosphate reabsorptive capacity (Fig. 9–3).

The plasma levels of alkaline phosphatase may be elevated by increased activity of osteoblasts; radiographic changes of osteitis fibrosa (see discussion later in this chapter) may also be seen. These last two findings occur in only a small percentage of patients with primary hyperparathyroidism.

Hypercalcemia may rarely be found in patients with secondary hyperparathyroidism (see the discussion of hypocalcemia). This can occur either because of a reversal of the cause of secondary hyperparathyroidism (i.e., following a kidney transplant) or because of massive parathyroid hyperplasia, with parathyroid cells so numerous that they are poorly responsive to changes in blood Ca.

Malignant Disease

Malignant disease is a common cause of hypercalcemia, which may be associated with metastases to bone (80% of cases) or can develop in the absence of apparent skeletal metastases. When hypercalcemia appears in the absence of detectable metastatic disease, hypercalcemia is thought to arise from various humoral factors including (1) the production of PTH or a PTH-like peptide by the tumor, (2) the stimulation of prostaglandin generation by the tumor, and (3) the generation of "osteoclast activating factor" (OAF). OAF is a peptide that produces bone resorption in vitro; it has been identified in cases of multiple myeloma and malignant lymphoma. In the presence of bone metastases, hypercalcemia is usually ascribed to an osteolytic action of the tumor cells in bone, although other humoral and local factors may be operative. Evidence also suggests that parathyroid adenomas may exist more frequently than expected in patients with malignant disease. For this reason, one should not ignore a possible coexistence of malignant disease and primary hyperparathyroidism.

Vitamin D Overdosage or Overaction

Vitamin D or one of its metabolites can cause hypercalcemia due to enhanced intestinal Ca absorption and increased bone resorption. Overactivity of vitamin D is seen in patients receiving vitamin D treatment for hypoparathyroidism and in uremic patients receiving vitamin D sterols. With vitamin D overdosage, plasma levels of 25(OH)D are substantially elevated, while levels of $1,25(OH)_2D_3$ are normal. This finding and the observation that large amounts of 25(OH)D can mimic the actions of $1,25(OH)_2D_3$ suggest that the high levels of plasma 25(OH)D are responsible. The prolonged circulating half-life of 25(OH)D of 20 to 25 days is consistent with the course of hypercalcemia that occurs with vitamin D overdosage. This hypercalcemia is best managed by discontinuing therapy with vitamin D and, in urgent cases, by the administration of glucocorticoids.

Sarcoidosis and Other Granulomatous Diseases

Hypercalcemia may occur with sarcoidosis and other granulomatous diseases. Patients with sarcoidosis demonstrate increased intestinal absorption of Ca, and the hypercalcemia can be aggravated by sunlight exposure or by the administration of small quantities of vitamin D. That the serum levels of $1,25(OH)_2D_3$ are often elevated suggests increased generation of $1,25(OH)_2D_3$. Where this occurs is uncertain, but it may originate in the granulomatous tissue itself. The hypercalcemia of sarcoidosis is sensitive to the administration of glucocorticoids, perhaps because steroid therapy reduces the generation of $1,25(OH)_2D_3$.

Recovery Phase of Acute Renal Failure

Hypercalcemia may develop during the diuretic phase of acute renal failure, particularly that caused by rhabdomyolysis. During the oliguric phase, marked hypocalcemia is common in such patients because of marked hyperphosphatemia and is due in part to the deposition of Ca salts in the damaged muscle and other soft tissues. With persistence of the secondary hyperparathyroidism arising from the hypocalcemia and the appearance of hypophosphatemia during the diuretic phase, the generation of $1,25(OH)_2D_3$ may be increased to cause the subsequent hypercalcemia. Increased levels of $1,25(OH)_2D_3$ may be found because a recovery of the endocrine function of the renal tubule takes place in the presence of high levels of iPTH and low serum PO_4 levels.

Thiazide Diuretics

The administration of thiazide diuretics can cause mild hypercalcemia. This hypercalcemia is most commonly seen in patients with an underlying problem causing rapid bone turnover, i.e., multiple myeloma, uremic bone disease, and hyperparathyroidism. The mechanisms underlying such hypercalcemia include (1) hemoconcentration due to the sodium diuresis produced by thiazides, (2) a reduced urinary excretion of Ca as a consequence of the diuretic's effect, and (3) potentiation of the action of parathyroid hormone on bone. In patients with no disorder of calcium metabolism, thiazide diuretics may cause a transient, small rise in serum Ca, but the level usually remains within the normal range. Patients who develop frank hypercalcemia while receiving thiazide diuretics should be evaluated for a coexistent disorder affecting calcium or bone metabolism.

Immobilization

With total immobilization and prolonged bed rest, the net balance between the rate of bone formation and bone resorption is disturbed, with resorption exceeding formation. An increase in urinary calcium and hypercalcemia are common when trauma or other illness necessitates total immobilization in young patients who have intrinsically higher rates of bone turnover as well as in patients with Paget's disease.

cyclase; this failure is caused by a deficiency of the guanine nucleotide regulatory protein (also called N-protein), which aids in binding of the PTH-receptor complex to adenylate cyclase itself. Pseudohypoparathyroidism type II is believed to be due to defective intracellular action of cyclic AMP. Renal insufficiency, either acute or chronic, may cause impaired end-organ action of PTH. The pathogenesis is complex, but may arise from altered metabolism of vitamin D (see next section). Severe Mg depletion, besides impairing the secretion of PTH, may also inhibit the response of bone to normal levels of PTH. Thus, if a patient is hypocalcemic and hypomagnesemic, the hypocalcemia cannot be corrected until the Mg deficit is first corrected.

Disturbances of Vitamin D

A deficiency or reduced action of the active form of vitamin D, $1,25(OH)_2D_3$, may cause hypocalcemia. Vitamin D deficiency can arise from a defect in vitamin D metabolism at any step from its intestinal absorption or synthesis in the skin to the final action of $1,25(OH)_2D_3$ on the end organs (see Fig. 9–1). It is convenient to classify vitamin D deficiency in terms of the step of vitamin D metabolism that is affected. These include altered availability of vitamin D_3, reduced $25(OH)D_3$, and decreased availability or action of $1,25(OH)_2D_3$.

Altered Availability of Vitamin D

Vitamin D may not be available if there is reduced vitamin D intake or absorption in combination with little or no exposure to ultraviolet irradiation from sunlight. With the fortification of foods such as milk and bread with vitamin D in the United States, nutritional vitamin D deficiency is unusual. Consequently, gastrointestinal disease with malabsorption of this fat-soluble vitamin is now the most frequent cause of vitamin D deficiency.

Impaired absorption of vitamin D_3 is seen in patients with fat malabsorption, including those with celiac disease, chronic pancreatitis, Crohn's disease, hepatic dysfunction, and after gastrectomy and small bowel operations.

Reduced 25-Hydroxy-Vitamin D_3

Vitamin D is readily converted to $25(OH)D$ in the liver. Therefore, reduced plasma levels of $25(OH)D$ can indicate decreased availability of vitamin D_3, as previously described. In the face of normal availability of D_3, decreased levels of $25(OH)D$ may develop if there is an increased metabolism of $25(OH)D$ to inactive metabolites. This process may occur during treatment with phenobarbital, phenytoin, and glutethimide, which may induce a hepatic microsomal enzyme causing the rapid breakdown of $25(OH)D$. The plasma $25(OH)D_3$ levels may be reduced in the nephrotic syndrome because of excessive urinary loss of $25(OH)D_3$, which is bound to a specific vitamin D binding protein in plasma. Certain liver diseases, in particular biliary cirrhosis, may be associated with decreased synthesis of $25(OH)D_3$ or may impair the normal enterohepatic circulation of $25(OH)D_3$.

Decreased Availability or Action of 1,25(OH)-Vitamin D_3

Reduced plasma levels of $1,25(OH)_2D_3$ have been identified in chronic renal insufficiency owing to a reduction of the functioning renal parenchymal tissue, in an hereditary defect (vitamin D dependency rickets), in Fanconi's syndrome, and in osteomalacia associated with mesenchymal tumors. Plasma levels of $1,25(OH)_2D_3$ are lower than expected in sex-linked hypophosphatemic rickets. Except for chronic renal insufficiency, these disorders are unusual.

Finally, there are children with features of vitamin D dependency rickets who have end-organ insensitivity to $1,25(OH)_2D_3$.

Removal of Calcium from Serum

Hyperphosphatemia

Hypocalcemia may be caused by hyperphosphatemia. The mechanism responsible for this lowering of Ca is not well understood. The most common explanation is that the solubility product of $CaHPO_4$ is exceeded, leading to the deposition of Ca in soft tissues and bone. Hyperphosphatemia is a principal factor in the hypocalcemia of chronic or acute renal disease (see discussion to follow). Hyperphosphatemia also sometimes develops after excessive intake of PO_4, either by oral or intravenous administration, or by a PO_4-containing enema. Severe hyperphosphatemia is rare unless there is impaired renal function with the reduced excretion of the PO_4.

Hypocalcemia is more likely to develop when serum PO_4 increases rapidly. Acute hyperphosphatemia from rapid cell lysis can occur with rhabdomyolysis or in the treatment of certain lymphoproliferative diseases.

Calcium Deposition in Bone

Hypocalcemia may develop as a consequence of the rapid deposition of Ca into bone. This phenomenon is seen in osteoblastic metastases, particularly with tumors of the prostate, breast, and lung. Marked and protracted hypocalcemia can appear following the removal of a parathyroid adenoma, with the rapid uptake of Ca by bone. Such a problem can be anticipated preoperatively by the finding of increased plasma alkaline phosphatase and by bone roentgenograms that show severe subperiosteal resorption. This postoperative hypocalcemia may be reduced by pretreatment with vitamin D.

Increased Renal Excretion of Calcium

The kidney is believed to play a role in the regulation of serum Ca concentration in man; consequently, increased urinary losses of Ca can contribute to hypocalcemia. Increased urinary loss is rarely the only factor causing hypocalcemia; instead, it is usually a contributing factor. An example is hypoparathyroidism, where the absence of circulating PTH leads to increased urinary Ca and contributes to the hypocalcemia.

The administration of furosemide or ethacrynic acid can inhibit renal tubular Ca reabsorption and can increase urinary Ca. Similarly, the intravenous infusions of large volumes of saline solution or other sodium-containing fluids can enhance the renal excretion of Ca. These effects of saline and furosemide make them useful in the treatment of hypercalcemia (see previous discussion). Mild hypocalcemia is also common in the syndrome of inappropriate ADH (see Chap. 10). This syndrome may be due both to a reduced plasma albumin and to the expansion of ECF volume caused by the increase in total body water, which leads to sodium diuresis accompanied by increased urinary Ca.

Renal Failure

Hypocalcemia is common in renal insufficiency, either acute or chronic, and certain evidence exists that some decrease in ionized Ca can develop early in the course of mild renal insufficiency. In renal failure, the major mechanisms responsible for hypocalcemia include (1) phosphate retention, (2) altered vitamin D metabolism, and (3) impaired skeletal action of parathyroid hormone.

It has been postulated that minimal phosphate retention, occurring as a consequence of reduced renal function, may result in a slight rise in serum PO_4 and in a small reciprocal fall in serum Ca. The consequent secretion of PTH then causes phosphaturia, which lowers serum PO_4; this change results in the return of serum Ca to normal, but only at the expense of an increased blood PTH. This process is believed to repeat itself during progressive renal insufficiency until renal failure reaches such a degree of severity that hyperphosphatemia is persistent. This series of events is postulated as a major cause of the secondary hyperparathyroidism of renal insufficiency.

Another cause of hypocalcemia is impaired metabolism of vitamin D. With the kidney as the only source for the generation of $1,25(OH)_2D_3$, availability of this sterol may be reduced. Decreased $1,25(OH)_2D_3$ impairs Ca absorption with an attendant decrease in blood Ca; PTH is thereby stimulated. PTH may increase the renal generation of $1,25(OH)_2D_3$ until more advanced renal failure prevents this compensatory mechanism. The PO_4 retention and altered vitamin D metabolism may be related, in that PO_4 retention may decrease the generation of $1,25(OH)_2D_3$.

Finally, evidence suggests that the skeleton fails to release Ca normally in response to PTH in renal insufficiency; the result would be a lower blood Ca for any given level of PTH. Although the mechanism is unclear, it may be related to altered vitamin D metabolism. The dominant mechanism leading to a low blood Ca in renal failure is disputed, but more than one mechanism probably accounts for the parathyroid hyperplasia so commonly observed in chronic renal insufficiency.

Hypocalcemia is not invariable in uremic patients, particularly those undergoing long-term dialysis treatment; indeed, hypercalcemia may occasionally be encountered, perhaps owing to marked parathyroid hyperplasia. Under such circumstances, the improvement of uremia with dialysis, a normal or high Ca intake, an increase in Ca level in dialysate, or the administration of an active vitamin D sterol may contribute to the appearance of hypercalcemia. Moreover, blood Ca may increase during marked PO_4 deprivation.

Miscellaneous Causes of Hypocalcemia

Pancreatitis

Hypocalcemia is a well-known manifestation of pancreatitis. Most patients have a reduced total serum Ca, and virtually all have a reduction of the ionized fraction. The pathogenesis of this hypocalcemia is not well understood, but local precipitation of Ca salts of fatty acids, reduced PTH secretion, and resistance to PTH action have been suggested.

Neonatal Hypocalcemia

Serum Ca levels normally decline in the neonate during the first 3 days of life. When the Ca level falls below 8.0 mg/dl at term or below 7.0 mg/dl in the premature infant, the hypocalcemia is pathologic. Several pathogenetic mechanisms have been suggested, including vitamin D deficiency, parathyroid hypofunction, Mg deficiency, and hyperphosphatemia due to a high content of PO_4 in cow's milk.

Citrate Administration

Citrate, present in transfused blood, can bind ionized Ca, and a fall in Ca is occasionally seen after multiple transfusions with citrated blood.

Clinical Features of Hypocalcemia

Hypocalcemia is potentially dangerous, with clinical manifestations caused by disturbances in neuromuscular function. Increased excitability of the motor nerves and lowering of the threshold of sensory nerves can occur and may lead to tetany. Symptoms of hypocalcemia include numbness and tingling or "pins and needles" sensation of the hands, feet, tongue, or circumoral area. Muscle spasms are commonly noted in the forearm and hand, with the elbow, wrist, and metacarpal-phalangeal joints flexed and abducted across the palm (carpal-pedal spasm). In extreme situations, generalized convulsions and laryngeal spasm may cause life-threatening respiratory embarrassment.

Two classic physical findings may be seen with hypocalcemia: Chvostek's sign, which consists of contractions of facial muscles after tapping over the facial nerve in front of the ear, and Trousseau's sign, which is the induction of carpal spasm by inflating a blood pressure cuff to a level of systolic pressure for three minutes. Both the Chvostek's and Trousseau's signs may be negative in hypocalcemic patients; therefore, negative tests do not exclude this diagnosis.

METABOLIC BONE DISEASES

In this consideration of metabolic bone disease, osteitis fibrosa, osteomalacia, osteoporosis, and Paget's disease of bone are discussed.

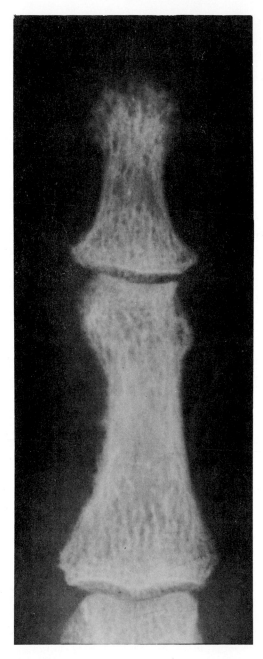

Figure 9–5. Hyperparathyroid bone disease. Roentgenogram of the index finger of the right hand, showing substantial erosions of both the distal tuft and the middle phalanx. The subperiosteal erosions are typically more marked on the radial (left) than on the ulnar surfaces of the phalanx and lead to the ragged, irregular appearance.

Osteitis Fibrosa

This pathologic process occurs in hyperparathyroidism, either primary or secondary. X-ray studies of bone may show subperiosteal resorption, detected most readily in the hands (Fig. 9–5), resorption or "loss" of the distal ends of the clavicles, a mottled, moth-eaten, or ground-glass appearance of the skull and cystic "brown tumors." Histologically, it is characterized by marked increases in osteoclastic activity, in numbers of osteoclasts, and in areas of osteoclastic resorption. The number of osteoblasts is also increased; wide rows of osteoblasts overlie areas of collagen deposition and new bone formation. Studies that permit evaluation of the rate of bone turnover indicate an accelerated rate. Moreover, a variable degree of peritrabecular fibrosis occurs, a finding that led to the original descriptive term, osteitis fibrosa.

Osteomalacia

This disorder is characterized by impaired mineralization of bone. The major criteria for its histologic identification are the finding of wide seams of mineralized protein matrix (i.e., osteoid) or the demonstration of delayed mineralization of such osteoid. The bone turnover is usually reduced, a finding that contrasts with osteitis fibrosa. Clinically, this disorder is manifested by bone pain, fractures, and x-ray evidence of demineralization and, occasionally, pseudofractures, which appear as lucent areas at the insertion of nutrient arteries. It should be noted that x-ray evidence of demineralization of bone is nonspecific and can occur with osteomalacia, osteoporosis, and, at times, osteitis fibrosa.

The causes of osteomalacia are numerous; they include (1) hypocalcemia and a deficiency of Ca, (2) a deficiency of PO_4, and (3) either a deficiency of, abnormal metabolism of, or defective action of vitamin D. Thus, the pathogenic factors leading to osteomalacia may be the same as those causing hypocalcemia (see previous discussion). In addition, substances that may inhibit the mineralization of bone are present; they include excess fluoride, aluminum accumulation, cadmium, and certain diphosphonates. Osteomalacia can also develop as a consequence of profound phosphate deficiency and hypophosphatemia. In the United States, the most common causes of osteomalacia are the malabsorption syndromes, which lead to a deficiency of vitamin D and/or Ca.

Osteoporosis

This is the most common clinical disorder affecting skeletal metabolism, especially in women over age 50. It can most easily be defined as a condition with "too little bone;" osteomalacic bone is abnormal, whereas osteoporotic bone is normal but simply reduced in amount. In certain types of osteoporosis, bone turnover may be enhanced; in others, there is no increase and bone formation lags behind bone resorption. Osteoporosis may occur secondary to a variety of diseases and situations, including Cushing's disease, hyperthyroidism, acromegaly, rheumatoid arthritis, immobilization, multiple myeloma, and osteitis imperfecta. The cause of osteoporosis is unknown in most instances.

Backache is the most common symptom; on occasion, this symptom is aggravated by a crush fracture of a vertebral body. Patients may occasionally experience a loss of height, but the correlation between the severity of the disease, as evaluated by roentgenogram, and the symptoms is often poor. An organic diagnosis of osteoporosis is frequently given to middle-aged, depressed women with the nonspecific symptom of back pain. Osteoporosis is commonly detected because of fractures; vertebral crush fracture, Colles' fracture of the wrist, and intertrochanteric fractures of the femur are the most common. The diagnosis of osteoporosis is usually established by an x-ray study showing uniform rarefaction of the spine and pelvis in the absence of other causes of bone rarefaction. Accentuation of the end plates of vertebral bodies is noted; later, they become biconcave and resemble a typical "codfish spine." In the absence of fractures, the x-ray diagnosis is difficult because of the lack of reliable quantitative measurements of bone loss. It is estimated that 30 to 50% of bone Ca must be lost before osteoporosis is apparent radiologically. Another method, the absorption of photons by bone with the use of a specialized instrument, may provide a more precise measurement of mineral loss.

The major feature that separates osteoporosis from other metabolic bone diseases is the absence of abnormalities of serum Ca, P, and alkaline phosphatase; characteristic abnormalities are usually found with other types of metabolic bone disease (Table 9–3).

Because the diagnosis of osteoporosis is nonspecific, figures on its incidence are not precise. It has been estimated that 30% of women over age 55 and of men over age 60 may have sufficient mineral loss from bone to predispose them to fracture. It is best to consider such a loss of bone mineral in light of the normal course of bone mineral content. Thus, bone mineral content increases continuously to a peak at age 20 to 25; bone mass then remains stable until the fourth or fifth decade, when it decreases by 1 to 2% per year in both men and women. With the menopause, the rate of mineral loss is accelerated, although an age-related increase in bone loss occurs independent of estrogen status. Because of the progressive loss of bone with time, some have regarded osteoporosis not as a disease but as a reflection of aging.

Table 9–3.   Laboratory Findings in Metabolic Bone Disease

Disorder	Serum		
	Ca	P	Alk P'tase
Osteoporosis	N	N	N
Osteitis Fibrosa	I*	D,N	I
Osteomalacia	D	N,D	I
Paget's Disease	N	N	I

N, normal; I, increased; D, decreased; * indicates that levels may be normal or decreased in secondary hyperparathyroidism.

The pathogenesis of bone loss is unclear, and it is likely that many factors contribute to this syndrome. Population surveys reveal that patients with osteoporosis generally ingest lower amounts of Ca than those without osteoporosis and that they exhibit a greater degree of negative Ca balance. With Ca supplements, Ca absorption may increase and Ca balance may eventually become positive, although it is less clear that the status of the bone is improved. It is apparent that the risk of osteoporosis is increased by premature menopause, i.e., with castration without estrogen replacement. The role of estrogen replacement after menopause in the management or prevention of osteoporosis is controversial; evidence suggests that small quantities of estrogen given over a period of several years can reduce the rate of mineral loss after the menopause; however, it is uncertain whether this apparent "beneficial" effect is sustained.

Paget's Disease of Bone (Osteitis Deformans)

Paget's disease of bone is common, with an incidence reaching 4% in autopsy series of adults. Although asymptomatic lesions involving a single site are the most common, the disease can be generalized, with thickening of the skull and deformities of the long bones, particularly bowing of the tibias. The roentgenographic findings can be specific, with the initial development of sharply circumscribed radiolucency followed by the appearance of areas of dense sclerosis. Histologic examination of affected bone discloses a marked increase in bone resorption adjacent to areas of intense new bone formation. The collagen deposited in the new bone is abnormal and has a blotchy mosaic or woven pattern. The new bone is poor in tensile strength, and fractures are common. The pathogenesis of the condition is unclear; certain ultrastructural studies reveal virus-like particles in areas of pagetic bone; thus, it has been suggested that this disorder may represent a "slow virus" infection.

The pain, which may or may not be prominent, does not correlate with the degree of skeletal involvement. Deafness can occur as a complication of Paget's disease of the skull; it is caused either by sclerosis of the bones of the middle ear or by entrapment of the acoustic nerve within the diseased temporal bone. Areas of pagetic bone often show increased blood flow, with an increase in blood flow in overlying soft tissues as well. High cardiac output, presumably largely due to arteriovenous fistulas, can lead to high-output heart failure. In addition to the deformities of bone, examination may reveal tissue warmth overlying the affected bone. The laboratory features include normal levels of serum Ca and PO_4, with alkaline phosphatase values elevated to levels higher than are seen with other conditions. Increased urinary excretion of Ca and hydroxyproline are evidence of increased bone turnover.

Treatment with calcitonin, which causes a prompt decrease in osteoclastic bone resorption, may be associated with substantial symptomatic improvement and a decrease in the serum alkaline phosphatase toward normal, although the roentgenograms remain abnormal. The diphosphonates presumably act by decreasing bone turnover and are also useful in the management of patients with severe Paget's disease.

CLINICAL PROBLEMS

Patient 1. A 53-year-old man was found to have a serum Ca concentration of 12 mg/dl on a routine laboratory analysis taken at the time of his retirement from the Air Force. A physical fitness buff, he successfully completed the Boston Marathon at age 50. He was entirely without symptoms, and he consumed no medications, vitamins, or tonics. Skeletal roentgenograms and evaluation for malignant disease were entirely negative.

LABORATORY DATA. Calcium, 12.0 to 12.4 mg/100 ml; PO_4, 3.0 mg/dl; chloride, 104 to 106 mEq/L; creatinine, 1.0 mg/100 ml; tubular reabsorption of phosphorus, 80% on regular diet; Tm_{PO}/GFR, 2.4 mg/dl; alkaline phosphatase, normal.

Because he was without symptoms, the patient refused neck exploration. He was followed with serial calcium determinations for 12 months as an outpatient. At the last 4 determinations, the calcium levels were between 13 and 13.5 mg/100 ml, but the patient remained entirely well. Because of the apparent trend in calcium concentration, he acquiesced to an operation. A single 250-mg parathyroid adenoma was resected, and the patient's serum Ca returned to normal.

QUESTIONS

1. Was it appropriate to delay operation on this man with unequivocal hyperparathyroidism?
2. What specific indications for surgical procedure should be sought in following a patient with hyperparathyroidism?

Patient 2. A 15-year-old boy is referred to you for evaluation of hypocalcemia. He has not been in good health since the age of 10, when he began to experience seizures and was found to have cataracts. At age 12 he underwent bilateral cataract surgery, and his vision has been reasonably good ever since. He has taken phenytoin, 200 mg/day, and phenobarbital, 15 mg twice daily, ever since his seizure disorder was discovered, and he has not experienced any seizures over the past 6 months. His only complaints are fatigue and muscle cramps.

PHYSICAL EXAMINATION. On examination you find a short, teenage boy in midpuberty. His height is 5 feet, 1 inch, and his weight is 120 pounds. His face is round, and bilateral dimples appear at the fourth metacarpal head when he makes a fist. Chvostek's sign is absent.

LABORATORY DATA. Calcium, 7.1 mg/100; albumin, 4 g/100 ml; phosphorus, 5.2 mg/100 ml; alkaline phosphatase, 110 IU (normal, up to 80 IU). Skeletal roentgenograms show generalized demineralization and a cystic lesion in the right humerus. Immunoreactive PTH, 3.4 ng/ml (normal, less than 0.5 ng/ml).

QUESTIONS

1. What is the diagnosis? How can your impression be confirmed?
2. What complicating feature is found in the management of his seizure disorder?
3. What further management is indicated?

Patient 3. This 54-year-old black man complains of back pain and fatigue. In good health until 6 months ago, he has worked as a stevedore for 30 years without missing a day of work.

PHYSICAL EXAMINATION. He is found to have pale conjunctivae, a resting pulse of 110, and an orthostatic drop in blood pressure from 115/80 to 80/70. Point tenderness of the spine appears at T12 and L4.

LABORATORY DATA. Hematocrit, 27; serum Ca, 11.2 mg/100 ml; alkaline phosphatase, 75 IU. Serum protein electrophoresis showed an abnormal globulin, which proved to be gamma D. Skeletal roentgenograms showed only diffuse osteopenia. Despite prompt initiation of chemotherapy and corticosteroids, the patient succumbed to sepsis on the fifth hospital day.

QUESTIONS

1. Is it surprising to find a normal alkaline phosphatase in a patient with obvious malignant disease in bone?
2. What are the causes of hypercalcemia in this patient?
3. How great should the suspicion of malignant disease be for a black patient with osteoporosis?

Patient 4. You are asked to evaluate a 24-year-old man for hypocalcemia. Patient was in good health until the age of 16, when he was diagnosed as having Crohn's disease. He has subsequently required 3 bowel resections with removal of 3 feet of ileum including the terminal ileum. He had been doing well until 3 weeks prior to admission when diarrhea began. He has noted some weakness and has not felt well. The patient is not receiving any medications.

PHYSICAL EXAMINATION. He is found to have a positive Chvostek's and Trousseau's sign.

LABORATORY DATA. Calcium, 6.2 mg/100 ml; albumin, 4.0 g/100; PO$_4$, 4.0 mg/100 ml; creatinine, 1.0 mg/100 ml.

QUESTIONS

1. What additional laboratory information is needed?
2. What is the mechanism for the hypocalcemia?
3. Does the level of serum PO$_4$ give you a clue to the diagnosis?

SUGGESTED READING

Bone Physiology

Avioli, L.V., and Krane, S.M. (eds.): Metabolic Bone Disease. 2 Vol. London, Academic Press, 1978.

Calcium, Parathyroid Hormone, Vitamin D

Coburn, J.W., Kurokawa, K., and Kleeman, C.R.: Divalent ion metabolism. *In* Contemporary Metabolism. Edited by N. Freinkel. New York, Plenum Publishing, 1979.

Gallagher, J.C., et al.: Intestinal calcium absorption and serum vitamin D metabolites in normal subjects and osteoporotic patients. J. Clin. Invest., *64*:729, 1979.

Habener, J.F., and Potts, J.T.: Parathyroid physiology and primary hyperparathyroidism. *In* Metabolic Bone Disease. Edited by L.V. Avioli and S.M. Krane. Vol. 2. London, Academic Press, 1978.

Haussler, M.R., and McCain, T.A.: Basic and clinical concepts related to vitamin D metabolism and action. N. Engl. J. Med., *297*:974, 1041, 1977.

Hypercalcemic Disorders

Mallette, L., et al.: Primary hyperparathyroidism clinical and biochemical features. Medicine, *53*:127, 1974.

Mundy, G.R.: Calcium and cancer. Life Sci., *23*:1735, 1978.

Seyberth, H.W., et al.: Prostaglandins as mediators of hypercalcemia associated with certain types of cancer. N. Engl. J. Med., *293*:1278, 1975.

Walton, R.J., and Bijovet, O.L.M.: Nomogram for derivation of renal threshold phosphate concentration. Lancet, 2:309, 1975.

Hypocalcemic Disorders

Nagant, D.E., Deuxchaisnes, C., and Krane, S.M.: Hypoparathyroidism. *In* Metabolic Bone Disease. Edited by L.V. Avioli and S.M. Krane. Vol 2. London, Academic Press, 1978.

Nusynowitz, M.L., Frame, B., and Kolb, F.O.: The spectrum of the hypoparathyroid states. Medicine, *55*:105, 1976.

Metabolic Bone Disease

Evans, I.M.A.: Calcitonin treatment of Paget's disease. Lancet, 2:1232, 1979.

Frame, B., and Parfitt, A.M.: Osteomalacia: current concepts. Ann. Intern. Med., *89*:966, 1978.

Ibbertson, H.K., et al.: Paget's disease of bone: assessment and management. Drugs, *18*:33, 1979.

CHAPTER 10

Disorders of Water Metabolism

Richard E. Weitzman and Charles R. Kleeman

Every living organism from the simplest unicellular form to the most complex mammal has developed mechanisms to guard the total solute content or osmolality of its body fluids. The more complex the organism the more complex the system must be for controlling osmolality, and the narrower is the range of osmolality consistent with normal cell function. This process occurs despite wide variations in fluid intake. When one deliberately ingests a large quantity of water over a short period of time, the body responds by excreting this water load as dilute urine over a few hours and any sensation of thirst is dissipated. Conversely, a period of 16 to 24 hours of water restriction is associated with profound thirst and the production of a small volume of the most concentrated urine. The body has responded appropriately to both these perturbations in order to maintain its osmolality and volume within a narrow range.

The physiologic control system responsible for this stability includes both receptors that sense the osmotic pressure of body fluids as well as those that are responsive to changes in the volume and/or pressure in certain anatomic areas of the circulation. In nearly all clinical circumstances, both receptor systems function simultaneously to regulate the volume and tonicity of body fluids (Fig. 10–1).

OSMOTIC CONTROL

Water diffuses rapidly and freely along osmotic gradients across all cell membranes. Therefore, the specialized neuronal cells of the hypothalamic neurohypophyseal tract and the thirst centers of the hypothalamus immediately sense changes in the effective osmolality of the extracellular fluid. Only the cells of the cortical and medullary collecting duct of the mammalian nephron vary their permeability to water in response to a given endogenous chemical, arginine vasopressin (AVP) or antidiuretic hormone (ADH). The osmorecep-

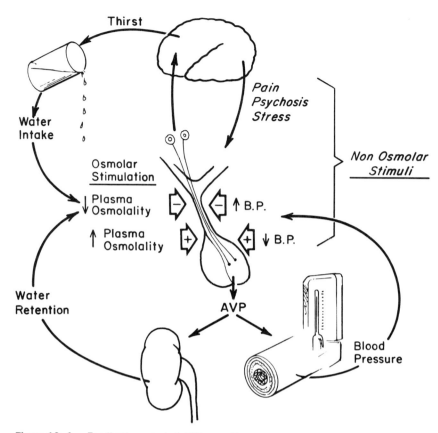

Figure 10–1. Feedback control of AVP secretion.

tor cells respond to as little as a 1 to 2% rise in plasma osmolality with an increase in the frequency of depolarization. This increase results in the synthesis and release of ADH. Hypertonicity also results in the sensation of thirst. AVP facilitates the renal conservation of existing body stores of water, whereas thirst results in drinking additional fluid to return the hypertonicity of the body fluids to normal. Both the release of AVP and thirst are critical to the maintenance of water homeostasis. Without AVP, renal water excretion would assume such large proportions that the thirst mechanism would be constantly stressed to keep up with urinary losses. Absent thirst with intact AVP release results in chronic hypernatremia without polyuria.

While the anatomic and physiologic details of the control system are still being elucidated, it appears that the sequence approximates the following: free water losses in urine, stool, and sweat result in a rise in the concentration of solutes per unit weight of plasma (plasma osmolality). This stimulates the osmoreceptor centers in the hypothalamus to initiate the synthesis and release of AVP and also to bring about the sensation of thirst. These actions in turn result in water conservation and ingestion so that there is a return of plasma solute concentration to normal. At that point the stimulus to the osmoreceptor ceases; AVP secretion declines to a baseline level and thirst disappears. The system also functions to maintain plasma osmolality in the face of a water load. The ingestion of a liter or two of water would cause dilution of the plasma solute concentrations, and this dilution reduces the stimulus to the osmoreceptor, which in turn diminishes the secretion of AVP. A water diuresis results until the water load is eliminated and the plasma osmolality returns to normal. At that time AVP secretion is resumed. The dilution of the body fluid thus results in a negative feedback on AVP secretion.

AVP is an octapeptide with a molecular weight of 1084. It is found in all mammals except members of the suborder Suina, which includes pigs and the hippopotamus. This suborder secretes lysine vasopressin; the lysine is in the position of arginine. AVP is synthesized in magnocellular neurons located largely in the supraoptic nucleus of the hypothalamus. The hormone appears to be synthesized along with a carrier protein, neurophysin, and is packaged into neurosecretory granules. The vasopressin-neurophysin granules "trickle" down the axons by axoplasmic flow to be stored at the axons' terminals in the posterior lobe of the pituitary.

Osmotic or other stimuli not only induce increased de novo synthesis of AVP, but also result in the hormone's secretion into the circulation by the process of exocytosis. This process is rapid; large quantities of AVP can be measured in the systemic circulation within minutes after administration of hypertonic saline solution. There is no evidence that it remains bound to neurophysin after its secretion or that neurophysin has any role in its action. Once secreted, the hormone is rapidly inactivated by metabolic degradation in the liver and the kidney and about 10% of the active hormone is excreted in the urine. Estimates of its half-life in humans range from 15 to 20 minutes. The rapid stimulation and turnover of AVP are in accord with its physiologic function of quickly responding to small changes in plasma tonicity, blood pressure, or blood volume. Its action on the nephron and smooth muscle cells of the arterioles ceases almost simultaneously with its disappearance from the circulation.

NONOSMOLAR CONTROL

The release of AVP from the posterior lobe of the neurohypophysis is also responsive to nonosmotic factors. These factors are mediated mainly by receptors that respond to alterations in either the pressure or volume in the left atrium and the carotid sinus. The limb of the control system responsive to changes in volume or pressure appears to be less sensitive to small perturbations than the osmolar control system. Only a 1 to 2% rise in plasma tonicity stimulates AVP release, although it requires an approximately 10% reduction in plasma volume to obtain a similar response. However, the magnitude of the response, when elicited, is considerably greater than that induced by osmotic stimulation. This "hypersecretion" of AVP after hemorrhage seems to have two functions. First, it acts synergistically with the renin-aldosterone system to restore plasma volume. Aldosterone conserves sodium while AVP conserves water; the combined effect is an increase in the extracellular fluid volume. Second, AVP is a potent pressor agent and may have pressure-elevating effects at the concentrations achieved after hemorrhage.

Recent studies indicate that AVP contributes to the support of blood pressure when cardiac output is acutely reduced and when pressures in the aortic arch and carotid sinus are lowered. AVP is even more potent than other vasoconstrictor substances such as norepinephrine and angiotensin.

The baroreceptors located predominantly within the left atrium have been designated as low-pressure receptors. Afferent impulses from these receptors are carried by the vagus nerve. They appear to respond to small reductions in central blood volume that are not associated with systemic hypotension. Other baroreceptors are present within the carotid body and the arch of the aorta. These receptors are designated the high-pressure baroreceptors, and their afferent impulses are carried by the glossopharyngeal nerve. At present, it appears that small changes in blood volume are perceived by the low-pressure receptors. These receptors tonically inhibit AVP release, and a decrease in their firing rate from diminished stretch results in increased AVP release. Severance of the vagi or carotid sinus nerves produces an antidiuresis. The relative importance of the low- and high-pressure receptor systems in the hypovolemic stimulation of AVP release has not been established.

Recent studies have suggested that many nonosmolar stimuli for AVP secretion are mediated by stimulation of the baroreceptors rather than having a direct effect on the hypothalamus. However, severe pain or emotional stress can evoke AVP release, presumably by direct neural connections from the cerebral cortex to the hypothalamus. Several drugs have been thought to act directly on the hypothalamus or posterior pituitary to release AVP, but confirmation using hormone measurements in peripheral blood has been lacking. Angiotensin has been shown to be a potent stimulus for thirst and AVP release when injected in minute quantities into the lateral and third ventricles of the central nervous system. At these sites it is in close proximity to the nuclei controlling both of these functions. The interrelationship of the renin-angiotensin system to AVP secretion is of interest because it suggests a supplementary reflex arc to mediate AVP release in hypovolemic or hypotensive states.

MECHANISM OF ACTION OF AVP

The major sites of action of AVP in the kidney appear to be the cortical and medullary collecting ducts. AVP binds to receptor sites on the apical side of the cells and activates adenylate cyclase. This action in turn results in intracellular accumulation of cyclic AMP, which activates protein kinase. The latter enzyme alters the permeability of the luminal membrane for water, the precise mechanism for which is undefined. Water but not solute passes through the membrane resulting in production of concentrated urine.

Altered water permeability of the tubular membrane by itself is not sufficient to produce a concentrated urine. The process is dependent upon an intact cortical-medullary concentration gradient for solutes because, even with maximal permeability, the urine can never be more concentrated than the surrounding interstitial tissue. The gradient is created by the active transport of chloride ions from the thick ascending limb of the loop of Henle. Sodium follows the electrochemical gradient across the membrane. Water, on the other hand, is unable to diffuse out of the ascending limb because of its limited water permeability under all conditions, so that the medulla becomes hypertonic to the tubular fluid. The effectiveness of the chloride pump in creating a high solute concentration in the medullary interstitium is enhanced by the countercurrent multiplier system. With this system the relatively small gradient of sodium and chloride in the medulla is greatly increased as a result of the anatomic juxtaposition of the vasa recti with the loop of Henle. The blood flow in the vasa recti serves to prevent the dissipation of the hypertonic gradient while urine flow in the loop of Henle creates the gradient. The back diffusion of water and urea across renal membranes and the variable permeability of these membranes then function to produce either dilute or concentrated urine.

As will be described in a later section, multiple factors can disrupt the generation of the cortical-medullary concentration gradient and in so doing can block the effect of AVP on increasing urinary concentration. For example, in sickle cell anemia, degeneration and destruction of the renal medulla with its vasa recti may be associated with inability to concentrate the urine. Occasional patients are known to ingest copious amounts of fluid, which "washes out" their medullary concentration gradient. Furosemide blocks chloride transport from the thick ascending limb of the loop of Henle and thus lowers the medullary solute concentration. All these circumstances cause impairment of the antidiuretic action of AVP independent of its cellular action.

CLINICAL EVALUATION OF ABNORMAL WATER BALANCE

The initial evaluation of body water balance begins with taking a pertinent history and performing a physical examination. The patient is asked about the sensation of thirst, the quantity of fluid intake, the frequency of voiding, and the volume of urine excreted. The patient is examined for signs of water depletion such as tachycardia, orthostatic hypotension, dry mucous membranes and decreased skin turgor, or signs of excess water such as edema. However, most if not all edema is due to both salt (NaCl) and water retention. Pure water retention can be marked, with proportionate hypo-osmolality of body fluids and little or no pitting edema.

The laboratory evaluation includes estimation of the plasma concentration of osmotically active solute. A valid approximation can be made by measuring plasma sodium concentration. Potassium, glucose, and urea also contribute to plasma osmolality but to a lesser degree. The formula $2 (Na^+) + (glucose)/18 + (BUN)/2.8$ is useful under most circumstances to approximate the plasma osmolality. Osmolality can be determined directly by measuring the depression of the freezing point of plasma samples. The normal range is from 280 to 290 mOsm/kg of plasma water.

Isotopic dilution studies can provide a more direct assessment of plasma volume, extracellular fluid volume, or total body water, but these studies are not generally available and are not clinically practical. Reliable laboratory clues to body water status are the BUN (blood urea nitrogen) and serum uric acid, which in otherwise normal people are low in states of water retention and high with dehydration. The action of AVP on the nephron can be assessed indirectly by determination of either the specific gravity or osmolality of the urine. These two measurements correlate well with each other unless the urine contains large amounts of molecules such as sugars (glucose or mannitol), protein, or some pharmacologic agents such as the radiopaque contrast materials used for angiograms or pyelograms. All these may greatly increase the specific gravity out of proportion to their effect on osmolality. An even better approximation of AVP action would come from calculating the free water clearance by determining the urinary flow rate in milliliters per minute. The osmolar clearance is then calculated as the product of the urinary osmolality times the volume of urine collected divided by the plasma osmolality times the interval in minutes over which the sample was collected. The difference between the flow rate and the osmolar clearance is the free water clearance ($C_{H_2O} = V - C_{osm}$). This calculation is a measure of the conservation or excretion of solute-free water by the kidney and thus reflects AVP action on water permeability.

Urinary sodium concentration does not parallel urinary osmolality. Its determination is useful to distinguish inappropriate AVP release with water retention causing hyponatremia from states of salt depletion with the same degree of hyponatremia. In both situations urinary tonicity may be elevated, but urinary sodium is high (50 to 100 mEq/L) in states of abnormal water retention and low (less than 25 mEq/L) in states of sodium depletion.

In Figure 10–2 the urine and plasma osmolalities for a variety of disease states are plotted. The data for diabetes insipidus tend to be grouped together with hypertonicity of the plasma in association with hypotonic urine. In contrast, patients with polyuria due to psychogenic water drinking have hypotonicity of both plasma and urine.

Steady-state observations are often insufficient to categorize borderline or partial disorders. In some circumstances it is necessary to stress the system. The type of stress used depends on the nature of the disorder. For polyuric disorders the patient is subjected to a dehydration test. Baseline body weight, urinary and plasma osmolality are obtained, and water is withheld from 8 to 16 hours (depending upon the rate of urinary water loss). Serial determinations are then made of urinary osmolality. Normal subjects are able to concentrate their urine to approximately 1000 to 1200 mOsm/kg without either excessive weight loss or elevation of plasma osmolality. The achievement of maximal endogenous urinary concentration is signified by a relatively stable or only a

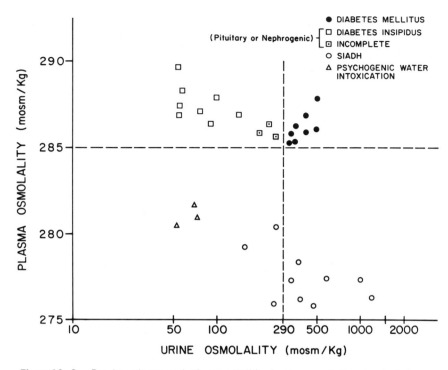

Figure 10–2.   Random plasma and urine osmolalities in diseases of altered water balance.

slight fall in urinary osmolality on 2 successive 1-hour collection periods. At this time, aqueous vasopressin (Pitressin) is given parenterally, or desamino-d-arginine (DDAVP), a potent synthetic analogue, may be given intranasally, and the urinary osmolality is measured. If the maximal concentration is low and is significantly improved (greater than 9%) by exogenous hormone, a defect in AVP secretion is likely. If, on the other hand, the urine is dilute after water restriction and fails to become further concentrated after exogenous hormone, a defect in renal response is likely.

Another approach uses hypertonic saline infusion to stimulate the release of AVP. When a water diuresis has been induced by oral water loading, a hypertonic saline infusion is given. Urinary volumes are measured on serial samples. An abrupt reduction of urinary volume or a decrease in free water clearance is interpreted as reflecting the release of AVP. This procedure is more tedious than the dehydration test described previously, but may be of value in special cases in which it is suspected that osmotic responsiveness of the neurohypophysis is selectively lost.

Dynamic studies may also be useful in differential diagnosis of hyponatremic disorders. Frequently the diagnosis of inappropriate AVP release is made based on the findings of dilute plasma, inappropriately concentrated urine, low BUN, high urinary sodium as well as normal thyroid and adrenal function, and the presence of a normal effective plasma volume. Disease states in which the effective plasma volume is reduced mimic the syndrome of inappropriate secretion of antidiuretic hormone (SIADH) in the difficulty of excreting a water load. In SIADH a small water load often provokes increased urinary excretion of sodium even if not present in the steady state. In contrast sodium conservation is seen in states of diminished effective plasma volume. Plasma renin activity is usually suppressed in SIADH while it is generally elevated in hypovolemic states.

Radioimmunoassay of plasma AVP is becoming more available. Generally the diagnosis of vasopressin deficiency or excess is easily made without resorting to direct hormone measurements. In some cases of SIADH, the plasma AVP is within the normal range although it is inappropriately high for the concomitant plasma osmolality.

DIABETES INSIPIDUS

Diabetes insipidus is a dramatic but relatively rare condition that involves an absolute or partial deficiency of AVP. This deficiency renders the kidneys unable to conserve free water, and a massive diuresis ensues. As a consequence, the plasma tonicity rises, and this occurrence stimulates osmoreceptors to relay a perception of thirst to the cerebral cortex. Subsequent water ingestion brings the plasma osmolality down to the normal range but this change is accomplished with considerable inconvenience to the patient. He must drink copiously and void as frequently as twice an hour during both the day and night. (There is commonly a preference for ice water.) In a small proportion of patients with diabetes insipidus, the sensation of thirst is also missing. Such patients are chronically hypernatremic and dehydrated. Their urines are not as dilute as those of patients with classic diabetes insipidus—not usually because of greater ability to secrete AVP but rather because of diminished ability to excrete free water owing to hypovolemia. In some cases the absent thirst can be restored by treatment with chlorpropamide. Patients with classic diabetes insipidus subjected to anesthesia or in a coma likewise lack the thirst reflex and are at risk of hypernatremia and dehydration.

The onset of polydipsia and polyuria in a patient raises two major questions. First, is it diabetes insipidus? The most common cause for this symptom complex is diabetes mellitus, but it is usually accompanied by weight loss and polyphagia. Certain patients get in the habit of ingesting large amounts of water, which depresses their plasma osmolality and inhibits AVP secretion, resulting in a water diuresis. They may be distinguished from patients with diabetes insipidus because their steady-state plasma osmolality is usually somewhat lower than normal (Figure 10–2). However, laboratory diagnosis is impeded because prolonged water ingestion washes out the renal medullary concentration gradient such that patients are unable to elaborate a concentrated urine in response to either endogenous or exogenous AVP. This factor may result in a false-positive diagnosis of nephrogenic diabetes insipidus. Another significant cause of polyuria is renal resistance to AVP. Hereditary nephrogenic diabetes insipidus is rare, but many disease states and several drugs interfere with the conservation of free water by the kidney. Some of these were mentioned earlier; other causes of renal resistance to AVP include post-obstructive nephropathy, Sjögren's syndrome, hypokalemia, hypercalcemia, and the diuretic phase of acute renal failure. The diagnosis in these conditions is established by the persistent production of hypotonic urine and by noting the failure of exogenous vasopressin to concentrate the urine.

Once the diagnosis of hypothalamic-pituitary diabetes insipidus is established, it is important to look for a specific origin. Causes of hypothalamic-pituitary diabetes insipidus include:

1. Idiopathic
2. Familial
3. Granulomatous
    eosinophilic granuloma, sarcoidosis, tuberculosis
4. Infections (encephalitis, meningitis)
5. Tumors
    pituitary tumors
    craniopharyngiomas
    metastatic tumors
6. Traumatic
7. Postsurgical (iatrogenic)

Although at least half the cases have no obvious cause, it is important to evaluate the patient thoroughly for tumors or granulomas infiltrating the hypothalamic centers for vasopressin secretion. Frequently these lesions are so circumscribed that other hypothalamic functions, such as regulation of anterior pituitary hormone secretion, are only minimally involved. It is useful, therefore, to carefully evaluate visual fields, olfaction, and temperature regulation as well as anterior pituitary hormone reserve and appearance of skull roentgenograms. Computed tomographic scans may even be necessary.

Treatment consists of either replacement of the deficient hormone or use of drugs to augment its peripheral action. Vasopressin can be given in the form of long-lasting injections of Pitressin tannate in oil or by intranasal use of DDAVP. DDAVP, a synthetic modification of the AVP molecule, causes a much longer antidiuresis than lysine vasopressin (LVP) after intranasal administration. Furthermore, it has a higher ratio of antidiuretic-to-pressor action than either AVP or LVP and thus has fewer side effects. Its average duration of action is 12 to 14 hours.

Several drugs such as chlorpropamide, clofibrate, and carbamazepine have been noted to decrease urinary volume in patients with diabetes insipidus. Their effectiveness is limited to those patients whose neurohypophysis is still able to secrete some AVP. These patients usually have a milder form of the disease. It has been speculated that the drugs work by increasing pituitary release of AVP, but direct hormone measurements have shown conflicting results. Chlorpropamide has been shown to potentiate the effect of AVP on water transport at the renal tubule. Thiazide diuretics are effective in reducing urinary volume in either pituitary or nephrogenic diabetes insipidus by inducing mild extracellular volume depletion, which in turn enhances proximal tubular reabsorption of salt and water. This action reduces volume delivered to the more distal nephron segments and thus inhibits free water excretion.

HYPO-OSMOLAR STATES

Hyponatremia is a frequent laboratory finding, particularly in hospitalized patients with multiple medical problems. It may cause gradual obtundation and even coma. In the evaluation of such patients, one must first determine whether the hyponatremia is caused by water retention due to impaired ability to excrete water. If excessive AVP is indeed responsible for the water retention, it must be shown that this release of the hormone is inappropriate and is not caused by sustained stimulation of the low- and high-pressure baroreceptors in the thorax. When the presence of excessive AVP in the circulation is due to inappropriate nonphysiologic causes, this state is called the syndrome of inappropriate antidiuretic hormone or SIADH.

The causes of SIADH are as follows:

Central Nervous System
    Infectious: meningitis, abscess, encephalitis
    Tumor
    Post-traumatic
    Subarachnoid hemorrhage
    Acute intermittent porphyria
Pulmonary
    Pneumonia
    Tuberculosis
    Abscess
Ectopic Production by Tumor
    Carcinoma of the lung, duodenum, pancreas, prostate
    Thymoma, acute myeloid leukemia
Drugs
    Chlorpropamide
    Vincristine
    Thiazide diuretics
    Nicotine
    Carbamazepine
    Clofibrate
    Cyclophosphamide
    Morphine derivatives
    Isoproterenol
    ? Antidepressants
Others*
    Idiopathic
    Pneumoencephalography
    Postoperative
    Positive pressure breathing
    Postmitral commissurotomy

In some patients body fluids are lost through vomiting or gastrointestinal suction. The sodium-rich fluid is replaced by either oral tap water or, in the hospital, by intravenous dextrose and water. This replacement results in a

---

*Cirrhosis, congestive heart failure, nephrosis, Addison's disease, and myxedema all involve impaired renal water handling, due in part to ADH stimulated by decreased effective plasma volume.

state of hyponatremic dehydration in which the patient is both volume depleted and salt depleted, but the degree of salt depletion is greater than the water loss. In such cases the urinary sodium is low and the BUN is elevated. Decreased skin turgor and orthostatic hypotension may be present. This condition is in contrast to states of dilutional hyponatremia. In such circumstances total body sodium is normal, but total body water increases because of inability to excrete free water, which may be seen in adrenal insufficiency and hypothyroidism. Both of these diseases can cause hyponatremia in the Brattleboro rat, which lacks AVP, thus indicating that AVP is not required to mediate the abnormal water retention in these states. Other disease states such as congestive heart failure, liver disease, and nephrosis can also cause water retention. The pathogenesis is more complicated in these conditions. Part of the problem is a reduction in effective plasma volume. This situation enhances proximal tubular reabsorption of sodium, which in turn impairs production of free water. The reduced effective plasma volume may also stimulate the baroreceptors to release AVP. The secretion of AVP in such circumstances is appropriate for the hypovolemia but not for the concomitant hypo-osmolality. It appears that under such circumstances the volume stimulus overrides the osmotic stimulus. Various drugs can also cause hyponatremia by directly interfering with renal free water excretion, as with thiazides, by stimulating AVP release, as with vincristine, or by greatly enhancing the action of a small amount of AVP in the circulation, as with chlorpropamide.

With so many disease states causing hyponatremia, the diagnosis of SIADH is in part a diagnosis of exclusion. The diagnosis can be made if there is hypotonicity of the plasma in the presence of urine that is not appropriately dilute, along with the additional criteria discussed previously. The syndrome may be due to nonsuppressible pituitary release of AVP such as that seen after head trauma, central nervous system infections, and major surgical procedures. It may also be due to AVP ectopically secreted by malignant tumors. In ectopic AVP secretion, the hyponatremia may be more severe and more difficult to treat.

Treatment usually consists of water restriction. Water losses through the skin, feces, and urine are allowed to exceed water intake until the plasma osmolality returns to normal. Recurrence of the syndrome is avoided by restricting fluid intake to a level commensurate with renal losses. In severe cases of hyponatremia bordering on coma, furosemide may be given intravenously. This drug's action blocks solute transport in the ascending limb of the loop of Henle and results in formation of dilute urine. The resulting electrolyte losses are replaced quantitatively with hypertonic saline solution. Hypertonic saline solution by itself may be beneficial, but its effect is short-lived because of the elevated sodium excretion in this syndrome. On rare occasions, particularly associated with ectopic production of AVP from tumors, it may be desirable to prescribe a drug to interfere with the action of AVP on the kidney. Both demeclocycline and lithium can be effective; demeclocycline is preferable because of its fewer side effects. These drugs appear to interfere with the generation of cyclic AMP, probably by blocking AVP stimulation of adenylate cyclase.

CLINICAL PROBLEMS

Patient 1, Part 1. A 5-year-old boy started drinking large quantities of fluids and complained of being thirsty all the time. This condition began rather abruptly over 2 to 3 days. He had nocturnal enuresis after a lapse of a year and a half. His past history was normal except that he had not had any noticeable growth in height over the past 6 months.

LABORATORY DATA. Plasma osmolality, 289 mOsm/kg; sodium, 140 mEq/L; BUN 18 mg/100 ml; urine osmolality, 108 mOsm/kg; serum thyroxine, 5.5 µg/100 ml. Plasma growth hormone (GH) drawn before and after administration of L-dopa was less than 3 ng/ml. Lateral skull roentgenogram showed a normal sella turcica, with a small calcification noted above the region of the sella.

A 6-hour water deprivation test resulted in a rise of the plasma osmolality to 294 mOsm/kg while the urine osmolality rose to 140 mOsm/kg. The urine osmolality rose to 760 mOsm/kg after 5 U of aqueous vasopressin (posterior pituitary extract).

QUESTIONS

1. What is the most likely diagnosis?
2. What is the significance of the lack of growth?
3. What disease processes would be considered in the differential diagnosis of this case?

Patient 1, Part 2. After the boy described in Part 1 had been evaluated, he was started on DDAVP but was lost to follow-up. He discontinued his medication after 6 months with no obvious ill effects. At a reevaluation 2 years later, his parents stated that he rarely drank fluids except as part of a meal.

LABORATORY DATA. Serum sodium, 180 mEq/L; potassium, 4.4 mEq/L; bicarbonate, 28 mEq/L; and chloride, 140 mEq/L. Random urine osmolality was 420 mOsm/kg, which rose to 580 mOsm/kg with dehydration. It further rose to 1140 mOsm/kg after intranasal DDAVP.

QUESTIONS

1. Why did the patient not develop polyuria after discontinuing his vasopressin?
2. How was he able to concentrate his urine after the dehydration test in the hospital?

Patient 2. A 44-year-old man comes to the emergency room with mild obtundation. He has been a heavy drinker in the past but stopped drinking 5 days earlier. The family states that he has been quite nauseated and has been vomiting frequently. There is no history of hematemesis or melena.

PHYSICAL EXAMINATION. His pulse is 100 and rises to 120 when he sits up. Supine BP is 96/70. He is responsive to painful stimuli. His chest is clear. The liver is palpable 5 cm below the right costal margin. No edema is noted and skin turgor is decreased.

LABORATORY DATA. Sodium is 118 mEq/L; potassium, 2.8 mEq/L; Cl, 77 mEq/L; CO$_2$, 24 mEq/L; BUN, 32 mg/100 ml; plasma osmolality, 258 mOsm/kg; urine osmolality, 220 mOsm/kg; and urine sodium, 9 mEq/L.

QUESTIONS

1. Is the hyponatremia due to water retention or salt loss?
2. What is the explanation for the low urinary sodium with the high urinary osmolality?
3. What is the diagnostic significance of the BUN?

Patient 3. A 59-year-old steel mill employee is brought to the emergency room because of mental confusion. His family thinks he has been ill for about 6 months. During this time he has lost 35 pounds because of chronic anorexia. He complains of excessive fatigue, weakness, and a chronic nonproductive cough. About 2 weeks ago he was found to be unusually irritable and became irrational. He has been confused and disoriented for the last 2 days. He drinks about 6 bottles of beer a day and smokes 2 packs of cigarettes per day. The remainder of his history is unremarkable.

PHYSICAL EXAMINATION. On examination he is a disoriented, irritable, chronically ill appearing man who has obvious signs of weight loss. His BP is 140/80 mm Hg supine and does not change with standing. His pulse is 100/minute, respiration 18/minute and temperature 101° F. Cardiovascular exam is normal and chest exam unremarkable. A hard 3×2 cm lymph node is palpable in the left supraclavicular fossa. The liver, palpable 4 cm below the right costal margin, is firm, smooth, and 17 cm in overall length. Extremities show early clubbing of the fingernails but no edema. Except for confusion, bilaterally decreased deep tendon reflexes and extensor toe reflexes, the neurologic examination is unremarkable.

LABORATORY DATA. Urinalysis shows specific gravity 1.020, pH 7.0, negative for glucose, acetone and protein, sediment unremarkable; fasting glucose, 90 mg/100 ml; BUN, 8 mg/100 ml; creatinine, 0.9 mg/100 ml; Na, 115; K, 3.8; Cl, 80; bicarbonate, 20 mEq/L; Ca, 9.2; phosphorus, 3.1 mg/100 ml; total protein, 6.1 g/100 ml; serum cortisol, 10 μg/100 ml; urine 17-OHCS, 11 mg/24 hours; 17-KS, 9 mg/24 hours; chest roentgenogram, 2×3 cm mass in left lower lobe; skull roentgenogram, normal; ECG, nonspecific ST-T wave changes; serum osmolality, 235 mOsm/kg; urine osmolality, 210 mOsm/kg; 24-hour urine sodium excretion, 150 mEq. Left supraclavicular node biopsy showed oat cell carcinoma.

QUESTIONS

1. What is the most likely explanation for the hyponatremia in this patient?
2. If the patient is given a large saline load, what would happen to the serum sodium concentration?
3. What is the probable source of hormone production in this patient?

Patient 4. A 48-year-old woman has had mild polydipsia and polyuria of 2 months' duration. She has a positive family history for diabetes mellitus. She is a food faddist and eats a restricted diet. There is no history of head trauma or neurologic symptoms. Physical examination is unremarkable.

LABORATORY DATA. A glucose tolerance test showed a fasting glucose of 104, 1 hour of 190, and 2 hours of 150 mg/100 ml with trace glycosuria at 1 hour. A random plasma osmolality was 290 mOsm/kg and the urine osmolality was 150 mOsm/kg. BUN was 18 mg/100 ml and creatinine 1.2 mg/100 ml. The patient was deprived of water for 16 hours. Her maximal urinary osmolality was 490 mOsm/kg and rose to 520 after 5 U of subcutaneous aqueous vasopressin. Renal biopsy showed nephrocalcinosis.

On further questioning the patient admitted to ingestion of "large numbers" of vitamin D-calcium tablets each day.

QUESTIONS

1. Which diseases might play a role in her polyuria?
2. What was the significance of the response to aqueous vasopressin?
3. Why was the plasma osmolality normal?
4. What other conditions could cause a similar response to exogenous vasopressin?

SUGGESTED READING

Bartter, F.C.: The syndrome of inappropriate secretion of antidiuretic hormones (SIADH). D.M., November, 1973.

Dunn, F.L., et al.: The role of blood osmolality and volume in regulating vasopressin secretion in the rat. J. Clin. Invest., *52*:3212, 1973.

Goetz, K.L., Bond, G.C., and Bloxham, D.D.: Atrial receptors and renal function. Physiol. Rev., *55*:157, 1975.

Hays, R.M., and Levine, S.D.: Vasopressin. Kidney Int., *6*:307, 1974.

Hayward, J.N.: Neural control of the posterior pituitary. Annu. Rev. Physiol., *37*:191, 1975.

Hendricks, S.A., Lippe, B., Kaplan, S.A., Paul Lee, W.–N.: Differential diagnosis of diabetes insipidus: use of DDAVP to terminate the seven hour water deprivation test. J. Pediatr., *98*:244, 1981.

Miller, J., et al.: Recognition of partial defects in antidiuretic hormone secretion. Ann. Intern. Med., *73*:721, 1970.

Schrier, R.W., and Berl, T.: Non-osmolar factors in renal water excretion. N. Engl. J. Med., *292*:81, 1975.

Schrier, R.W., and Goldberg, J.P.: The physiology of vasopressin release and the pathogenesis of impaired water excretion in adrenal, thyroid, and edematous disorders. Yale J. Biol. Med., *53*:525, 1980.

Weitzmann, R., and Kleeman, C.R.: Water metabolism and the neurohypophyseal hormones. *In* Clinical Disorders of Fluid and Electrolyte Metabolism. 3rd Ed. Edited by M. Maxwell and C.R. Kleeman. New York, McGraw-Hill, 1980.

CHAPTER 11

Hyperlipidemia

Alan M. Fogelman

BIOCHEMISTRY AND PHYSIOLOGY OF CHOLESTEROL AND THE TRIGLYCERIDES

Function

Cholesterol is the precursor of the steroid hormones and the bile acids. It is also a constituent of every mammalian cell's membranes, and thus an important determinant of membrane fluidity.

The triglycerides (more properly named triacylglycerols) are the esterified form of fatty acids and glycerol.

Synthesis

Cholesterol can be synthesized by virtually every cell in the body. The rate-controlling enzyme in humans as in other species is 3-hydroxy-3-methyl-glutaryl Co-enzyme A reductase (HMG CoA reductase) (Fig. 11–1). The synthesis of cholesterol is expensive in terms of energy required.

Until recently, it was thought that in mammals synthesis of mevalonate (the product of the HMG CoA reductase reaction) was a committed step (i.e., once formed, it had to be used for the synthesis of cholesterol or related compounds). It is now known that a pathway exists to shunt some of the carbon atoms passing through the mevalonate step away from cholesterol biosynthesis and back to acetyl CoA and acetoacetyl CoA. This process does not occur by reversal of the step catalyzed by HMG CoA reductase but through intermediates that are as yet unidentified. This "shunt" is particularly active in the kidneys. Additionally, mevalonate is important in the synthesis of isoprenoid units for dolichol, ubiquinone, and a compound that regulates DNA replication.

While every cell can synthesize cholesterol, the plasma cholesterol is largely derived from the secretions of the liver and the intestine.

In the liver and in adipose tissue the glycerol skeleton is synthesized from glucose or glycogen through the Embden-Meyerhof pathway, and yields di-

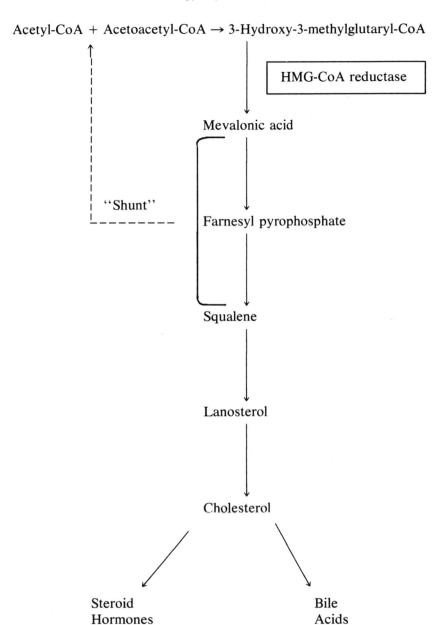

Acetyl-CoA + Acetoacetyl-CoA → 3-Hydroxy-3-methylglutaryl-CoA

HMG-CoA reductase

Mevalonic acid

"Shunt"

Farnesyl pyrophosphate

Squalene

Lanosterol

Cholesterol

Steroid
Hormones

Bile
Acids

Figure 11–1. Schematic diagram of the cholesterol biosynthetic pathway.

hydroxyacetone phosphate, which is then converted to L-α-glycerophosphate (Fig. 11–2). Alternatively, in the liver glycerokinase can act directly on glycerol to form L-α-glycerophosphate. Subsequently, two molecules of fatty acyl-CoA react with each molecule of L-α-glycerophosphate to yield phos-

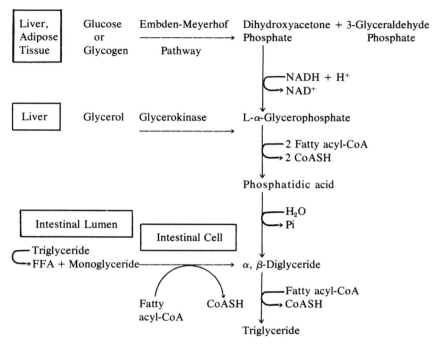

Figure 11–2. Schematic diagram of triglyceride biosynthesis.

phatidic acid. The phosphate group is then removed to produce α,β-diglyceride, the immediate precursor of triglyceride. In the intestinal lumen the hydrolysis of dietary triglyceride generates monoglycerides that can diffuse into the intestinal cell and react with a molecule of fatty acyl-CoA to yield the diglyceride. In all tissues, the free primary hydroxyl group of the diglyceride is then esterified with another molecule of fatty acyl-CoA to yield the triglyceride.

Transport

Cholesterol and the triglycerides are virtually insoluble in aqueous solutions. Their transport is dependent on their inclusion in water-soluble molecules called lipoproteins. The plasma lipoproteins are grouped into four major classes according to their density in the ultracentrifuge: the chylomicrons, very low density lipoproteins (VLDL), low-density lipoproteins (LDL), and high-density lipoproteins (HDL). The largest, the chylomicrons, consist (by weight) of 80 to 95% exogenous triglycerides, 2 to 7% cholesterol, 3 to 6% phospholipid, and 1 to 2% protein. These particles are synthesized in the intestinal cells and carry the dietary triglycerides through the thoracic duct into the venous circulation.

The VLDL are the next largest particles. Sixty to 80 % of the VLDL molecule is composed of endogenous triglycerides that are synthesized and packaged into the lipoprotein in the liver. Both the chylomicrons and VLDL are acted upon in the capillaries of muscle and adipose tissue by lipoprotein lipase, an enzyme distinguished from other lipases by its requirement for an apolipoprotein activator (Apo C-II). Lipoprotein lipase acts in a variety of tissues to remove the triglyceride from the lipoprotein and hydrolyze it to yield glycerol and free fatty acids, which can then diffuse across the cell membranes and be utilized for energy or stored.

After the administration of intravenous heparin, several lipase activities are released into the plasma. A hepatic lipase can be differentiated from lipoprotein lipase by assays based on differences in sensitivity to ionic strength or protamine and the requirement for Apo C-II. The exact function of the hepatic lipase in vivo is unknown.

The fragment resulting from the removal of triglyceride and some protein from the VLDL molecule is called intermediate density lipoprotein (IDL). IDL is processed further, possibly in the liver, by a lipase, and within 2 to 6 hours the remaining molecule is identifiable in the plasma as LDL. By weight LDL contain about 50% cholesterol (mostly esterified cholesterol) and 25% protein. Approximately half of the plasma cholesterol is found in LDL.

The heaviest lipoprotein is called HDL. It contains 30% phospholipid, 20% cholesterol, and approximately 50% protein. HDL is secreted by the liver and modified in the circulation by an interaction with the enzyme lecithin: cholesterol acyl transferase (LCAT). This enzyme generates cholesteryl esters from free cholesterol and lecithin. Apo A-I is an activator of the LCAT reaction. LCAT and HDL may be important in the modification of the chylomicrons and VLDL as they are acted upon by lipoprotein lipase (Table 11–1).

The apoproteins of the lipoproteins are under intensive study, and changes in the nomenclature are to be expected. At present, the most commonly used system designates the two major proteins of HDL as Apo A-I and Apo A-II. Apo B is found in the chylomicrons and VLDL and is the major protein of plasma LDL. Apo C-I, Apo C-II, and Apo C-III are the small molecular weight proteins present in chylomicrons, VLDL, and HDL. In the plasma the C proteins move, in either direction, between chylomicrons or VLDL and HDL. Apo D or a similar protein may participate in the removal of cholesterol from the tissues. Free cholesterol is esterified by a complex in plasma that contains Apo A-I, LCAT, and Apo D. The newly esterified cholesterol is then transferred by Apo D to LDL or VLDL. Apo E is found in chylomicrons, VLDL, LDL, and HDL.

The lipoproteins are recognized and cleared from the circulation as a function of their apoproteins. Apo B and Apo E are recognized by the LDL receptor. Apo E may also be recognized by a liver receptor different from the LDL receptor. Apo C may inhibit the recognition of Apo E.

In addition to the serum lipoproteins, several intracellular proteins seem capable of carrying cholesterol and some of its precursors through the aqueous portions of the cell. The earliest cholesterol precursor that has been shown to bind to these carrier proteins is squalene.

Degradation

Approximately one-third of the LDL in the plasma of normals is cleared by the LDL receptor pathway. LDL is first bound at the cell surface in rapidly internalizing areas called coated pits. The internalized LDL is carried to lysosomes, and the receptor is recycled to the cell surface. In the lysosome, the protein portion of the LDL is degraded and the cholesteryl esters are hydrolyzed. The liberated free cholesterol regulates microsomal enzyme activities, down regulating HMG-CoA reductase and activating acyl cholesterol: acyl transferase (ACAT), the enzyme that reesterifies the cholesterol. This reesterification yields cholesteryl oleate, while the LDL contained cholesteryl linoleate. Cholesteryl oleate is the predominant storage form for excess intracellular cholesterol. The cyle is completed by the hydrolysis of the cholesteryl oleate by a neutral cytoplasmic cholesteryl ester hydrolase. The cholesteryl ester content of the cells is determined by the amount of free cholesterol available to ACAT. The cholesterol that is released from the degradation of LDL and the other lipoproteins can be lost from the body only along with desquamating cells (particularly the skin) and from the gastrointestinal tract in bile either as cholesterol or as bile acids. Mammalian cells cannot degrade the sterol nucleus, but bacteria in the intestinal lumen can break the ring structure and utilize the carbon atoms.

The removal of triglycerides from the circulation via the lipoprotein lipase mechanism has already been discussed.

Storage

As previously noted, cholesterol is "stored" in cells in the form of cholesterol esters that can be hydrolyzed to allow use of the free cholesterol that is needed for cell membranes. The cholesterol content of most cells is closely regulated, and cells such as normal human smooth muscle cells and macrophages contain little "stored" cholesterol (cholesterol esters).

Triglycerides are stored primarily in adipocytes where they are held until required for energy.

Control Mechanisms

Western man absorbs dietary cholesterol inefficiently such that even on diets rich in cholesterol, only 20 to 40% of the plasma cholesterol is derived from the diet. Human populations such as the Masai in Africa absorb more cholesterol from their diet, but they synthesize less and maintain lower serum cholesterol levels than Western men who are eating similar diets.

At the cellular level, the loss of cholesterol from the cell into its environment stimulates the induction of HMG CoA reductase and increases the number of LDL receptors, presumably as a homeostatic mechanism to maintain sterol content. In the whole animal, including man, this action can be demonstrated by feeding cholestyramine. This drug interrupts the enterohepatic circulation and causes a significant loss of cholesterol from the body; this loss leads to the induction of HMG CoA reductase, increased cholesterol synthesis, and increased LDL receptor activity.

In addition to lipoprotein lipase, a "hormone-sensitive lipase" in adipose tissue catalyzes the hydrolysis of triglyceride in response to a variety of hormones including epinephrine. These hormones convert the enzyme from an inactive to an active form probably by the stimulation of adenylate cyclase and the formation of an active protein kinase that phosphorylates the inactive form of the lipase. Insulin inhibits the activity of this lipase. Hormone-sensitive lipase is present in the active form in the adipose tissue of fed mammals, but at a low level. In fasted mammals the activity is much higher and produces a greater hydrolysis of triglycerides.

CLINICAL TESTS

The ninety-fifth percentile values (these values approximate two standard deviations above the mean) estimated for sex- and age-adjusted plasma lipids in a Seattle control population were 285 mg/100 ml for cholesterol and 165 mg/100 ml for triglycerides. This population was chosen from the spouses of persons who survived myocardial infarction. While these values are representative of persons living in Seattle, they were not derived from an exclusively normal population. A useful rule of thumb for the upper limits of cholesterol concentrations for persons over the age of 20 is to add 200 to the age in years (e.g., a person 30 years old with a plasma cholesterol concentration of less than 230 mg/100 ml would be considered normal). If the measured value exceeds this level, further evaluation is warranted. The upper limit for triglycerides measured in persons over the age of 20 is between 150 and 175 mg/100 ml depending on age, sex, and laboratory technique.

Lipoproteins can be separated by electrophoresis as well as in the ultra-centrifuge. In the usual electrophoretic system, the chylomicrons remain at the origin. LDL remain next closest to the orgin and are referred to as the β-lipoproteins. VLDL migrate further from the origin and are referred to as the pre-β lipoproteins. HDL migrate the greatest distance from the origin and are referred to as the α-lipoproteins. A nomenclature popularized by Fredrickson, Levy, and Lees was based on lipoprotein electrophoresis (Table 11–2). It was hoped that this clinically applicable procedure would yield information of a genetic nature. Unfortunately, it did not; hence its usefulness is limited.

Measurement of the total plasma cholesterol predicts accurately the LDL cholesterol concentration. Because the LDL cholesterol concentration is directly correlated with the risk for atherosclerosis, one can effectively use the total plasma cholesterol level in the diagnosis and treatment of most hyper-cholesterolemias. The exception is in broad β disease (Type III hyperlipo-proteinemia). This disorder is due to a deficiency of one of the subclasses of Apo E; there is E_3 deficiency. At present, except for this one rare disease, the measurement of the total plasma cholesterol and triglyceride concentrations is sufficient to establish the presence of hyperlipidemia, and lipoprotein electrophoresis is not necessary in routine clinical practice. The blood samples should be taken after a 12- to 14-hour fast. If the triglyceride levels are increased, the presence of chylomicrons can be detected by lipoprotein electrophoresis or more simply by observing the formation of a cream layer on

Table 11–1.　The Lipoproteins

Lipoprotein Class	Possible Physiologic Role	Site of Synthesis	Site of Degradation
Chylomicrons	Transports dietary triglycerides	Intestine	Acted upon by lipoprotein lipase in the peripheral tissues; remnant may be processed by liver
VLDL	Transports endogenous triglycerides	Liver and intestine	Acted upon by lipoprotein lipase in the peripheral tissues; remnant may be processed by liver, and may accumulate in broad beta disease; normally the remnant (IDL) is further processed, possibly by the liver to yield LDL
LDL	Transports majority of plasma cholesterol; regulates HMG CoA reductase activity; regulates lymphocyte responsiveness	(see Degradation of VLDL)	Extrahepatic tissues and liver
HDL	Physiologic role unknown; may transport cholesterol from tissues to liver for further processing	Secreted from liver and then modified in plasma, possibly by LCAT; also may be formed as a degradation product from chylomicron catabolism	?

Table 11–2. Classification of Hyperlipidemia Based on
Lipoprotein Electrophoresis

Type	Chylomicrons	LDL	VLDL	Floating β-Lipoproteins
I	+			
IIa		+		
IIb		+	+	
III				+
IV			+	
V	+		+	

+ = excess lipoproteins.

plasma left overnight in the refrigerator. In order to detect a genetically determined hyperlipidemia, the physician should obtain lipid values from as many first-degree relatives as possible. This procedure should be done while they are eating a normal American diet and are off all drugs that are known to affect lipid levels. One should not attempt to measure the plasma lipids during the course of an acute myocardial infarction. Within 24 hours after the acute event, the plasma cholesterol concentration often drops precipitously. (The reason for this fall in the cholesterol level is not known.) One should usually wait until 3 months after the infarction before measuring the plasma lipids.

Epidemiologic studies suggest an independent and inverse relationship between HDL levels and atherosclerotic events. The usual measurement of HDL cholesterol is subject to considerable technical variation. Most often, chylomicrons are removed and the remaining proteins containing Apo B are precipitated. The cholesterol content of the supernatant is taken as a measure of HDL cholesterol. Since most plasma cholesterol is contained in LDL and VLDL, failure to precipitate these Apo B-containing lipoproteins completely will give falsely high values for HDL cholesterol.

SECONDARY HYPERLIPIDEMIAS

Hyperlipidemia that is due to a drug or another disease is defined as secondary hyperlipidemia. Its causes follow.

Disease States
1. Diabetes (severe,[T] moderate, mild)
2. Obstructive liver disease[C]
3. Nephrotic syndrome
4. Hypothyroidism
5. Dysglobulinemia
6. Gout[T]
7. Chronic renal failure[T]
8. Porphyria[C]
9. Glycogen storage disease[T]
10. Acromegaly
11. Cushing's syndrome
12. Gram-negative septicemia[T]

13. (Pregnancy)

Drugs
1. Estrogens[T]
2. Alcohol[T]
3. Corticosteroids (high dose,[T] low dose)
4. Dilantin[C]
5. Thiazides[C]
6. Vitamin D intoxication[C]

C = Associated mainly with an elevation in the plasma cholesterol concentration.
T = Associated mainly with an elevation in the plasma triglyceride concentration.

This definition implies that withdrawal of the drug or correction of the primary disease leads to correction of the hyperlipidemia and that the diagnosis of primary hyperlipidemia can only be made after excluding drugs and other diseases as the cause of the hyperlipidemia. In the case of hypothyroidism, the mechanism of the hypercholesterolemia appears to be due to a failure of the LDL receptor pathway that is corrected when thyroid is administered. Patients can have more than one primary disease. For example, hypertriglyceridemia is commonly associated with hyperuricemia and gout. However, the correction of the hyperuricemia with uricosuric drugs or allopurinol almost never leads to a total correction of the hypertriglyceridemia. It is assumed then that two primary diseases are coexisting and perhaps are coinherited. Although this assumption is the current thinking, the possibility exists that both the hyperuricemia and the hypertriglyceridemia are secondary to an as yet unidentified but more basic defect. Hypertriglyceridemia occurs in a significant fraction of adults with normal fasting blood sugars but with mild glucose intolerance (such as an abnormal blood sugar response to food or glucose). These individuals frequently are obese and have hyperinsulinism presumably because of insulin resistance in peripheral tissues. Correction of the glucose intolerance with oral hypoglycemic agents does not correct the hypertriglyceridemia, nor will correction of the hypertriglyceridemia with hypolipidemic drugs correct the glucose intolerance or hyperinsulinemia. However, weight reduction corrects the glucose intolerance, hyperinsulinemia, and the hypertriglyceridemia. In such patients it is thought that the hyperinsulinism causes an overproduction of triglycerides by the liver. In severe diabetes, the lack of insulin impairs lipoprotein lipase function and can lead to impaired removal of chylomicrons and VLDL from the plasma. In moderate diabetes some patients demonstrate a normal increase in plasma lipoprotein lipase activity when first given an infusion of heparin, but later show a decreased lipoprotein lipase activity during the continued heparin infusion. By contrast, normal subjects sustain a high plasma lipoprotein lipase activity throughout the heparin infusion. The basis for the hypertriglyceridemia in such patients may be a defect in the removal of chylomicrons and VLDL.

PRIMARY HYPERLIPIDEMIAS

The primary hyperlipidemias can be divided into those that are genetic and those that are not.

Genetic
1. Monogenic
   a. Familial hypercholesterolemia
   b. Familial hypertriglyceridemia
   c. Familial combined hyperlipidemia
   d. Broad β disease
   e. Lipoprotein lipase deficiency
2. Polygenic hypercholesterolemia
Sporadic

The genetically determined hyperlipidemias can be further divided into those that are monogenic (i.e., caused by a single genetic defect) and those that are polygenic (i.e., caused by the interaction of more than one gene). Table 11–3 summarizes the plasma lipid abnormalities in these disorders.

Monogenic Hyperlipidemias

Familial Hypercholesterolemia

This autosomal dominant disorder has complete penetrance in childhood. By one year of age, 50% of the children will have hypercholesterolemia with normal triglyceride levels. Both the cholesterol and triglyceride levels are normal in the other 50% of the family members. Familial hypercholesterolemia occurs in the heterozygote form in the general population at a frequency in the range of one to two per thousand. The homozygote form is rare, occurring in no more than one per million.

This primary hyperlipidemia is the only one in which a cellular defect has been identified. Three forms of this disease have been identified: (1) receptor negative—these persons lack a functional LDL receptor; (2) receptor defective—these persons have defective binding to the LDL receptor, so that their LDL receptor activity is only 10 to 15% of normal; and (3) internalization

Table 11–3. Summary of Plasma Lipids in Primary Hyperlipidemia

	Cholesterol	Triglycerides	Appearance of refrigerated plasma
Familial hypercholesterolemia	↑ *	N*	Clear
Familial hypertriglyceridemia	N	↑	Turbid (rarely with cream layer)
Familial combined hyperlipidemia	N or ↑	N or ↑	Clear or turbid (rarely with cream layer)
Broad β disease	↑	↑	Turbid (often with cream layer)
Lipoprotein lipase deficiency			Cream layer with
without increased VLDL	↑	↑ ↑ ↑	clear infranatant
with increased VLDL	↑	↑ ↑	turbid infranatant
Polygenic hypercholesterolemia	↑	N	Clear
Sporadic hypertriglyceridemia	N	↑	Turbid

* ↑ = increased
  N = normal

defective—this is a rare form in which LDL binds normally but is not internalized.

The incidence of atherosclerotic events in males affected with the heterozygous form is 40 times normal. The incidence of clinical atherosclerotic events is less in affected females. The homozygotic individuals frequently die of atherosclerotic complications before the age of 20.

Clinically the excess cholesterol accumulates in the plasma, blood vessels, eyelids (xanthelasma), cornea (arcus corneae), and tendons (tendon xanthomas). The Achilles tendons and the extensor tendons of the hand are commonly involved. Subperiosteal accumulations below the knee or over the olecranon process also occur. Approximately half the affected families have one or more hypercholesterolemic members with tendon xanthomas. The plasma cholesterol levels in homozygotes is in the range of 800 to 1000 mg/100 ml; in heterozygotes it ranges between 300 and 600 mg/100 ml. Almost all the increased plasma cholesterol is found in LDL.

Familial Hypertriglyceridemia

This autosomal dominant disorder has incomplete penetrance in childhood. Hypertriglyceridemia is rarely detected in children (approximately 10%) from such families, but 50% of the adults have hypertriglyceridemia with normal plasma cholesterol levels. The other 50% of the adult family members over the age of 30 have a normal cholesterol and triglyceride concentration. The incidence of the heterozygous form in the general population may be as high as one per hundred. The incidence of atherosclerotic events in affected persons may be higher than in the general population, but the relative risk for myocardial infarction is low compared to familial hypercholesterolemia or familial combined hyperlipidemia. The physical examination is usually not revealing but if the levels of plasma triglyceride are high (over 1500 mg/100 ml), eruptive xanthomas (papules with a yellow center and a reddish base) may be present. The hypertriglyceridemia is endogenous in origin and usually is on the order of 250 to 300 mg/100 ml with normal plasma cholesterol concentrations. Oral contraceptives, estrogen treatment, alcohol, or untreated diabetes can lead to high triglyceride concentrations and even chylomicronemia in these patients.

Familial Combined Hyperlipidemia

This autosomal dominant disease has incomplete penetrance in childhood (approximately 10%). When the children have hyperlipidemia, it almost always is hypertriglyceridemia. Among the adults, half of the family members have normal plasma cholesterol and triglyceride concentrations. The other half of the adults have an elevation of either triglyceride or cholesterol concentration or of both. Of the affected adults, approximately one-third have hypercholesterolemia, one-third have hypertriglyceridemia, and one-third have elevations of both the cholesterol and triglyceride concentrations. The frequency of the gene for this disorder in the general population may be as high as 1%. The risk for atherosclerotic events in affected males is 10 times normal. The physical examination is not diagnostic. Tendon xanthomas are rarely found in this disorder.

Epidemiologic evidence suggests that the basic defect may be in triglyceride metabolism and the hypercholesterolemia is somehow secondary.

In affected individuals, the plasma cholesterol concentrations often are on the order of 300 mg/100 ml and the triglyceride concentrations often are on the order of 250 mg/100 ml.

Although these three monogenic disorders occur in no more than 2% of the general population, they are found in approximately 20% of persons under the age of 60 who have suffered a myocardial infarction and survived.

Broad β Disease

This autosomal disorder probably occurs in not more than 1 per 5000 of the general population. It is characterized by the presence of increased circulating levels of IDL (the cholesterol-rich remnant created by the action of lipoprotein lipase on VLDL). IDL are rarely found in normals and are rarely if ever found in affected children, though 4% of children from affected families may have hypertriglyceridemia. The incidence of premature atherosclerosis is clearly elevated in affected family members, but whereas peripheral vascular disease is uncommon in familial hypercholesterolemia, it is present in more than a quarter of persons with broad β disease. Xanthomas (palmar, tendinous, tuberous, or eruptive) are found in approximately three-quarters of affected persons. More than half have xanthoma striata palmaris (yellow deposits in the palmar creases). Palmar xanthomas are not pathognomonic for broad β disease, being also found in homozygous familial hypercholesterolemia, obstructive liver disease, and dysglobulinemia. The plasma cholesterol concentration is often on the order of 450 mg/100 ml with plasma triglycerides in the range of 600 to 700 mg/100 ml. Frequently, there are swings in the lipid levels in these patients, but the ratio of the cholesterol concentration to the triglyceride concentration usually remains on the order of 1:1 regardless of the absolute lipid levels. The diagnosis is suggested by a broadly staining band on lipoprotein electrophoresis. This area occurs between the β band (LDL) and the pre-β band (VLDL). The diagnosis is made by demonstrating Apo E_3 deficiency. The Apo E_3 deficiency apparently prevents the IDL from being recognized by the liver receptor, and hence there is an accumulation of these "remnant" particles in the plasma.

Lipoprotein Lipase Deficiency

Two forms of this rare disease show a defective removal of chylomicrons; one form shows an accumulation of VLDL as well. The best-studied form is inherited as an autosomal recessive and appears in childhood with eruptive xanthomas, lipemia retinalis, hepatosplenomegaly, episodic abdominal pain, and bouts of pancreatitis. The plasma looks like "cream-of-tomato soup," and the plasma triglyceride concentration on a regular diet is often in the range of 3000 to 7000 mg/100 ml, while the plasma cholesterol concentration is often in the 300 to 450 mg/100 ml range. Plasma left in the refrigerator overnight shows a cream layer with a clear infranatant layer. Lipoprotein electrophoresis also demonstrates that the excess lipid is in chylomicrons. These chylomicrons are derived from dietary fat, and the clear infranatant layer reflects the minor increase in VLDL levels. (Plasma left overnight in the refrigerator appears turbid if VLDL are present in excess.) The disease appears to be due to a deficiency of lipoprotein lipase activity, which results in a failure to remove chylomicrons from the circulation. The most common clinical measurements of lipoprotein lipase activity are made after the administration of heparin—the post heparin lipolytic activity (PHLA). In normal subjects, lipoprotein lipase activity increases. In this disorder, it remains low even after heparin administration. Glucose tolerance is normal and there is no evidence of increased risk for atherosclerosis.

A less well-defined variant of the clinical picture just described usually begins in the third decade of life and may be characterized by bouts of abdominal pain, pancreatitis, hepatosplenomegaly, lipemia retinalis, eruptive xanthomas (when the triglyceride concentrations exceed 1500 mg/100 ml), a higher than normal prevalence of diabetes, and hyperuricemia without clear evidence for premature vascular disease. The PHLA is usually not as low as that seen in the form that begins in early childhood. Both plasma VLDL and chylomicron concentrations are elevated, in contrast to the form that begins in childhood. When left overnight in the refrigerator, the plasma shows a cream layer with a turbid infranatant layer (the result of an elevation in both chylomicrons and VLDL). The plasma triglyceride concentration ranges between 400 and 6500 mg/100 ml, and the plasma cholesterol concentrations range between 150 and 1300 mg/100 ml. The mean values for triglycerides are approximately 2500 mg/100 ml and for cholesterol, about 450 mg/100 ml.

The mode of inheritance is not clear and is often difficult to ascertain because of the frequent appearance of this phenotype in persons with diabetes, alcoholism, renal disease, hypothyroidism, and dysglobulinemia as well as in persons receiving estrogen treatment or high-dose corticosteroid therapy. One subset of this disorder, however, has now been demonstrated to be due to an autosomal recessive disease leading to Apo C II deficiency. Only the homozygotes manifest that disorder. Apo C II is required for the activation of lipoprotein lipase, and therefore its deficiency causes a failure of this critical enzyme.

Polygenic Hypercholesterolemia

This disorder is caused by the action of multiple genes possibly interacting with environmental factors. Unlike the monogenic autosomal dominant disorder, familial hypercholesterolemia, in which half the family is normal and half abnormal (a bimodal distribution), polygenic hypercholesterolemia has a unimodal distribution of cholesterol levels but with a mean that is higher than normal. Polygenic hypercholesterolemia and sporadic hypertriglyceridemia are the most common hyperlipidemias, one or the other occurring in perhaps 3 or 4% of the population. In polygenic hypercholesterolemia, it is uncommon for tendon xanthomas to be found in persons under the age of 60. The incidence of atherosclerotic events is higher in persons with polygenic hypercholesterolemia than in matched normolipidemic individuals, but the events tend to occur later in life and often after the age of 60, in contrast to persons with familial hypercholesterolemia or familial combined hyperlipidemia.

Sporadic Hypertriglyceridemia

This disorder is defined as hypertriglyceridemia for which no genetic component or other disease state or drug can be found to explain the disorder. Its exact frequency in the general population and its presence as a risk factor of significance in atherosclerosis remain to be determined.

TREATMENT

Even in the monogenic hyperlipidemias, evidence suggests that other risk factors enhance an already great propensity to atherosclerosis. Therefore, it is especially important to eliminate cigarette smoking and to control hypertension in these individuals. Sudden death occurs in young people from atherosclerotic coronary artery disease often because neither the patient nor his physician was aware of the presence of one of the monogenic hyperlipidemias and its propensity to premature atherosclerosis. Consequently, symptoms that should have been interpreted as ominous were ignored until the final, fatal event. It is particularly important in persons with monogenic hyperlipidemia to look for early signs of significant atherosclerosis carefully by such measures as periodic treadmill exercise tests.

The principles of therapy are based on the hope that lowering the lipid levels will lower the risk for atherosclerosis. It is possible, however, that LDL itself is not atherogenic, but some derivative of LDL that is present in small amounts or some other abnormal lipoprotein is required to produce atherosclerosis. Evidence does indicate that lowering the lipid levels of persons under the age of 65 by dietary means reduces the incidence of atherosclerotic events. None of the evidence suggests that lowering the lipid levels with any of the currently available drugs reduces the incidence of atherosclerotic events. I only use these agents in persons in whom diet therapy has failed, who are under 65 years of age, and who are at particularly high risk for an atherosclerotic event, or who are symptomatic from their hyperlipidemia (eruptive xanthomas or pancreatitis).

Diet

Except in lipoprotein lipase deficiency, in which the removal of exogenous fat from the diet is mandatory, the dietary regimen for lowering lipids is essentially the same. The diet is low in cholesterol and low in saturated fatty acids (though it is not necessary to supplement the diet with polyunsaturated fatty acids). Initially the diet is low in calories until a lean body weight is achieved; then it is isocaloric to maintain ideal body weight. This diet produces a decrease in both the plasma cholesterol and triglyceride concentrations. In persons with hypertriglyceridemia, it may be useful to limit alcohol and possibly simple sugars.

Pharmacologic Agents

Clofibrate

Clofibrate used to be the most commonly prescribed hypolipidemic agent. It primarily produces a lowering of the plasma triglycerides with a less dramatic and less sustained effect on the plasma cholesterol concentration. It has a half-life of 12 hours and is excreted in the urine as the glucuronide. It increases the excretion of cholesterol in the bile (and may lead to an increased incidence of gallstones) without a concomitant increase in cholesterol synthesis. The effect on triglycerides is probably mediated through its inhibitory actions on fructose-1, 6-diphosphate aldolase, citrate cleavage enzyme, acetyl CoA carboxylase, and glucose 6-phosphate dehydrogenase, thus interfering with the synthesis of the glycerol skeleton and the fatty acids. Clofibrate is not effective in the lipoprotein lipase deficiency that produces dietary chylomicronemia without appreciable elevations in VLDL, nor is it effective in familial hypercholesterolemia. It may be effective in any of the other hyperlipidemias. Recent studies have demonstrated, however, that the use of clofibrate is associated with a decreased life expectancy. Therefore, I only use this agent as a last resort in patients with hyperlipidemia and pancreatitis.

Nicotinic Acid

Nicotinic acid is also known as niacin. This vitamin is used in the treatment of pellagra. It lowers both cholesterol and triglyceride levels. The effect seems to be to decrease the synthesis of VLDL and consequently LDL as well. The therapeutic dosage is 3 to 6 g/day given in divided doses after meals. Cutaneous flushing and pruritus initially occur 1 to 2 hours after each dose, but in 85% of patients these symptoms disappear after 2 weeks. Moreover, the administration of 300 mg aspirin 30 minutes before the nicotinic acid often prevents these prostaglandin-mediated side effects. In order to minimize the initial symptoms, the drug is usually started in a dose of 250 mg 3 times a day. Rarely, serious hepatic injury can be caused by nicotinic acid. Nicotinic acid may be effective in any of the hyperlipidemias except the lipoprotein lipase deficiency that results in dietary chylomicronemia without significant VLDL elevation. Nicotinic acid is especially useful in combination with cholestyramine or colestipol in the treatment of familial hypercholesterolemia.

Cholestyramine and Colestipol

Cholestyramine is the chloride salt of a basic anion exchange resin. This large polymer contains quaternary ammonium groups attached to a styrene divinylbenzene skeleton. It binds bile salts tightly, thus interfering with the enterohepatic circulation and causing the loss of bile acids and neutral sterols. Colestipol is similar in its mode of action. This leads to a compensatory increase in HMG CoA reductase; hence the drug becomes effective only in a dose that overwhelms the body's maximum capacity to synthesize cholesterol. There is also an increase in hepatic LDL receptor activity. The effect on triglycerides is variable, without a dramatic change in either direction. The usual effective dose of cholestyramine is 24 to 32 g/day given in 2 doses. The usual dose of colestipol is 15 to 30 g/day given in 2 doses. The main side effects are related to the gastrointestinal tract where it can produce cramps, constipation, or diarrhea. Cholestyramine and colestipol are the drugs of choice in familial hypercholesterolemia. The use of such agents has been shown to increase LDL receptor activity in heterozygote familial hypercholesterolemic patients. The addition of nicotinic acid often lowers the LDL levels of heterozygotes into the low-normal range.

CLINICAL PROBLEMS

Patient 1. A 34-year-old woman complains of left arm pain since delivering her third child 18 months ago. The pain is poorly related to exertion. Moving the arm through a full range of motion does not reproduce the pain nor aggravate it if it is already present. Her father died at age 68 of a myocardial infarction. He had his first infarction at age 40. The family physician treated him for "high cholesterol." The patient's 40-year-old sister has "high cholesterol." Her 3 other siblings were normal as far as she knew. At age 17 the patient first noticed "bumps" on her knuckles. She smokes 2 packs of cigarettes each day and has done so for 15 years.

PHYSICAL EXAMINATION. On examination tendon xanthomas were found on the extensor tendons of the hands and on the Achilles tendons. The remainder of the physical examination was normal.

LABORATORY DATA. Routine laboratory tests were likewise normal except for a plasma cholesterol concentration of 450 mg/100 ml; the plasma triglyceride concentration was 100 mg/100 ml. Blood lipids were obtained from her siblings, and three were normal with respect to both the plasma cholesterol and triglyceride concentration. The 40-year-old sister had a plasma cholesterol concentration of 436 mg/100 ml with triglyceride concentration of 95 mg/100 ml. On physical examination the sister had Achilles tendon xanthomas. Blood lipid values were obtained from the patient's 3 children—a boy 13 years old, a boy 10 years, and a girl 18 months old. The values for plasma cholesterol were 350 mg/100 ml, 400 mg/100 ml, and 300 mg/100 ml, respectively. The plasma triglyceride concentrations were all normal.

QUESTIONS

1. What is the mode of inheritance?
2. What is the diagnosis?
3. What tests would you do to further evaluate the arm pain?
4. What general measures would you prescribe?
5. What specific measures would you advise for the patient and her children?

Patient 2. A 51-year-old woman was referred by her dentist because he noticed that her blood looked "milky" when she bled during a dental procedure. She had been taking clofibrate for several years for "high fat in the blood" and was taking tolbutamide for diabetes and estrogens for menopausal symptoms. The family history was unremarkable.

PHYSICAL EXAMINATION. This examination was normal except for mild obesity.

LABORATORY DATA. A fasting blood sugar was 308 mg/100 ml, and a 2-hour postprandial blood sugar was 564 mg/100 ml. Her T_4 was 13.5 µg/100 ml. The plasma cholesterol was 512 mg/100 ml, and the triglycerides were 5000 mg/100 ml. The plasma showed a cream layer with a turbid infranatant layer after standing in the refrigerator overnight. All medications were stopped, and an oral glucose tolerance test with insulin levels was performed. The results are shown below:

	Glucose (mg/100 ml)	Insulin (μU/ml)	
Fasting (hr)	234	18	(Fasting normal 4–24)
1	484	22	
2	448	18	
3	392	19	
4	235	21	
5	197	17	

QUESTIONS

1. Does this patient have primary or secondary hyperlipidemia?
2. What factors may be contributing to the elevated plasma lipids?
3. What would you advise regarding her diet?
4. What would you advise regarding her present medications?
5. What new medications would you prescribe?

Patient 3. A 68-year-old man had his first myocardial infarction 3 months ago.
PHYSICAL EXAMINATION. On the follow-up visit the physical examination was normal.
LABORATORY DATA. The laboratory examination was normal except for a plasma cholesterol of 312 mg/100 ml. The triglycerides were 145 mg/100 ml. Plasma lipid values were obtained from her 3 brothers, ages 55, 57, and 60. The plasma cholesterol concentrations were 260 mg/100 ml, 268 mg/100 ml, and 271 mg/100 ml. The triglycerides were high normal. Examination of 10 adult children from these 4 siblings revealed high normal to slightly elevated cholesterol concentrations (range, 230 to 265 mg/100 ml) with normal triglyceride concentrations, except for 2 young women in their 20's who were taking oral contraceptives and had triglyceride concentrations of 178 and 187 mg/100 ml.

QUESTIONS

1. Does the 68-year-old have primary or secondary hyperlipidemia?
2. What is the mode of inheritance?
3. What is the relative risk for an atherosclerotic event in this family?
4. What therapy would you prescribe for the 68-year-old man and his brothers?
5. What therapy would you prescribe for the children?

Patient 4. A 55-year-old executive is found to have a triglyceride concentration of 230 mg/100 ml on a routine evaluation.
PHYSICAL EXAMINATION. His examination was normal except for excess weight estimated to be on the order of 10 pounds.
LABORATORY DATA. Other routine fasting laboratory tests were normal. He is referred to you. He is taking no medications, and the family history is negative except for a maternal uncle and a paternal aunt who had adult onset diabetes that was detected in their early 70's. His family lives in another city and his children are away at school and unavailable for testing at this time. You confirm the physical examination and order repeat lipid levels and an oral glucose tolerance test. The cholesterol concentration is 247 mg/100 ml and the triglycerides are 238 mg/100 ml. The fasting blood glucose was again normal, but the oral glucose tolerance was abnormal with a 2-hour value of 220 mg/100 ml. (He had been given a special diet in preparation for this glucose challenge.)

QUESTIONS

1. Does this patient have primary or secondary hyperlipidemia?
2. What do you think is the pathophysiology of his hyperlipidemia?
3. What therapy would you prescribe?

Patient 5. A 45-year-old man is referred to you 6 months after a coronary bypass operation for angina pectoris. The operation was successful and he is taking no medications.

PHYSICAL EXAMINATION. Except for the surgical scar, the physical examination is normal.

LABORATORY DATA. The laboratory examination is likewise normal except for a cholesterol of 298 mg/100 ml and a triglyceride concentration of 242 mg/100 ml. He has two children, a daughter age 18 and a son age 23. The daughter's plasma cholesterol was 147 mg/100 ml and her triglyceride was 75 mg/100 ml.. The son, who was neither obese nor diabetic, had a cholesterol concentration of 210 mg/100 ml and a triglyceride concentration of 195 mg/100 ml. The patient's 48-year-old brother was examined and found to have a cholesterol concentration of 300 mg/100 ml with a triglyceride concentration of 150 mg/100 ml. The man's 20-year-old son had low normal serum lipids. His 27-year-old daughter, who was not diabetic and did not take oral contraceptives, had a plasma cholesterol concentration of 300 mg/100 ml and triglyceride of 223 mg/100 ml. Her 2 children, ages 3 and 5, had normal plasma lipids.

QUESTIONS

1. Does this patient have primary or secondary hyperlipidemia?
2. What is the mode of inheritance?
3. What is the diagnosis?
4. What further tests would you request?
5. What general measures would you advise?
6. What specific therapy would you prescribe?

SUGGESTED READING

Biochemistry and Physiology of Cholesterol and Triglycerides

Brown, M.S., and Goldstein, J.L.: Receptor-mediated endocytosis: insights from the lipoprotein receptor system. Proc. Natl. Acad. Sci. USA, *76*:3330, 1979.

Fielding, P.E., and Fielding, C.J.: A cholesteryl ester transfer complex in human plasma. Proc. Natl. Acad. Sci. USA, *77*:3327, 1980.

Fogelman, A.M., et al.: Malondialdehyde alteration of low density lipoproteins leads to cholesteryl ester accumulation in human monocyte-macrophages. Proc. Natl. Acad. Sci. USA, *77*:2214, 1980.

Goldstein, J.L., Anderson, R.G., and Brown, M.S.: Coated pits, coated vesicles, and receptor-mediated endocytosis. Nature, *279*:679, 1979.

Goldstein, J.L., and Brown, M.S.: The low-density lipoprotein pathway and its relation to atherosclerosis. Annu. Rev. Biochem., *46*:897, 1977.

Havel, R.J., Goldstein, J.L. and Brown, M.S.: Lipoproteins and lipid transport. *In* Metabolic Control and Disease. 8th Ed. Edited by P.K. Bondy and L.E. Rosenberg. Philadelphia, W.B. Saunders, 1980.

Mahley, R.W., et al.: Cholesteryl ester synthesis in macrophages: stimulation by B-very low density lipoproteins from cholesterol-fed animals of several species. J. Lipid Res., *21*:970, 1980.

Shechter, I., et al.: The metabolism of native and malondialdehyde altered low density lipoproteins by human monocyte-macrophages. J. Lipid Res., *22*:63, 1981.

Shepherd, J., Bicker S., Lorimer, A.R., and Packard, C.J.: Receptor-mediated low density lipoprotein catabolism in man. J. Lipid Res., *20*:999, 1979.

Clinical Tests

Goldstein, J.L., et al.: Hyperlipidemia in coronary heart disease. I. Lipid levels in 500 survivors of myocardial infarction. J. Clin. Invest., *52*:1533, 1973.

Hazzard, W.R., et al.: Hyperlipidemia in coronary heart disease. III. Evaluation of lipoprotein phenotypes of 156 genetically defined survivors of myocardial infarction. J. Clin. Invest., *52*:1569, 1973.

Rhoads, G.G., Gulbrandsen, C.L., and Kagan, A.: Serum lipoproteins and coronary heart disease. N. Engl. J. Med., *294*:293, 1976.

Secondary Hyperlipidemias

Bierman, E.L.: Insulin and hypertriglyceridemia. Isr. J. Med. Sci., *8*:303, 1972.

Bierman, E.L., and Porte, D., Jr.: Carbohydrate intolerance and lipemia. Ann. Intern. Med., *68*:926, 1968.

Bluestone, R., Lewis, B., and Mervart, I.: Hyperlipoproteinemia in gout. Ann. Rheum. Dis., *301*:134, 1971.

Olefsky, J., Reaven, G.M., and Farquhar, W.: Effects of weight reduction on obesity. J. Clin. Invest., *53*:64, 1974.

Thompson, G.R., e al.: Defects of receptor-mediated low density lipoprotein catabolism in homozygous familial hypercholesterolemia and hypothyroidism in vivo. Proc. Natl. Acad. Sci. USA, *78*:2591, 1981.

Primary Hyperlipidemias

Breslow, J.L., and Zannis, V.I.: Characterization of a unique human apolipoprotein E variant associated with type III hyperlipoproteinemia. J. Biol. Chem., *255*:1759, 1980.

Brunzell, J.D., et al.: Myocardial infarction in the familial forms of hypertriglyceridemia. Metabolism, *25*:313, 1976.

Cox, D.W., Breckenridge, W.C., and Little, J.A.: Inheritance of apolipoprotein C-II deficiency with hypertriglyceridemia and pancreatitis. N. Engl. J. Med., *299*:1421, 1978.

Goldstein, J.L., et al.: Hyperlipidemia in coronary heart disease. II. Genetic analysis of lipid levels in 176 families and delineation of a new inherited disorder, combined hyperlipidemia. J. Clin. Invest., *52*;1544, 1973.

Hazzard, W.R.,O'Donnell, T.F. and Lee, Y.L.: Broad β disease (type III hyperlipoproteinemia) in a large kindred. Ann. Intern. Med., *82*:141, 1975.

Morganroth, J., Levy, R.I., and Fredrickson, D.S.: The biochemical, clinical, and genetic features of type III hyperlipoproteinemia. Ann. Intern. Med., *82*:158, 1975.

Motulsky, A.G: The genetic hyperlipidemias. N. Engl. J. Med., *294*:823, 1976.

Treatment

Bierman, E.L.: Dietary carbohydrates and hyperlipidemic states in man. Nutr. Metab. (Suppl. I), *18*:108, 1975.

Dayton, S., et al.: A controlled clinical trial of a diet high in unsaturated fat in preventing complications of atherosclerosis. Circulation (Suppl. II) *40*:II–1, 1969.

Kane, J.P., et al.: Normalization of low-density lipoprotein levels in heterozygous familial hypercholesterolemia with a combined drug regimen. N. Engl. J. Med., *304*:251, 1981.

Levy, R.I., et al.: Dietary and drug treatment of primary hyperlipoproteinemia Ann. Intern. Med., *74*:267, 1972.

Shepherd, J., et al.: Cholestyramine promotes receptor-mediated low-density-lipoprotein catabolism. N. Engl. J. Med, *302*:1219, 1980.

Answers to Questions in Clinical Problems

CHAPTER 2

Patient 1

1. Pituitary infarction and necrosis due to hypotension and vasoconstriction have led to loss of anterior pituitary function. The specific hormonal deficiencies have produced failure to lactate, hypotension, and amenorrhea.

2. GH, PRL, ACTH, LH, and FSH are deficient. Neither GH nor ACTH responded to insulin hypoglycemia, and prolactin showed only a minimal response to TRH. Although no specific stimulation test of gonadotropin release was performed, serum LH and FSH were both inappropriately low in the face of a hypogonadal serum estradiol concentration. TSH secretion is intact, based on a normal serum thyroxine concentration and a normal TSH response to TRH.

3. Metyrapone, by inhibiting the patient's already deficient secretion of cortisol, could provoke a severe hypoadrenal crisis with hypotension and cardiovascular collapse.

4. The patient's limited capacity to secrete cortisol was insufficient to meet the stress of the pneumoencephalogram, and the features of acute hypoadrenalism developed. Emergency treatment would include large intravenous doses of hydrocortisone and volume expansion with physiologic saline solution. Considering the clear clinical history of postpartum shock and the small sella turcica, the pneumoencephalogram was probably not indicated. Pneumonoencephalography would be expected to be normal in this patient, but aids in the evaluation of suspected pituitary tumors.

Patient 2

1. This patient has probably had acromegaly for at least 20 years; additionally, several clinical features of hypopituitarism have been present for 8 years.

2. Pituitary apoplexy (hemorrhage into his tumor) occurred acutely.

3. Features of acromegaly noted to be present include the increase in shoe and ring size, as well as enlargement of the facial features, tongue, and soft tissues of the extremities. The elevated serum GH is somewhat supportive of the diagnosis of acromegaly, although the stress of the acute illness might raise serum GH to this level in a normal subject.

   The slow growth of the pituitary tumor has enlarged the sella turcica. While some visual field abnormalities may have resulted from the tumor alone, the subsequent pituitary hemorrhage undoubtedly expanded the sellar contents and further compressed the optic chiasm. Lateral expansion accounts for the third cranial nerve palsy.

   Hypogonadism is revealed by the history of decreased libido and beard growth, by the physical findings of scanty hair and atrophic testes, and by the low serum testosterone and LH. Hypothyroidism is suggested by the history of fatigue and cold intolerance, by the dry skin and delayed reflexes on physical examination, and by the low serum thyroxine and TSH. Deficient ACTH secretion may have produced poor tanning of the skin, orthostatic hypotension, and hyponatremia; the increased number of eosinophils seen on the white cell differential count may also be a result of hypoadrenalism. The low serum cortisol in the face of major stress supports the diagnosis of hypoadrenalism.

4. Elevated serum PRL is a common finding with pituitary tumors. This symptom may result either from direct production by the tumor or by interruption of the hypothalamic-pituitary portal vessels by the expanding tumor, with resultant decrease in PRL inhibiting factor at the pituitary.

5. A transfrontal hypophysectomy was probably done; this approach is traditionally used when significant suprasellar extension accompanies compression of the optic chiasm. The transsphenoidal route is used when there is less need for suprasellar dissection. Although radiation therapy might have been appropriate at any prior time in the patient's course, it would not be useful in the present situation since it would not produce the rapid decompression of the tumor needed to preserve vision. Treatment with glucocorticoid was given before, during, and after the operation. When the patient had recovered from the operation, it would be reasonable to begin replacement therapy with L-thyroxine and testosterone, and to continue hydrocortisone.

6. The elevated serum calcium raises the possibility that this patient may also have hyperparathyroidism; acromegaly and other pituitary tumors may occur with hyperparathyroidism and pancreatic islet-cell tumors in the familial syndrome of multiple endocrine neoplasia, type 1. The patient's parathyroid status (such as measurement of plasma parathyroid hormone and renal tubular reabsorption of phosphate) should be further investigated. Serum gastrin and fasting blood sugar should also be measured (gastrin, insulin and glucagon may be produced by islet-cell tumors of the pancreas).

7. In many cases of pituitary apoplexy in acromegaly, enough tumor is destroyed to cure the acromegaly; thus, the serum GH might fall to normal levels over several days or weeks following the acute infarction and hemorrhage. If the serum GH remained elevated, either surgical or radiation therapy could be given.

Patient 3

1. In normal men and prepubertal children, GH responses to provocative testing are sometimes inadequate. Brief pretreatment with large doses of estrogens will enhance GH responses to all stimuli and will thus help separate normal from abnormal responses. Estrogens also increase the production of serum cortisol-binding globulin, the carrier for circulating cortisol. In a normal individual, these extra binding sites are rapidly filled with additional cortisol; thus, this patient's relatively low serum cortisol concentration after estrogen administration and the deficient rise in cortisol after hypoglycemia suggest that cortisol production is impaired.

2. GH deficiency is not yet established. Since hypothyroidism impairs GH responses to provocative tests, the practical approach is to give replacement thyroid hormone, if necessary, before evaluating GH secretion.

3. Since serum TSH rose adequately following TRH administration, the pituitary's capacity to secrete TSH appears to be intact. Thus, the low basal TSH in the face of hypothyroidism is probably due to TRH deficiency producd by hypothalamic disease. The delayed and prolonged peak of TSH following TRH also supports the diagnosis of hypothalamic hypothyroidism.

Patient 4

1. TSH secretion capability appears to be intact, as judged by normal serum T_3, T_4, and TSH levels. Both serum GH and plasma cortisol showed normal increments following

hypoglycemia, and plasma deoxycortisol rose appropriately after metyrapone, demonstrating normal pituitary GH and ACTH reserve. Deficient LH and FSH secretion are suggested by low or normal serum LH and FSH in the presence of a low serum estradiol concentration.

2. The inappropriately low LH and FSH may be due to compression or destruction of pituitary gonadotrophs by the tumor. Alternatively, the elevated PRL concentrations may have suppressed gonadotropin secretion through a poorly understood action of prolactin on the pituitary or hypothalamus.

3. Although it is difficult to make a positive diagnosis, the patient's history of disordered menses since age 14 suggests the disease process began at that time.

4. Following neurosurgical procedures on or near the hypothalamus, it is common for transient diabetes insipidus to develop; this is presumably due to minor reversible damage to the vasopressin-producing nuclei. This patient did not have *complete* diabetes insipidus at evaluation in late 1974, since she could concentrate her urine to some extent, but she may have had a *partial* defect in vasopressin secretion. A water deprivation test would be necessary to assess the capacity for maximal urinary concentration.

CHAPTER 3

Patient 1

1. Her loss of memory and slow speech indicate reduced cerebration, which is subtle and difficult to quantitate. A history of reduced ability to perform familiar work, such as calculation and memory of names and numbers, is a helpful clinical index. Surprisingly, children with acquired hypothyroidism may get good school grades because they are "quiet." The ataxia could arise from cerebellar involvement, peripheral neuropathy, or muscle weakness.

2. The greatly elevated serum TSH indicates that the woman has primary hypothyroidism rather than pituitary or hypothalamic disease. A skull roentgenogram is not necessary to make this differentiation. A significant proportion of patients with primary hypothyroidism have an enlarged sella turcica, presumably related to pituitary enlargement from hyperplasia of the thyrotrophs; recently, the sellar enlargement has been positively correlated with the serum TSH concentration.

3. Hashimoto's thyroiditis is the most likely cause. Significantly elevated titers of antithyroglobulin and antimicrosomal antibodies would confirm the diagnosis. Unfortunately, diagnostic titers are not found in one-fourth of patients. The high titers are more likely to occur when patients have thyroid enlargement.

4. Her macrocytic anemia could be due either to pernicious anemia, which coexists in about 10% of patients with Hashimoto's disease, or to hypothyroidism alone. Work-up for pernicious anemia is indicated, as is a more detailed neurologic evaluation for coexisting subacute combined degeneration, which could also explain her ataxia.

Patient 2

1. She has classic Graves' disease with hyperthyroidism clinically. However, her oral contraceptive will also elevate the serum T_4 and serum T_3 levels. This factor is an indication for measuring the T_3 uptake; her value was 40%, the mean normal being 30% (range 25 to 35%).

2. Her FT_4I is:

$$22 \times \frac{40\%}{30\%} = 29.3$$

3. The pulmonic flow murmur, common in hyperthyroidism, is due to the increased cardiac output. The thyroid bruit indicates increased blood flow to the thyroid.

4. Because of the tachycardia and nervousness, propranolol is indicated. Her definitive therapy would be long-term propylthiouracil. When the hyperthyroidism is controlled by the antithyroid drug, propranolol can be stopped.

    After treatment with propylthiouracil for 1 year, she has about a 50% chance for a long-term remission. Her large goiter (more than $2^1/_2$ times normal) is an unfavorable prognostic factor for long-term remission, but the short duration of symptoms (less than 1 year) is a favorable prognostic factor. Because she is young, destructive forms of treatment are best avoided; therapy with ^{131}I or surgical thyroidectomy may be reconsidered if she relapses after stopping propylthiouracil.

    The prognosis concerning the exophthalmos is not predictable. Although most patients have significant improvement, some become steadily worse.

5. Yes, but this contraindication is relative. The antithyroid drugs can be transmitted across the placenta to cause hypothyroidism and goiter in the fetus. Graves' thyroid-stimulating IgG's are also transmitted across the placenta and can cause neonatal hyperthyroidism. Pregnancy should be postponed for 1 year with the anticipation that the Graves' disease will be inactive, or at worst that the hyperthyroidism will be controlled on a low dose of antithyroid drug at that time.

Patient 3

1. The patient has all the clinical features of subacute thyroiditis; the tender enlarged thyroid is the key to the diagnosis. Presumably, the cause is the antecedent viral pharyngitis.

2. The inflammation of the thyroid gland interferes with normal function (trapping of iodide and oxidative iodination). In addition, the release of hormone suppresses TSH secretion and lowers the thyroid uptake.

3. Her serum thyroglobulin would be considerably elevated.

4. Features suggestive of hyperthyroidism could be explained in part by the local inflammatory disorder. However, her elevated serum T_4 and serum T_3 concentrations indicate chemical hyperthyroidism. These measurements, as carried out presently, are not influenced by iodoprotein, such as thyroglobulin.

5. Because the disorder is usually self-limited, only moderate rest, aspirin, and observation are indicated at this time. If the hyperthyroidism gets worse, propranolol may be helpful. Corticosteroids reduce the inflammation of the thyroid and are given in worse cases in doses of 20 to 30 mg prednisone per day for 1 to 3 weeks.

Patient 4

1. She had Hashimoto's lymphocytic thyroiditis with goiter and high antithyroglobulin titer.

2. In this disorder, some patients have a defect in organic binding; iodine will be trapped, but does not remain in the gland so that early uptakes are higher than 24-hour uptake. The perchlorate discharge test in this situation will be abnormal.

3. The elevated serum TSH and the serum T_4 at the lower limit of normal indicate thyroid disease. The high TSH stimulates the trapping of iodide (high 6-hour uptake); there is also compensation in the form of relatively greater thyroidal secretion of T_3.

4. Apparently, she has recovered. A significant proportion of adolescents with mild Hashimoto's thyroiditis do recover. When the hypothyroidism is more profound, the possibility

for recovery is poor. For her, the long-term prognosis is unclear. She may develop recurrent goiter, hypothyroidism, or even hyperthyroidism of Graves' disease.

5. Associated with Hashimoto's thyroiditis are other autoimmune endocrine diseases, including Addison's disease, hypoparathyroidism, ovarian failure, and diabetes mellitus. (The autoimmune basis of the diabetes is not established.) These diseases are rare compared with Hashimoto's disease.

Patient 5

1. The myxedema was caused by the potassium iodide. In some patients, iodide interferes with the biosynthesis of thyroid hormone, probably by blocking the peroxidase enzyme system. In normal individuals, escape from this blocking effect occurs within a few days, but in a small number of patients, escape does not occur. The inhibition of biosynthesis eventually results in hypothyroidism, the serum TSH rises, and compensatory thyroid enlargement occurs. Presumably, these patients have an underlying thyroid disorder that predisposes them to this condition. Goiter may also occur without hypothyroidism. A second effect of excess iodide is inhibition of release of thyroid hormone, but this effect is probably not the major one in patients with iodide-induced goiter and hypothyroidism. In this patient, the abnormal perchlorate discharge test showed that organic binding of iodine was blocked. (In normal individuals, perchlorate causes less than a 10% reduction of the uptake in the gland.) The normal perchlorate discharge 3 weeks later showed no underlying defect in the peroxidase enzyme system.

   The goiter caused the "lump in the throat." As normal biosynthesis took place, TSH fell, the goiter shrunk, and the symptom disappeared.

2. Iodine is used for treatment of hyperthyroidism. Its block of biosynthesis is helpful, but its rapid reduction of serum thyroxine levels is mainly attributed to the slowing of hormone release from the gland due to iodine's inhibition of proteolysis.

Patient 6

1. All causes of thyroid nodules must be considered. The most common lesions in such instances are adenomas or differentiated carcinomas of the thyroid.

2. The history of radiation to the neck in childhood is important because of the neoplasia that may develop 10 to 40 years later. In similar patients, 40 to 50% have been found to have papillary or follicular carcinoma. The other lesions are adenomas. In some patients, the palpable nodule is an adenoma, but the other lobe (or another area) may harbor a carcinoma.

3. Fine-needle aspiration biopsy. This showed evidence of a follicular lesion; carcinoma could not be ruled out.

4. Thyroidectomy is recommended. At surgical procedure, a benign follicular adenoma was found and a left lobectomy was performed. The right lobe was entirely normal to inspection and was not removed. Becuse of the multicentricity of the lesions, some advocate total thyroidectomy in patients with similar lesions who have received radiation. The counter argument is that microscopic carcinoma (possibly in the right lobe) does not alter the long-term prognosis. To prevent recurrent nodule formation by suppression of TSH secretion, this patient was placed on "permanent" therapy with 0.2 mg L-thyroxine.

CHAPTER 4

Patient 1

1. Symptoms of anorexia, nausea, vomiting, abdominal cramping, and weight loss result from cortisol deficiency in the cells of the gastrointestinal tract. Somnolence and fatigue

result from cortisol deficiency in brain cells, and extreme weakness results from lack of cortisol effect in muscle cells. Constipation probably resulted from an essentially liquid diet. Light-headedness, palpitations, dyspnea, and fullness in the ears on standing upright are the result of total body sodium and volume depletion from aldosterone deficiency and also lack of the normal response of arterioles to the vasoconstrictor effect of catecholamines in cortisol deficiency. Dry skin probably is due to both volume depletion and lack of cortisol in the skin and appendage cells. Alopecia of the head and vitiligo are probably a result of autoimmune-mediated disease of the melanocytes and hair follicles, and loss of axillary and pubic hair is the result of adrenal androgen deficiency. Increased skin pigmentation and freckling are caused by chronic elevation of ACTH and LPH.

2.   The diagnosis of primary adrenal insufficiency is made by the low serum cortisol, which does not respond to ACTH stimulation, the elevated plasma ACTH level, and the low urinary 17-OHCS and 17-ketosteroids. Low serum aldosterone is also consistent with primary rather than secondary adrenal insufficiency. The cause of the adrenal disease is most likely autoimmune adrenalitis resulting in adrenal atrophy. Vitiligo is associated with idiopathic adrenal atrophy in 17% of patients. A negative tuberculin skin test and positive serum antiadrenal antibodies would confirm the diagnosis. Hashimoto's thyroiditis is suggested by the thyroid examination. The diagnosis would be confirmed by finding a significant titer of antithyroid antibodies in the serum.

3.   Idiopathic hypoparathyroidism, pernicious anemia, diabetes mellitus, thyroiditis (Hashimoto's and Graves' disease), and ovarian atrophy are all associated with idiopathic (but not tuberculous) adrenal atrophy.

4.   The patient's chronic adrenal insufficiency will be corrected by replacement doses of glucocorticoid (prednisone 7.5 mg daily, or hydrocortisone, 30 mg daily) and mineralocorticoid (9 α-fluorocortisol, 0.1 mg daily).

5.   Increasing circulating levels of T_4 and T_3 with thyroxine therapy may precipitate an adrenal crisis in the patient with chronic adrenal insufficiency by increasing the body's cortisol need. It is important to correct cortisol deficiency prior to therapy with T_4.

Patient 2

1.   Elevated urinary 17-ketosteroids and pregnanetriol, elevated urinary sodium excretion and decreased potassium excretion in the presence of decreased serum sodium and elevated serum potassium confirm the diagnosis of congenital adrenal hyperplasia.

2.   Salt loss occurs from a failure to secrete adequate quantities of aldosterone, particularly when salt intake is diminished as a result of intercurrent illness and sodium conservation does not occur. Failure to secrete adequate quantities of aldosterone occurs with 21-hydroxylase deficiency, 3β-dehydrogenase deficiency and 20,22-desmolase deficiency. Retention of sodium occurs in 11-hydroxylase deficiency and in 17-hydroxylase deficiency, because of increased secretion of 11-deoxycorticosterone, a potent mineralocorticoid.

3.   17α-hydroxyprogesterone is the precursor in the plasma of pregnanetriol in the urine, and is increased in 21-hydroxylase deficiency. Plasma progesterone is excreted as pregnanediol.

4.   The patient is tall because of excessive growth stimulation by androgenic substances such as testosterone produced by the adrenals. Because his bone age is 15 years, he only has 3 years of skeletal maturation left before his epiphyses fuse completely to arrest growth. His height is average for a 12 year old at a chronologic age of 9 years. He will be short as an adult.

5.   The ''testicular tumor'' is composed of cells that are frequently found in the testes and that increase in size and number when stimulated by ACTH. Histologically, they resemble

Leydig cells, but functionally they appear to have properties of adrenocortical cells. These testicular masses tend to occur in children with congenital adrenal hyperplasia that is poorly controlled. Similar masses may be found in the adrenal glands themselves.

Patient 3

1. In this patient, the abnormality is 11-hydroxylase deficiency, which leads to increased formation of 11-deoxycortisol (compound S) and 11-deoxycorticosterone (DOC). In normal individuals, compound S levels in the serum are virtually undetectable and are generally reported by the laboratory as being less than 2 μg/100 ml, the lower limit of sensitivity of the assay usually employed. Concentrations as high as 13 to 25 μg/100 ml are seen only in this type of adrenal hyperplasia and in testing for adrenocortical reserve by administration of metyrapone. Compound S is physiologically inert, but excessive amounts of DOC lead to sodium retention and hypertension. Typical of the 11-hydroxylase type of defect is the excretion of increased amounts of 17-ketosteroids and tetrahydro S in the urine. The latter represents a more polar, reduced derivative of compound S, which is more readily excreted. On the other hand, the amounts of pregnanetriol excreted are not much increased.

2. The commonest cause of progressive virilization in a female child is congenital adrenal hyperplasia. Rarer causes are adenomas and carcinomas of the adrenals and ovaries.

3. Hypertension in congenital adrenal hyperplasia occurs in association with 11-hydroxylase and 17-hydroxylase defects. Hypertension is largely a consequence of excessive elaboration of 11-deoxycorticosterone. Virilization occurs in association with the 11-hydroxylase defect but not with 17-hydroxylase defect because deficiency of 17-hydroxylase impairs secretion of adrenal androgens and gonadal testosterone.

Patient 4

1. Thinning of skin, muscle weakness, mild hypertension, centripetal fat deposition, bruises, light facial hair, altered facial appearance, and poor healing result from chronic excessive glucocorticoid secretion.

2. Cushing's syndrome was diagnosed by lack of circadian rhythm of plasma cortisol, lack of cortisol suppression by the low-dose dexamethasone test, and elevated urinary 17-hydroxycorticosteroids. Mildly elevated plasma ACTH and greater than 50% suppression of urinary 17-hydroxysteroids by the high dose of dexamethasone are indicative of Cushing's disease.

3. At operation, the left adrenal gland weighed 10 g; the right, 11 g (normal, 5 g each). Histologic examination revealed hyperplasia of the adrenal cortex with widening of the zona reticularis. Pathologic diagnosis was bilateral adrenocortical hyperplasia.

4. Skull roentgenograms and sellar tomograms are useful to estimate the volume of the sella. Examination of visual fields and CT scan of the head test for significant suprasellar extension of a pituitary tumor.

Patient 5

1. Moderate hypertension combined with muscle weakness, cramps, and nocturia suggest mineralocorticoid excess.

2. Chronic sodium retention from aldosterone excess results in hypertension. Potassium depletion from persistent mineralocorticoid action at the distal tubule of the nephron causes inability to concentrate the urine, muscle weakness, and cramps.

3. Basal urinary K^+ greater than 40 mEq/24 hours in the presence of hypokalemia (K^+ less than 3.5) indicates mineralocorticoid excess. Increased Na^+ delivery to the distal tubule

in the presence of nonsuppressible aldosterone secretion enhances urinary K^+ excretion and induces further hypokalemia, whereas in the normal state Na^+ load does not alter K^+ excretion markedly.

4. The most useful tests are dexamethasone-suppressed adrenal scan, ^{131}I-19-iodocholesterol, and adrenal venography with bilateral adrenal vein sampling for aldosterone levels. If aldosterone levels were elevated and similar bilaterally and the venogram confirmed bilateral hyperplasia, or if both adrenals were visualized on dexamethasone-suppressed adrenal scan, medical therapy would be recommended; whereas if an aldosteronoma were localized by unilaterally elevated aldosterone levels and an adrenal tumor on venogram, the patient would potentially be cured by surgical removal of the tumor.

Patient 6

1. Episodic catecholamine secretion is suggested by sudden headache, sweating, tachycardia, and tightness in the chest precipitated by change in position. Chronic catecholamine excess produces postural drop in blood pressure, nausea, and obstipation.

2. Secretion of 30% of catecholamines as epinephrine is characteristic of a pheochromocytoma located in the adrenal gland because the synthesis of epinephrine requires high concentrations of cortisol.

3. Basal and calcium-stimulated calcitonin measurements would screen for associated medullary carcinoma of the thyroid. Parathormone and calcium levels would exclude hyperparathyroidism. A work-up for a central nervous system tumor, such as may occur in the associated neuroectodermal syndromes, would be done only if the patient had symptoms and signs referable to such a lesion.

4. Propranolol blocks β receptors and thus blocks the vasodilating effect of catecholamines. This β blockade in the presence of elevated plasma catecholamines results in unopposed α-mediated vasoconstriction and strongly noticeable increase in blood pressure.

Patient 7

1. The high cortisol level is a result of ectopic ACTH secretion by the carcinoma. Cortisol in high concentration (greater than 50 $\mu g/100$ ml in this case) has mineralocorticoid activity resulting in sodium retention, edema, and urinary potassium loss. Other mineralocorticoids such as 11-deoxycorticosterone released by chronic ACTH stimulation may contribute to edema and hypokalemia.

2. Metyrapone, by blocking conversion of 11-deoxycortisol by cortisol, would decrease cortisol production in spite of persistent stimulation by ACTH.

3. Under constant ACTH stimulation, the adrenals produce compound S instead of cortisol when metyrapone blockade occurs. This patient may have compound S levels of 50 $\mu g/$ 100 ml in response to metyrapone. This elevation of compound S does *not* indicate that the pituitary has increased ACTH secretion in response to decreased cortisol feedback but reflects the adrenal response to autonomous ACTH secretion by the carcinoma. The hypothalamus and pituitary are chronically suppressed by the elevated cortisol and unresponsive to metyrapone in this disease.

CHAPTER 5

Patient 1

1. Based on the initial physical examination showing ambiguity with a probable left scrotal gonad, simple virilization of an otherwise normal female baby was essentially ruled out. Simple incomplete masculinization of a male was also unlikely. Therefore, a complex diagnostic problem existed and immediate gender assignment was impossible. While the situation is hard to explain to parents, it is more important not to identify the baby wrongly than to wait. Therefore, an explanation based on the fact that the infant had not yet finished developing (rather than was maldeveloped) is in order, as are rapid studies of its blood and organs in order to tell them how it will finish developing. This kind of explanation needs continued reinforcement from all doctors associated with the child.

2. If the parents want to name the baby prior to gender assignment, a "neuter" name such as Frances can be used. However, the parents should be encouraged to wait for gender assignment so they can use the name they had already chosen for their child. This name will be much more real to them in the future than a "neuter" name.

3. No, it is not necessary to file a birth certificate immediately. This procedure can be postponed until gender assignment is made. It is virtually impossible to change the sex on this certificate once filed.

4. Urogenital sinus.

5. Bladder.

6. Vagina.

7. Uterine cavity (uterus).

8. A hemiuterus or uterine structure.

9. The physical examination of partial virilization with asymmetric external genitalia and one scrotal gonad, combined with a vagina and uterus (or hemiuterus) on contrast studies and the XO/XY karyotype, best describes asymmetric or mixed gonadal dysgenesis. In this condition, germ cells of an XO composition migrated to one genital ridge while those with an XY composition migrated to the other—thus, the mixed picture. It is postulated that the gonadal ovarian streak is found on the XO side. Since no testicular tissue exists on this side, müllerian regression substance is *not* produced; therefore, a fallopian tube and hemiuterus connected to the upper part of the vagina develop. On the contralateral side, the XY cells have induced the gonad (testicle) which is incarcerated. Müllerian regression substance was produced so no uterine structure is found.

10. The swelling in the left scrotal fold was an incarcerated gonad. On biopsy, testicular tissue was evident. Its attachments were traced to a blind-ending vas deferens. A laparotomy was performed and a right-sided hemiuterus was identified, associated with a right-sided fallopian tube. No gonad was identified although a shiny streak was seen.

11. Since the anatomy and the karyotype confirm ambiguity secondary to chromosomal mosaicism, rather than an enzymatic or biochemical defect, the infant has the potential to respond appropriately to either androgen or estrogen in the future. Thus, the decision for gender assignment is based on the physician's assessment of the best possible *cosmetic* and *functional* result that can be achieved from operations and hormone therapy.

    For male assignment, one considers the number and complexity of the reconstructive surgical procedures needed to create a functional phallus with a phallic urethra, the need for hysterectomy and vaginectomy, and the future need to implant a testicular prosthesis.

    For female assignment, one considers clitoroplasty and reconstruction of the external genitalia so that the vaginal introitus is adequate, gonadectomy (removal of the testis and the streak), and future hormonal therapy. Hormonal therapy with estrogen gives good breast development, and cyclic therapy will result in menstruation (even a small uterus or hemiuterus usually responds well).

In general, the female gender is assigned when the phallus is inadequate and multiple urologic procedures over many years are required. Creation of a vaginal introitus in the infant with a vagina and uterus is usually quite satisfactory and requires fewer surgical procedures. Additionally, although it might be argued that the testis present would be a future natural source of male hormone, there is little chance for fertility (as the vas is usually blind ending) in either case.

Patient 2

1. Past heights and weights would be helpful in deciding whether the child is exhibiting a recent growth spurt or has always been tall. A recent growth spurt suggests systemic estrogenization. Heights of the parents are also helpful in evaluating the stature of any child.

2. Since the initial differential diagnosis included isosexual precocity and premature the-larche, lesions associated with conditions causing isosexual precocity should be sought. These lesions include the irregular café-au-lait spots found in McCune-Albright's poly-ostotic fibrous dysplasia, the smaller, regular café-au-lait spots found in neurofibromatosis, or dermal neurofibromas themselves. Darkly pigmented areola might suggest exogenous estrogen exposure (diethylstilbestrol).

3. The majority of cases of true isosexual precocity found in girls are ''idiopathic;'' that is, no lesion of the central nervous system is found to account for the activation of the hypothalamic-pituitary-gonadal axis. This lack of lesions is in contrast to the male, where as many as 50% of cases are due to identifiable central nervous system lesions (usually gliomas, teratomas, or hamartomas). Therefore, in the absence of any positive neurologic or central nervous system findings, extensive neuroradiologic evaluation of girls is usually deferred. In males, however, the high incidence of central nervous system lesions makes further investigation mandatory regardless of the finding of an initially normal neurologic examination.

4. The laboratory studies suggest true idiopathic isosexual precocity. Gonadotropins are elevated as is estradiol. The bone age is advanced and the skull series is normal. Had the estradiol been elevated and the gonadotropins been low (suppressed), an autonomous source of estrogen would have had to be sought. In that case, the ultrasound visualization of the ovaries would have been helpful in identifying an ovarian tumor (asymmetry of the ovaries would be checked). If the ovaries were both small, an intravenous pyelogram and adrenal imaging technique (ultrasound) might have been necessary to look for a feminizing adrenal lesion.

Patient 3

1. The patient grew slowly in the first 3 years of life but has grown at a normal rate since. Therefore, she is unlikely to be hypothyroid, or her growth retardation would have continued and she would be much shorter with a much more retarded bone age by this time. Therefore, while a normal T_4 would confirm that she was not hypothyroid, this diagnosis has a low probability.

2. The same holds true for growth retardation from acquired hypopituitarism. Growth rates usually fall to less than 5 cm/year, and progressive deviation from the normal growth pattern is noted. Therefore, extensive radiologic investigation is not in order.

3. Her lack of puberty goes along with her retarded bone age and represents the concomitant conditions of growth and pubertal delay. If gonadal dysgenesis were responsible for her

short stature and failure to develop puberty by age 13, she would have high gonadotropin concentrations. Her low gonadotropins tend to rule out a gonadal problem, making chromosome studies unnecessary.

4. She does not appear to have gonadal failure, so that condition is not responsible for her short stature and pubertal delay, and her good growth rate over the past 10 years tends to rule out deficiency of T_4 (therefore, of pituitary TSH) and GH (therefore, most causes of panhypopituitarism). Then the 2 most likely diagnoses are: (1) constitutional growth and pubertal delay or (2) isolated idiopathic or acquired gonadotropin deficiency. In the absence of a positive family history of delay, it is hard to make the first diagnosis for sure, but the poor growth in the first 3 years followed by normal growth thereafter is most suggestive of growth delay. Gonadotropin deficiency on the other hand is rare. Dynamic testing to distinguish the two is most difficult as there are no reliable stimulation tests for delayed hypothalamic-pituitary gonadotropin secretion. Such a patient is usually followed. A female patient with delay and a bone age of 10 to 11 could expect to develop signs of puberty within the year (as she advances to bone age 11 to 12) while gonadotropin deficiency would cause a stationary bone age.

CHAPTER 6

Patient 1

1. Yes. Since this patient lacks an X chromosome, any X-linked disorder that is present on the remaining chromosome may be fully expressed.

2. No. Since this patient's karyotype is 45 XO, there is no increased risk of the development of gonadal tumors in the dysgenetic gonads. However, if a Y chromosome were found during the analysis, the gonads should be removed because of the increased potential for neoplastic transformation.

3. No. If estrogen therapy had been instituted earlier, her height may have been further compromised because an earlier closure of the epiphyses of the long bones would have resulted. The goal in beginning estrogen therapy in these patients is to wait as long as possible before giving estrogens during adolescence in order to allow the slow growth to continue before inducing epiphyseal closure. However, one must also consider the psychosocial consequences of delaying the patient's sexual maturation; in many instances these considerations outweigh the small gain in height that results from withholding the estrogens until the mid- to late teenage years.

Patient 2

1. The high levels of glucocorticoids that were secreted by the adrenocortical carcinoma suppress the pituitary and hypothalamus; therefore, pituitary ACTH levels would be expected to be low. Administration of more glucocorticoid in the form of dexamethasone does not suppress the ACTH any further, so that there will be no fall in cortisol or other 17-hydroxysteroids after the dexamethasone.

2. In this patient with a rapid onset of virilization, the diagnosis of an adrenal or ovarian neoplasm should be considered no matter what the family history is.

3. The only androgen measured in this patient's serum was testosterone; therefore, it is conceivable that the other 17β-hydroxysteroids may have been elevated. The adrenal gland's secretion of large amounts of androgen precursors may have resulted in the hair follicle's direct conversion of these precursors to more potent androgens that would not be measured in the blood. Although her serum levels of testosterone were less than twice the upper limit of normal, her particular levels may have been up to 8 times normal if her testosterone level was at the lower limits of normal prior to development of the adrenal carcinoma.

4. Male infants may demonstrate genital macrosomia, while female infants may have ambiguous genitalia. In both sexes, the fetal adrenal glands may be suppressed because of transplacental passage of large amounts of glucocorticoids that would suppress the fetal pituitary-hypothalamic-adrenal axis.

Patient 3

1. This patient is likely to have residual tumor because her prolactin levels are markedly elevated. However, the patient may have had some damage to her hypothalamus or pituitary stalk during the transsphenoidal operation, and this damage may have resulted in a decreased secretion of prolactin-inhibiting factor (PIF), hyperprolactinemia, and galactorrhea.

2. Bromocriptine may be useful in decreasing the prolactin levels, eliminating the galactorrhea, and inducing normal cyclicity of the patient's gonadotropins. If this therapy fails, direct stimulation of the ovaries with human menopausal gonadotropin containing LH and FSH, and human chorionic gonadotropin that has an LH-like activity, may be necessary in order to induce ovulation. During pregnancy, the gonadotropes of the normal pituitary hypertrophy, and pituitary vascularity also increases. Pituitary tumors may increase in size, sometimes suddenly, during pregnancy. This increase may lead to compression of the optic chiasm or optic nerves as well as to pituitary apoplexy. It is important to treat the tumors before the patient conceives. This patient should be followed closely during the pregnancy for symptoms of pituitary insufficiency and for visual acuity and visual field changes.

3. The normal cortisol rise after insulin-induced hypoglycemia and the normal rise in compound S (11-deoxycortisol) eliminates adrenal insufficiency as the cause of this patient's complaint of orthostatic dizziness.

CHAPTER 7

Patient 1

1. Klinefelter's syndrome is the most likely diagnosis. It occurs in about 0.2% of male births.

2. Examination of a buccal smear for the presence of Barr bodies.

3. If the patient had true Klinefelter's syndrome (XXY karyotype), you might expect him to have the same percentage of Barr bodies as a normal female because he has the same number of X chromosomes as a normal female. In practice, this reasoning does not hold true, though many Klinefelter's patients have Barr body counts in the normal female range. This intermediate value for Barr body count may suggest the presence of a mosaic in which not all cells have the same sex chromosome composition. This possibility could be further evaluated by obtaining a peripheral blood karyotype.

4. Klinefelter's syndrome is not hereditary, so the brother should be expected to have the same chance of having Klinefelter's syndrome as anyone else in the population. However, because Klinefelter's syndrome is associated with advanced parental age at the time of conception, a younger brother of a patient with Klinefelter's syndrome would have a slightly higher than normal chance of having the disorder. An eight-year-old with Klinefelter's syndrome would be difficult to diagnose on the basis of laboratory tests, since testosterone is normally low in prepubertal children and the gonadotropins may not become elevated in patients with Klinefelter's syndrome until puberty.

5. With the information available, a skull roentgenogram is not indicated. The finding of elevated levels of LH and FSH rules out a primary pituitary disorder as cause for the patient's hypogonadism.

6. Fertility has rarely been documented in patients with true Klinefelter's syndrome. Patients with mosaic chromosome composition have a better chance of attaining fertility.

7. The patient's low serum testosterone, combined with a normal or elevated level of serum estrogen, indicates an increase in the estrogen/androgen ratio acting on the breast to produce gynecomastia.

8. Because of the episodic secretion of LH by the pituitary, single samples of serum assayed for LH may vary by 50 to 100% from values obtained at a different time in the same patient. Though individual values of serum LH might be in the normal range, determination of the mean of several samples obtained at different times would give a truer picture of the serum LH level. To economize, it is preferable to measure LH in a pool of 3 serum samples drawn at 20-minute intervals.

9. Thyroid abnormalities and diabetes mellitus are more common in patients with Klinefelter's syndrome than in the general population.

10. Because the patient has a low serum testosterone, he has less inhibition of his pituitary and hypothalamus. Thus, his plasma LH will increase to a greater degree after LRH administration than does the LH in a normal male.

11. Because the testis is intrinsically defective in Klinefelter's syndrome, it cannot respond normally to exogenous stimulation by HCG. Thus, the increase in plasma testosterone after HCG administration in patients with Klinefelter's syndrome is subnormal even if their basal value of testosterone is normal.

Patient 2

1. The most likely possibilities are Kallmann's syndrome (hypogonadotropic hypogonadism and anosmia), craniopharyngioma, or constitutional delay in puberty. The subsequent finding that the patient in this case was unable to smell established the diagnosis of Kallmann's syndrome. The finding of visual field defects would strongly suggest the presence of a pituitary tumor or craniopharyngioma.

2. A skull roentgenogram is necessary because pituitary tumors constitute an important and treatable cause of delayed puberty and short stature.

3. The bone age would be retarded because normal advancement of bone age depends on the increased sex steroid production that occurs during puberty, which would not be present in this patient.

4. The relative slowdown in growth rate at age ten is due to absence of the pubertal increase in sex steroids, which is responsible for the normal growth spurt at the time of puberty. However, the patient will continue to grow; since his bone age will not advance and his epiphyses will not fuse because he cannot increase his sex steroid output, he will end up being tall if left untreated.

5. Since Kallmann's syndrome seems to be either a sex-linked recessive disorder or an autosomal dominant with incomplete penetrance, his younger brother has a high probability of being affected.

6. Kallmann's syndrome is thought to be a disorder of the hypothalamus. Though the pituitary is intrinsically normal, it has not been normally stimulated by endogenous LRH, and thus has poor reserve capacity to synthesize and secrete LH. Thus, plasma LH increase after LRH will be subnormal. Long-term pulsatile administration of LRH will restore to normal the synthetic and secretory ability of the pituitary, yielding a normal LH rise after LRH.

7. The testis, like the pituitary, is intrinsically normal in Kallmann's syndrome. Like the pituitary, it has not been normally stimulated by its tropic hormone, in this case LH.

Thus, reserve capacity of the testis is subnormal, and increase of the plasma testosterone after two injections of HCG is also subnormal. Long-term treatment with HCG restores to normal both the reserve capacity of the testis and the plasma testosterone increase after HCG.

CHAPTER 8

Patient 1

1. Fasting hypoglycemia, which is characterized by symptoms and signs occurring after not eating all night rather than after ingesting a (high carbohydrate) meal.

2. Ethanol and exercise.

   Ethanol (potentiation by alcohol can be inferred by the history of difficulty of arousal following a party)—interferes with hepatic gluconeogenesis probably because its catabolism uses nicotinamide-adenine dinucleotide (NAD), which is required for rate-limiting steps of gluconeogenesis.

   Exercise—increases muscle utilization of glucose, which potentiates any tendency to hypoglycemia. Insulin binding increases after exercise. In addition, increased concentrations of insulin have been demonstrated in the venous circulation draining an exercising limb. This finding suggests that some insulin may be nonspecifically bound and not exerting any metabolic effect under usual conditions, but, when released during exercise, it stimulates glucose transport into muscle.

3. Drugs, ethanol ingestion, hepatic failure, adrenal insufficiency, extrapancreatic neoplasm, and insulinoma.

   Drugs—especially insulin and sulfonylurea agents; propranolol, aspirin and MAO inhibitors must also be considered. In view of negative drug history, this diagnosis is unlikely.

   Ethanol ingestion—potentiates his basic problem but probably not the primary diagnosis.

   Hepatic failure—no evidence.

   Adrenal insufficiency—no historic or physical evidence for either primary or secondary adrenal insufficiency, but this diagnosis must be considered.

   Extrapancreatic neoplasm—a 3-year history, so this diagnosis is unlikely.

   Insulinoma—must always be considered in patients with documented hypoglycemia.

4. The normal value for urinary 17-OH steroids rules out both primary and secondary adrenal insufficiency. Although the insulin level of 35 μU/ml is not high considering this man's obesity (higher insulin concentrations are characteristic in obesity), it is inappropriately elevated for a plasma glucose of 23 mg/100 ml (glucose-insulin ratio = 0.66). Therefore, the patient probably has an insulinoma. (Factitious hypoglycemia secondary to the surreptitious injection of insulin is the only other possibility and is more likely to occur in patients connected with the medical profession.)

5. Multiple endocrine adenomatosis type I. This is a familial syndrome of multiple endocrine tumors of (1) pancreas—insulin-producing (insulinoma) or gastrin-producing (Zollinger-Ellison syndrome), (2) parathyroid glands, or (3) pituitary gland (chromophobe adenomas some of which may secrete growth hormone causing acromegaly). Hyperplasia of the involved endocrine glands rather than discrete tumors is the pathologic change usually seen. Occasionally an adrenal tumor is associated with this syndrome. Multiple lipomas are often present. It is inherited as an autosomal dominant. The hypercalcemia in this patient is the probable cause of his nocturia since high blood calcium levels impair the concentrating ability of the distal tubules in the kidney.

Patient 2

1. Each value would have been 15% lower (not 15 mg/100 ml).

2. Hyperalimentation (postgastric surgery), impaired glucose tolerance, idiopathic reactive hypoglycemia, adrenal insufficiency, and islet-cell tumor (insulinoma).

3. The curve should be characterized by a normal fasting glucose concentration, high one-half to 1-hour values, and hypoglycemia within 1 or 2 hours (early hypoglycemia).

4. The curve should be characterized by a normal to mildly elevated fasting glucose concentration, a 1-hour plasma glucose value of more than 200 mg/100 ml, a 2-hour value of between 140 and 200 mg/100 ml, and hypoglycemia between 3 and 5 hours after the OGTT (early hyperglycemia, late hypoglycemia).

5. The curve should be characterized by normal fasting, 1- and 2-hour glucose concentrations, and hypoglycemia between 3 and 5 hours after the test (normal early part of curve, late hypoglycemia).

6. Do symptoms occur at time of low plasma glucose level? Are symptoms quickly (10 to 20 minutes) relieved by carbohydrate snack? Does this pattern (i.e., symptoms consistent with hypoglycemia and quickly relieved by carbohydrate intake) occur on a regular basis?

7. The mainstay of treatment for the first 3 causes listed in answer 2 is a high-protein, low-carbohydrate diet (35% of total calories from carbohydrate with avoidance of mono- and disaccharides). Multiple feedings are sometimes necessary, especially in patients with hyperalimentation. Occasionally drugs such as anticholinergic agents, propranolol, phenytoin, or diazoxide may be necessary. Adrenal insufficiency and insulinoma are rare causes of reactive hypoglycemia. Glucocorticoid replacement is the specific treatment for adrenal insufficiency. If an insulinoma is not cured by surgery, oral diazoxide or streptozotocin (if the tumor is malignant) should be tried.

8. Normal asymptomatic person. "Low" glucose levels 2 to 5 hours following an oral carbohydrate challenge are common in the normal population. In young and overweight persons, the prevalence approaches 25 to 30%. For this reason, once low glucose levels are documented (usually less than 50 mg/100 ml for plasma or 40 mg/100 ml for whole blood), the 3 other criteria listed in answer 6 should be met before a diagnosis of idiopathic reactive hypoglycemia is made.

Patients 3 and 4

Hyperglycemia is the common denominator in both diabetic ketoacidosis and hyperosmolar nonketotic coma. This condition causes an osmotic diuresis by the kidneys that can only lead to the symptom of *polyuria*. Because more water than solutes is lost, the urine osmolality is hypo-osmolar to body fluids; this situation leaves a plasma osmolality that is hyperosmolar. The thirst center in the brain reacts to this hyperosmolar situation by signaling the person to drink more water; *polydipsia* then results. In the osmotic diuresis, tremendous amounts of sodium and potassium are lost causing *decreased total body sodium and potassium*. That loss combined with the fluid loss by the kidney also causes a *decreased plasma volume*. Because the osmolar state of the plasma is increased over normal, an *initial fluid therapy* of a hypo-osmolar content would be appropriate in both diabetic ketoacidosis and hyperosmolar nonketotic coma.

The following parameters are different in these 2 causes of coma for the following reasons:

Prodromal period—Acidosis supervenes quickly (1 or 2 days) when the effective insulin concentration becomes low; in hyperosmolar nonketotic coma, however, the chronic impairment of insulin action leads to a more gradual build-up of hyperglycemia over a much longer period of time. Since acidosis does not supervene, the patient can tolerate hyperglycemia for long periods of time and it may be weeks before the patient seeks medical care.

Respiratory rate—Because acidosis drives the respiratory center in an attempt to compensate by a respiratory alkalosis, the respiratory rate in diabetic ketoacidosis is much higher than in hyperosmolar nonketotic coma, where it is usually normal.

Neurologic examination—Although the depth of coma may be similar in the two situations, it is common to have focal neurologic changes in hyperosmolar nonketotic coma; indeed many of these patients are misdiagnosed initially as having cerebral vascular accidents.

Bicarbonate concentration—This level is low in diabetic ketoacidosis reflecting the metabolic acidosis.

pH—This level is low in diabetic ketoacidosis reflecting the metabolic acidosis; both pH and bicarbonate concentrations are normal in a "pure" case of hyperosmolar nonketotic coma.

Arterial P_{CO_2}—In diabetic ketoacidosis, this level will be low reflecting the compensatory respiratory alkalosis; in hyperosmolar nonketotic coma there is no acidosis and thus no need for a compensatory respiratory alkalosis, so P_{CO_2} (as well as arterial pH and serum bicarbonate concentrations) is normal.

Serum ketones—These levels are elevated in diabetic ketoacidosis and should be either nondetectable or only minimally detectable in hyperosmolar nonketotic coma. One reason that any ketone bodies at all may be detectable in the latter condition is that patients who have been unable to eat or to use glucose may have "starvation ketosis." In this situation, ketone bodies are positive in the undiluted serum but negative when the serum is diluted because the concentration is so low; by contrast, in diabetic ketoacidosis, tests remain positive as the serum is diluted. Probably a more common reason for the presence of ketone bodies is that most often these patients have aspects of both diabetic ketoacidosis and hyperosmolar nonketotic coma (high glucose levels and ketosis with a compensated acidosis).

Prognosis—The prognosis in diabetic ketoacidosis is usually much more favorable than in hyperosmolar nonketotic coma. In the former, mortality rates range from 3 to 30% (but are usually around the lower level) and depend on the age of the patient and the depth of coma. In hyperosmolar nonketotic coma, mortality rates have been approximately 50% in the past, owing to failure to recognize the situation in some cases; moreover, the patients are usually older and have more complicating illnesses.

Treatment after discharge—In diabetic ketoacidosis, therapy after discharge always includes insulin. (There may be a "honeymoon phase" in which over the next several months insulin requirements drop and may even disappear; however, in over 95% of the cases insulin is required again, usually within 4 to 6 months, occasionally after a period as long as a year or two.) In hyperosmolar nonketotic coma, a large percentage of these patients can be treated by diet alone or by diet with the addition of oral hypoglycemic agents; this regimen indicates that these patients can still secrete some insulin.

These cases represent each end of a spectrum. Often patients have some aspects of both, that is, high glucose levels and mild acidosis.

Patient 5

1. The answer is (b), type 1 diabetes mellitus. Starvation ketosis is the wrong answer because the patient has 2% glucosuria. Type 2 diabetes mellitus is not correct because he has ketosis. Diabetic ketoacidosis (DKA), although superficially a possibility, is not correct because the plasma shows only trace ketone bodies in the undiluted specimen. In DKA, the ketone body test is at least strongly positive in the undiluted specimen. Finally, hyperosmolar nonketotic coma is obviously incorrect because ketone bodies are present.

2. The correct answers are: b, e, and f. A 2600-cal American Diabetes Association diet is appropriate based on the patient's height and present weight. A small amount of NPH insulin is given to lower the glucose concentration by the next morning, and 5 U regular insulin are given immediately because the patient's blood sugar is nearly 400 mg/100 ml

and he still has to eat supper. Diabetic instruction is important in new diabetics and should be undertaken as soon as possible. Answer c is incorrect because the number of calories is too low. Although the 5 U NPH would be appropriate in answer d, because of the lag period, the glucose levels will go even higher after supper and therefore answer e is more appropriate.

3. The correct answer is a. Twenty units of NPH insulin (answer b) would be a doubling of his dose, and although he might need at least that much eventually, the approach outlined in this chapter is to increase the amount of insulin *gradually*. Although one could give 5 U regular insulin (answer c), my usual approach is to establish the NPH insulin dose first before adding short-acting insulin. Although sulfonylurea agents (answer d) have been shown to increase insulin receptors, currently the accepted approach to controlling insulin-dependent diabetics is to increase the insulin dose until control is obtained. If control is difficult to obtain, experiments are currently being carried out to ascertain whether adding the oral hypoglycemic agent will improve the situation. Ten units of NPH insulin is incorrect (answer e) because that amount of insulin the previous morning did not control the patient's glucose concentration before supper.

4. The correct answer is b. The amount of NPH insulin is appropriate because the fasting- and before-supper glucose concentrations are below 200 mg/100 ml. Because the patient has 2% glucosuria before lunch, it seems apparent that he will need some regular insulin in the morning. Answer a might be considered correct, except adding regular insulin at the time of discharge will save some time outside the hospital before the diabetes is brought under control. Answer c is incorrect because the patient's exercise outside the hospital will increase and will make him more sensitive to the injected insulin. Therefore, giving him more insulin on discharge might well lead to hypoglycemia. Answers d and e are incorrect because achieving tight control in the hospital may be an ''exercise in futility,'' owing to the different exercise, dietary, and emotional patterns following discharge.

Patient 6

In this situation, the patient is showing a Somogyi effect.

1-b. Patient already is receiving too much insulin and you are increasing it. His hormonal responses are not able to keep him out of trouble, so he goes into hypoglycemic coma at the time of maximal action of NPH insulin.

2-a. Sulfonylurea agent is completely ineffective, and as expected, nothing changes.

3-d. You have decreased his insulin (which is appropriate), but have done it too quickly. Therefore, he is underinsulinized, and though his symptoms of hypoglycemia, i.e., nocturnal sweating and morning headaches, disappear, a consistent pattern of positive urine tests appears.

4-c. Here you are on the right track; his hypoglycemic symptoms have disappeared and his urine tests have improved significantly.

CHAPTER 9

Patient 1

1. The majority of patients with hyperparathyroidism seen at present have mild or even intermittent hypercalcemia, and many of them are completely without symptoms or end-organ damage; thus, the clinician is faced with the dilemma of whom to treat and when. Recent studies suggest that a small fraction of asymptomatic hypercalcemia patients develop renal damage over a 2-year follow-up period. The true natural history of the mild illness is still not completely understood, however, and it is possible that a significant number will never develop either end-organ damage or progressive hypercalcemia.

2. Indications for surgical intervention include:

   a. Progressively increasing hypercalcemia
   b. Symptoms of early renal impairment, such as polyuria and polydipsia
   c. Hypertension
   d. Decreased glomerular filtration rate
   e. Refractory peptic ulcer symptoms
   f. Pancreatitis
   g. Parathyroid bone disease
   h. Stone disease
   i. Psychiatric complications

Patient 2

1. The most likely diagnosis is pseudohypoparathyroidism. The patient clearly is able to generate an exuberant PTH response to hypocalcemia, but he appears unable to maintain a Ca level in a range that leaves him symptom-free. There are two interesting aspects to this point:

   a. How did he go so long without the diagnosis? He may have struggled for years with hypocalcemia, never seeking additional medical help. However, many patients experience sustained periods of amelioration of the disorder, during which serum Ca may be maintained at the lower limits of normal; this description may characterize your patient.

   b. The finding of generalized demineralization of the skeleton suggests that lack of responsiveness to PTH may be restricted to or is more apparent in the kidney. This finding has been reported in several patients, some of whom showed osteitis fibrosis on skeletal biopsy. The implication of this finding is that renal calcium metabolism may be the major contributor to the normal maintenance of serum Ca. This point is a matter of some controversy. The diagnosis can be established by measuring urinary cyclic AMP in response to the administration of parathyroid hormone.

2. Your patient has been taking phenytoin and barbiturates for several years. Both drugs produce osteomalacia by increasing the degradation of 25(OH)D. The elevated alkaline phosphatase in the present case may reflect such a process. On the other hand, the normal range for alkaline phosphatase applies only to adults, because children who are undergoing linear bone growth have higher serum levels of the enzyme. To determine the normalcy of the present level, the value should be checked against normal values that are adjusted for age.

3. Management of this disorder consists of calcitriol $(1,25(OH)_2D_3)$ or pharmacologic doses of vitamin D. You should remember that either vitamin D sterol is potentially toxic, and hypercalciuria appears prior to hypercalcemia. Hypercalciuria itself is likely to occur since the protective action of PTH to enhance the tubular reabsorption of Ca is not operative, and a greater fraction of the filtered load of calcium is excreted in the urine. This creates a greater risk of kidney stones. The dose of vitamin D can vary from 25,000 to 300,000 U/day, and it should be titrated carefully against symptoms, urinary Ca excretion, and serum Ca concentration; calcitriol $(1,25(OH)_2D_3)$ may be easier to titrate because its actions are more predictable; moreover, the effect is rapidly dissipated if toxicity occurs.

Patient 3

1. Alkaline phosphatase reflects osteoblastic activity. It is, therefore, elevated in disorders associated with increased bone formation, such as Paget's disease, osteomalacia, and most metastatic carcinomas. However, involvement of bone by multiple myeloma, the diagnosis in this patient, is predominantly a disorder of bone resorption, with little if any compensatory osteoblastic activity. Therefore, a normal serum alkaline phosphatase is found in patients with myeloma.

2. Unlike the situation with certain solid tumors, bone resorption and hypercalcemia in multiple myeloma are not related to prostaglandin production by the malignant tissue. Instead, a peptide secretory product, called osteoclast activating factor (OAF), has been frequently implicated in the genesis of the metabolic abnormality. Moreover, direct invasion of bone by the tumor may result in local resorption and hypercalcemia.

3. A significant interracial difference in bone mineral exists, with black men and women showing a significant increase in mineral density throughout adult life over the levels in their white counterparts. Although mineral density decreases with age in the black population, it rarely declines to a degree sufficient to produce clinical or radiologic signs of osteoporosis. Therefore, osteoporosis in a black adult requires careful exclusion of a systemic illness, such as myeloma, which can decrease bone mineral content.

Patient 4

1. The serum magnesium level in this patient was 1.0 mg/100 ml. The cause of the hypomagnesemia was the malabsorption seen as part of Crohn's disease. Another characteristic of patients with hypomagnesemia and hypocalcemia is that the hypocalcemia cannot be corrected until the magnesium deficit is corrected.

2. Magnesium deficiency causes hypocalcemia by reducing PTH release from the gland and by inhibiting the action of PTH on bone.

3. One would expect secondary hyperparathyroidism in a patient with malabsorption and hypocalcemia. With normal renal function, one would expect a decrease in tubular reabsorption of PO_4 and a consequent decrease in serum PO_4. The high normal level of serum PO_4 provides a clue to the absence of PTH secretion.

CHAPTER 10

Patient 1, Part 1

1. Diabetes insipidus.

2. The lack of growth points to a defect in anterior pituitary function as well as posterior pituitary function. Thus, the diabetes insipidus is probably due to a hypothalamic or pituitary lesion.

3. Craniopharyngioma is the most likely cause of the syndrome in this patient in view of the suprasellar calcification. Hand-Schüller-Christian disease, granulomatous disease (such as sarcoidosis), and pituitary tumors could also be responsible. Idiopathic diabetes insipidus is much less likely because of the evidence of anterior pituitary involvement.

Patient 1, Part 2

1. He lost his sensation of thirst due to extension of his tumor. Without the sensation of thirst and subsequent increased water intake, he became chronically dehydrated and hypernatremic.

2. The chronic hypovolemia resulted in decreased glomerular filtration rate and enhanced proximal tubular reabsorption of sodium such that he was unable to excrete free water even in the absence of AVP.

Patient 2

1. Salt loss. Patients with recurrent vomiting, as is seen with alcohol withdrawal, may lose a considerable amount of sodium. The hyponatremia occurs when they replace the emesis fluid, volume for volume, with tap water.

2. The low urinary sodium is caused by intense renal conservation of sodium mediated by the renin-aldosterone system in patients with a diminished effective plasma volume. The urine osmolality tends to be high because of increased renal conservation of water.

3. The elevated BUN probably reflects prerenal azotemia due to hypovolemia.

Patient 3

1. Syndrome of inappropriate AVP production. Nothing suggests hypothyroidism, adrenal insufficiency, or renal disease; the urine is not maximally dilute in the face of hypo-osmolality of the plasma, and the urinary sodium excretion is elevated.

2. The serum sodium concentration might transiently rise, but would eventually fall again after the sodium was excreted in the urine.

3. The AVP is most likely being produced ectopically by the oat cell carcinoma. Metastases to the central nervous system could result in enhanced release of AVP by the pituitary, but this effect is less likely.

Patient 4

1. Nephrogenic diabetes insipidus secondary to vitamin D-induced hypercalciuria. Her glucose intolerance was only borderline and was unlikely to cause the polyuria.

2. Since the patient had only a 6% rise in urinary osmolality after exogenous vasopressin, she most likely had renal resistance to AVP.

3. Having an intact thirst mechanism, the patient was able to increase her fluid intake to keep up with her renal fluid losses.

4. Hypokalemia, Sjögren's syndrome, habitual water drinking, and sickle cell nephropathy.

CHAPTER 11

Patient 1

1. The pattern of inheritance is consistent with an autosomal dominant disorder.

2. A diagnosis of familial hypercholesterolemia was made.

3. The patient's treadmill exercise test was positive; her sister's was negative for ischemia. The patient underwent coronary arteriography, which revealed complete occlusion of the right coronary artery and 40 to 50% stenosis of the left main, circumflex, and left anterior descending coronary arteries.

4. After giving up cigarettes and going on a walking program, her treadmill test reverted to normal.

5. Diet was minimally effective in reducing the plasma cholesterol. Cholestyramine lowered the plasma cholesterol to 260 mg/100 ml. The addition of nicotinic acid lowered it further to 200 mg/100 ml. The children were treated with diet alone and had mild to modest improvement in their plasma cholesterol levels.

Patient 2

1. Secondary hyperlipidemia.

2. The normal increase in insulin following a glucose load was absent. The mechanism of her hyperlipidemia was felt to be a defect in the removal of VLDL and chylomicrons due to lipoprotein lipase deficiency secondary to the lack of insulin. The estrogens probably exaggerated the problem as did her obesity.

3. She was given a reducing diet.

4. All her medications were stopped for the glucose tolerance test, and she was advised not to resume taking these drugs.

5. Ten units of NPH insulin daily was prescribed. On this regimen her fasting blood sugar dropped to 135 mg/100 ml, her plasma cholesterol fell to 243 mg/100 ml, and her triglycerides fell to 229 mg/100 ml.

Patient 3

1. The physical and laboratory examinations exclude secondary hyperlipidemia.

2. The distribution of cholesterol values about a mean that is higher than normal suggests a polygenic mode of inheritance.

3. The relative risk for an atherosclerotic event in persons with polygenic hypercholesterolemia is higher than normal but much less than that with familial hypercholesterolemia or familial combined hyperlipidemia.

4. He was treated with a low cholesterol, low saturated fat diet. His plasma cholesterol concentration fell to 272 mg/100 ml. This response to diet was acceptable and no medications were prescribed. Dietary therapy was also advised for his 3 brothers.

5. The 2 women with hypertriglyceridemia were advised to use another method of birth control, and diet was prescribed for the children with elevated plasma cholesterol concentrations.

Patient 4

1. A presumptive diagnosis of secondary hyperlipidemia was made. (Without being able to study the family members, one cannot exclude primary hyperlipidemia as well.)

2. Presumably, he was over-producing VLDL in response to the hyperinsulinemia that is frequently found in such patients.

3. A reducing diet was prescribed, and over 3 months he lost the excess weight. Repeat glucose tolerance test and triglyceride determinations were normal.

Patient 5

1. The physical examination and the laboratory examinations, which are normal except for elevated blood lipids, exclude secondary hyperlipidemia.

2. Half the adult family members have either an elevated cholesterol concentration or an elevated triglyceride concentration, or abnormal levels of both plasma lipids. The other members have normal values. The pattern is bimodal and consistent with an autosomal dominant disorder.

3. The pattern of lipid levels is most consistent with familial combined hyperlipidemia.

4. A treadmill exercise test should be done for each affected person.

5. The 48-year-old brother and his daughter were strongly advised to stop smoking.

6. The patients and the affected family members were treated with diet alone. The lipid levels of the 2 children fell into the high normal range. The 48-year-old brother made little attempt to diet and his values did not significantly change. The patient's cholesterol level fell to 260 mg/100 ml and his triglyceride level decreased to 150 mg/100 ml.

Index

Page numbers in *italics* refer to illustrations; followed by a "t" refer to tables; followed by an "f" refer to footnote.